Thematic Collections
in Biomedical Research

Neuroimaging biomarkers *in* Alzheimer's disease.

Dr. Samuel Barrack

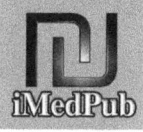
iMedPub

Title: *Neuroimaging biomarkers in Alzheimer's disease*

Autor: Samuel Barrack

ISBN-13: 978-1-49227-442-1
ISBN-10: 1492274429

Cover design and Layout: design@imedpub.com

Maquetación: David Márquez
david.maquetacion@gmail.com

Publisher: **Internet Medical Publishing**
info@imedpub.com
http://imedpub.com/

First edition: 2013

Preface for Biomarkers for Alzheimer's disease

In view of the growing prevalence of AD worldwide, there is an urgent need for the development of better diagnostic tools and more effective therapeutic interventions. Indeed, much work in this field has been done during last decades. As such, a major goal of current clinical research in AD is to improve early detection of disease and presymptomatic detection of neuronal dysfunction, concurrently with the development of better tools to assess disease progression in this group of disorders. All these putative correlates are commonly referred to as AD-related biomarkers. The ideal biomarker should be easy to quantify and measure, reproducible, not subject to wide variation in the general population and unaffected by co-morbid factors. For evaluation of therapies, a biomarker needs to change linearly with disease progression and closely correlate with established clinico-pathological parameters of the disease.

There is growing evidence that the use of biomarkers will increase our ability to better indentify the underlying biology of AD, especially in its early stages. These biomarkers will improve the detection of the patients suitable for research studies and drug trials, and they will contribute to a better management of the disease in the clinical practice. Indeed, much work in this field has been done during last decades. The vast number of important applications, combined with the untamed diversity of already identified biomarkers, show that there is a pressing need to structure the research made on AD biomarkers into a solid, comprehensive and easy to use tool to de deployed in clinical settings.

To date there are few publications compiling results on this topic. That is why when I was asked to address this task I accepted inmediately. I am happy to present you a bundle of the best articles published about biomarkers for Alzheimer's disease in recent times.

Signed
Dr Samuel Barrack

Contents

1

Diffusion Tensor Metrics as Biomarkers in Alzheimer's Disease

Julio Acosta-Cabronero[1]*, Stephanie Alley[2], Guy B. Williams[3], George Pengas[1], Peter J. Nestor[1,4]

1 Cognition, Memory and Language Group, Neurology Unit, Department of Clinical Neurosciences, School of Clinical Medicine, University of Cambridge, Cambridge, United Kingdom, 2 Department of Applied Mathematics and Theoretical Physics, Centre for Mathematical Sciences, University of Cambridge, Cambridge, United Kingdom, 3 Wolfson Brain Imaging Centre, Department of Clinical Neurosciences, School of Clinical Medicine, University of Cambridge, Addenbrooke's Hospital, Cambridge, United Kingdom, 4 German Center for Neurodegenerative Diseases (DZNE), Magdeburg, Germany

Abstract

Background: Although diffusion tensor imaging has been a major research focus for Alzheimer's disease in recent years, it remains unclear whether it has sufficient stability to have biomarker potential. To date, frequently inconsistent results have been reported, though lack of standardisation in acquisition and analysis make such discrepancies difficult to interpret. There is also, at present, little knowledge of how the biometric properties of diffusion tensor imaging might evolve in the course of Alzheimer's disease.

Methods: The biomarker question was addressed in this study by adopting a standardised protocol both for the whole brain (tract-based spatial statistics), and for a region of interest: the midline corpus callosum. In order to study the evolution of tensor changes, cross-sectional data from very mild (N = 21) and mild (N = 22) Alzheimer's disease patients were examined as well as a longitudinal cohort (N = 16) that had been rescanned at 12 months.

Findings and Significance: The results revealed that increased axial and mean diffusivity are the first abnormalities to occur and that the first region to develop such significant differences was mesial parietal/splenial white matter; these metrics, however, remained relatively static with advancing disease indicating they are suitable as 'state-specific' markers. In contrast, increased radial diffusivity, and therefore decreased fractional anisotropy–though less detectable early–became increasingly abnormal with disease progression, and, in the splenium of the corpus callosum, correlated significantly with dementia severity; these metrics therefore appear 'stage-specific' and would be ideal for monitoring disease progression. In addition, the cross-sectional and longitudinal analyses showed that the progressive abnormalities in radial diffusivity and fractional anisotropy always occurred in areas that had first shown an increase in axial and mean diffusivity. Given that the former two metrics correlate with dementia severity, but the latter two did not, it would appear that increased axial diffusivity represents an upstream event that precedes neuronal loss.

Citation: Acosta-Cabronero J, Alley S, Williams GB, Pengas G, Nestor PJ (2012) Diffusion Tensor Metrics as Biomarkers in Alzheimer's Disease. PLoS ONE 7(11): e49072. doi:10.1371/journal.pone.0049072

Editor: Wang Zhan, University of Maryland, College Park, United States of America

Received June 21, 2012; **Accepted** October 4, 2012; **Published** November 7, 2012

Funding: Medical Research Council, UK (to PJN); National Institute for Health Research, Cambridge Biomedical Research Centre, UK (to PJN); and Alzheimer's Research UK (to JAC and GP). The funders had no role in study design, data collection and analysis, decision to publish, or preparation of the manuscript.

Competing Interests: The authors have declared that no competing interests exist.

* E-mail: jac@cantab.net

Introduction

There is presently considerable interest in trying to expedite therapeutic development through the use of biomarkers to track change in Alzheimer's disease. To date, most biomarker work with magnetic resonance imaging (MRI) has focused on structural acquisitions to measure atrophy [1]. A potential strength of MRI, compared, for instance, to nuclear medicine imaging techniques, is that multiple types of data–offering complimentary information–can be acquired in a single scanning session. Diffusion tensor imaging (DTI) is one such method that offers information about white matter integrity. Early work using DTI in Alzheimer's disease focused particularly on fractional anisotropy or FA [2,3,4], though some studies have identified that this measure is insensitive to early white matter disruption in Alzheimer's disease [5,6]. This is because both axial (λ_1) and radial diffusivity (RD) increase and therefore FA, which is a function of the ratio of these two

measures, can remain relatively unperturbed. Conflicting results, however, have been reported in Alzheimer's disease; some studies show emphatic mean diffusivity (MD) differences, believed to be largely driven by λ_1 alterations [5,7,8]; some report stronger RD effects [7,9,10,11]–the former in limbic tracts only; and some show, in addition, highly-abnormal FA behaviours [2,4,7,10,12,13,14]. While these findings have helped define the landscape of diffusion changes in Alzheimer's disease, it is unclear how the various tensor metrics evolve over time, and, whether better understanding of such evolution may explain some of these apparently conflicting results. In order to address this issue, we used a common acquisition protocol to examine the evolution of tensor changes over the course of Alzheimer's disease by studying both cross-sectional data at differing dementia severities and longitudinal change over a 12 month period. We performed whole-brain analyses and also assessed a directly-visualised white matter tract that is known to be severely damaged in Alzheimer's

Table 1. Demographic summary including cognitive features for Alzheimer's disease patients and for a group of elderly controls.

		Control (N = 26)	Alzheimer's Disease (N = 43)	Very mild Alzheimer's disease (N = 21)	Mild Alzheimer's disease (N = 22)
General Demographics	Gender, M:F	11:15	26:17	13:8	13:9
	Age at imaging, years	68 (6)	70 (6)	72 (5)	69 (6)
Global Cognition	MMSE/30	29.1 (0.8)	23.7 (3.6)**	25.9 (1.6)**	21.7 (3.9)**^
	ACE-R/100	94.6 (3.0)	71.5 (11.9)**	81.4 (4.0)**	62.1 (8.8)**^
ACE-R Subscores	Attention & Orientation/18	17.9 (0.3)	15.4 (2.7)**	17.0 (1.4)*	13.9 (2.8)**^
	Memory/26	24.5 (1.9)	10.9 (4.3)**	13.7 (4.1)**	8.2 (2.4)**^
	Fluency/14	12.1 (1.7)	8.3 (3.2)**	10.6 (1.9)*	6.2 (2.6)**^
	Language/26	24.9 (0.9)	23.0 (2.6)**	24.6 (1.2)	21.5 (2.7)**^
	Visuospatial/16	15.4 (0.9)	13.7 (2.8)**	15.1 (1.2)	12.3 (3.1)**^

Disease severity (as measured by ACE-R) enabled a median split of the patient cohort into very mild and mild Alzheimer's disease subgroups.
Where appropriate, group values are given as mean (SD).
MMSE/30 = Mini-mental state examination score out of 30-point total; ACE-R/100 = Addenbrooke's cognitive examination-revised score out of 100-point total.
Wilcoxon rank-sum significance levels: *P<0.01 (Alzheimer's disease worse than controls, two-tailed); **P<0.05 (Alzheimer's disease worse than controls, two-tailed, Bonferroni-corrected on n = 28 tests); ^P<0.05 (Mild worse than very mild Alzheimer's disease, two-tailed, Bonferroni-corrected on n = 28).
doi:10.1371/journal.pone.0049072.t001

disease *i.e.* the corpus callosum [3,4,7,8,11,12,13,15,16]. The aim was to identify whether the various tensor metrics might show differential preference as biomarkers to track change or for early diagnosis, and if so, which are the best for each purpose.

Methods

Ethics Statement

The study was approved by the Cambridgeshire 2 Research Ethics Committee (Reference: 07/H0308/215) and by the National Hospital for Neurology and Neurosurgery & Institute of Neurology Joint Research Ethics Committee (Reference: 05/Q0512/12).

Written informed consent was obtained from all the participants. In the context of this study, although the target population were patients suffering from a degenerative brain condition, we expected them to have capacity to consent as only the mild stages of Alzheimer's disease were studied. Before inclusion, every patient was assessed by an expert cognitive neurologist to ensure capacity and this was indeed the case. Although we had ethical permission to scan patients who lacked capacity (with caregiver consent), this was not needed in the present study.

Subjects

Cross-sectional cohorts. Forty-three patients with early-stage probable Alzheimer's disease according to criteria from the National Institute of Neurological and Communicative Disorders and Stroke and the Alzheimer's Disease and Related Disorders Association (NINCDS-ADRDA) [17] were recruited from the memory clinic at Addenbrooke's Hospital (Cambridge, UK). For cross-sectional comparisons, 26 matched controls were also

Table 2. Cognitive profile evolution of a group of early-stage Alzheimer's disease patients that was followed-up for a period of 12 months.

Alzheimer's Disease (Longitudinal, N = 16)		Baseline	12 Months
General Demographics	Gender, M:F	8:8	
Global Cognition	MMSE/30	25.1 (2.0)	22.6 (4.9)§
	ACE-R/100	77.5 (7.3)	70.3 (13.6)**
ACE-R Subscores	Attention & Orientation/18	16.1 (1.1)	14.8 (3.5)
	Memory/26	13.5 (3.9)	9.8 (3.4)**
	Fluency/14	9.6 (2.5)	8.5 (3.8)
	Language/26	23.6 (1.8)	23.1 (2.5)
	Visuospatial/16	14.7 (1.5)	14.0 (2.9)

Cognitive measures are given as mean (SD).
MMSE/30 = Mini-mental state examination score out of 30-point total; ACE-R/100 = Addenbrooke's cognitive examination-revised score out of 100-point total.
Wilcoxon signed-rank significance levels: §0.01<P<0.05 (Alzheimer's disease: 12 months worse than baseline, two-tailed); **P<0.05 (Alzheimer's disease: 12 months worse than baseline, two-tailed, Bonferroni-corrected on n = 7).
doi:10.1371/journal.pone.0049072.t002

recruited and were screened to exclude neurological or major psychiatric illness. They performed normally on cognitive screening: mini-mental state examination or MMSE [18] and Addenbrooke's cognitive examination–revised or ACE-R [19]. The control exclusion criteria was ACE-R<88 (out of 100). Note that 25 patients (ACE-R = 69.5±12.5) and 12 elderly controls previously assessed [5] were also included in the present study.

Enabled by an ACE-R median split, patients were further subcategorised according to disease severity into very mild (best 50% ACE-R) and mild Alzheimer's disease cohorts (worst 50% ACE-R) (Table 1). The very mild patient group (N = 21) included 16 subjects who were diagnosed with the mild-cognitive impairment stage of Alzheimer's disease–*i.e.* these were patients scanned with mild-cognitive impairment that were subsequently shown to

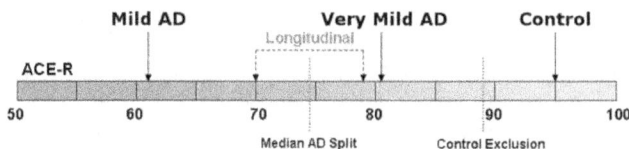

Figure 1. Cognitive status. Depiction of average cognitive profiles for all subject cohorts assessed in this study.
doi:10.1371/journal.pone.0049072.g001

have probable Alzheimer's disease by confirming progressive cognitive decline with longitudinal follow-up. Although significantly impaired overall on both global cognitive measures, the very mild Alzheimer's disease group was unimpaired on language and visuospatial subsections of the ACE-R at the time of scanning. The mild Alzheimer's disease group, however, was impaired in all subdomains of the ACE-R compared both to controls and to the very mild group of patients.

Longitudinal cohort. A subgroup of 16 Alzheimer's disease subjects –9 of which were diagnosed with mild cognitive impairment at baseline – was followed-up with scans and neuropsychology tests taking place 12 months apart. Serendipitously, the cognitive scores shown in Table 2 revealed a similar transition from baseline to 12 months as was seen in the cross-sectional data on the very mild Alzheimer's disease stage relative to controls (Table 1)–the memory subdomain of the ACE-R was also the most impaired, followed by statistical trends towards fluency and attention/orientation deficits; whereas in contrast, language and visuospatial abilities, despite being slightly reduced, remained comparatively preserved. Group-average cognitive profiles are summarised in Figure 1.

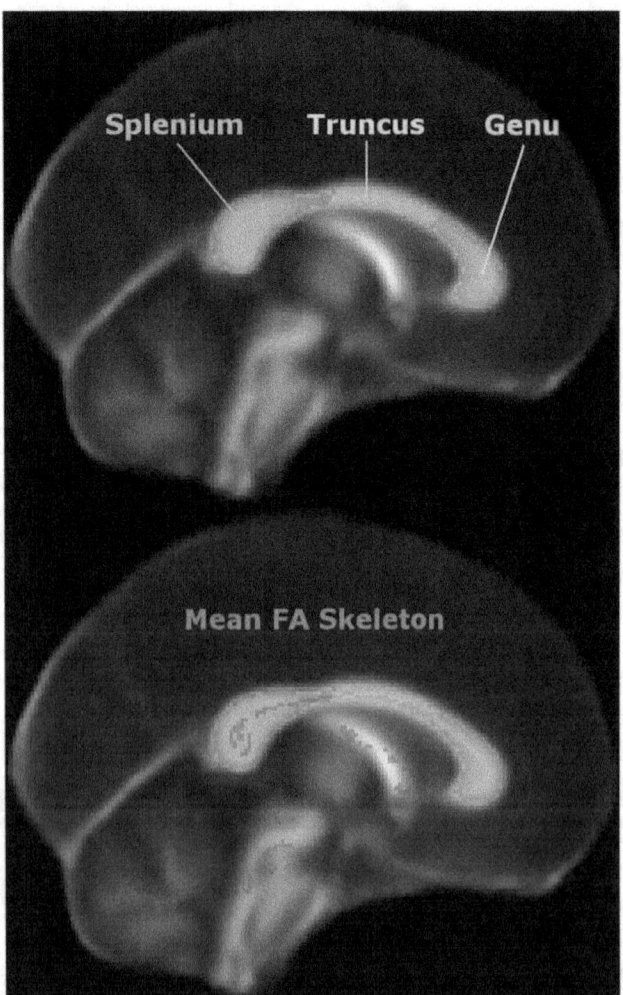

Figure 2. Corpus callosum subdivision. Depiction of the semi-automated callosal subdivision into splenium, truncus and genu (top), and their intersection with the mean FA skeleton inferred from N = 69 subjects–N = 43 Alzheimer's disease patients and N = 26 matched controls (bottom).
doi:10.1371/journal.pone.0049072.g002

Imaging

All patients were scanned within an average of 1.3 months (standard deviation = 1.9 months) from a cognitive assessment. MRI scans were performed on a Siemens Trio 3T system (Siemens Medical Systems, Erlangen, Germany) with gradient coils capable of 45 mT/m and 200 T/m/s slew rate. A standard 12-channel phased-array total imaging matrix head-coil (Siemens Medical Systems, Erlangen, Germany) was used to transmit/receive radiofrequency signals.

Diffusion tensor imaging. Diffusion datasets were acquired using a twice-refocused, single-shot, echo-planar imaging pulse sequence [20]: repetition time (TR)/echo time (TE)/number of excitations = 7800 ms/90 ms/1; matrix, 96×96; 63 contiguous axial slices; isotropic voxel resolution of $2×2×2$ mm^3; bandwidth of 1628 Hz/pixel and echo spacing of 0.72 ms. The tensor was computed using 63 non-collinear diffusion directions ($b = 1000$ s/mm^2) that were maximally spread by considering the minimal energy arrangement of point charges on a sphere, and one scan without diffusion weighting ($b = 0$ s/mm^2, b_0). We allowed for parallel acquisition of independently-reconstructed images using generalised, autocalibrating, partially-parallel acquisitions or GRAPPA [21]; acceleration factor of 2 and 39 reference lines. The total scan time was 8′44′′.

Volumetric T$_1$ imaging. T$_1$-weighted anatomical images were also acquired in the same session. The structural scan consisted of 3D magnetisation-prepared, rapid gradient-echo (MPRAGE) volumes with the following imaging parameters: TR/TE/inversion time/flip angle = 2300 ms/2.86 ms/900 ms/9°, 144 slices, 192×192 matrix dimensions and $1.25×1.25×1.25$ mm^3 voxel size. Receiver bandwidth and echo spacing were 240 Hz/pixel and 6.7 ms, respectively. The total scan time was 7′23′′.

Ultrafast T$_2$ imaging. Whole-brain, T$_2$-weighted, half-Fourier acquisition, single-shot turbo spin echo (HASTE) images were acquired to ensure that vascular pathology was not significant in any subject. The following scan parameters were used: TR/TE/flip angle/turbo factor = 2000 ms/89 ms/150°/205; matrix, 320×256; 25 axial slices (distance factor: 20%); voxel resolution, $0.7×0.9×4$ mm^3; 5/8-phase partial Fourier transform; bandwidth and echo spacing of 401 Hz/pixel and 5.58 ms, respectively. GRAPPA mode was enabled with an acceleration factor of 2 and 24 reference lines, resulting in a total scan time of 52 seconds.

In all acquisitions the field of view was aligned in stereotactic space: the axial plane was aligned to the anterior commissure–posterior commissure line, and the sagittal plane to the interhemispheric fissure. In addition to stereotactic alignment, in order to maximise acquisition consistency across subjects, the scanning bed was adjusted to co-localise the centre of the thalamus in the mid-sagittal plane with the scanner isocentre.

Data Processing and Analysis

Diffusion tensor parametric maps. The Oxford Centre for Functional MRI of the Brain (FMRIB) software library (FSL v4.1.2) [22] was used to correct for motion and eddy currents, fit the diffusion tensor and compute axial, radial and mean diffusivity as well as fractional anisotropy whole-brain maps. Initially, each diffusion-weighted volume was affine-aligned to its corresponding b_0 image using the FMRIB's linear image registration tool (FLIRT v5.4.2) [23]; this pre-processing step corrects for motion artefacts and eddy-current distortions. In addition, in order to eliminate spurious voxels, brain masks of each b_0 image were generated using the brain-extraction tool (BET v2.1) [24] with fractional threshold, $f = 0.1$, and vertical gradient, $g = 0$. The FMRIB's diffusion toolbox (FDT v2.0) was then used to fit the tensor and

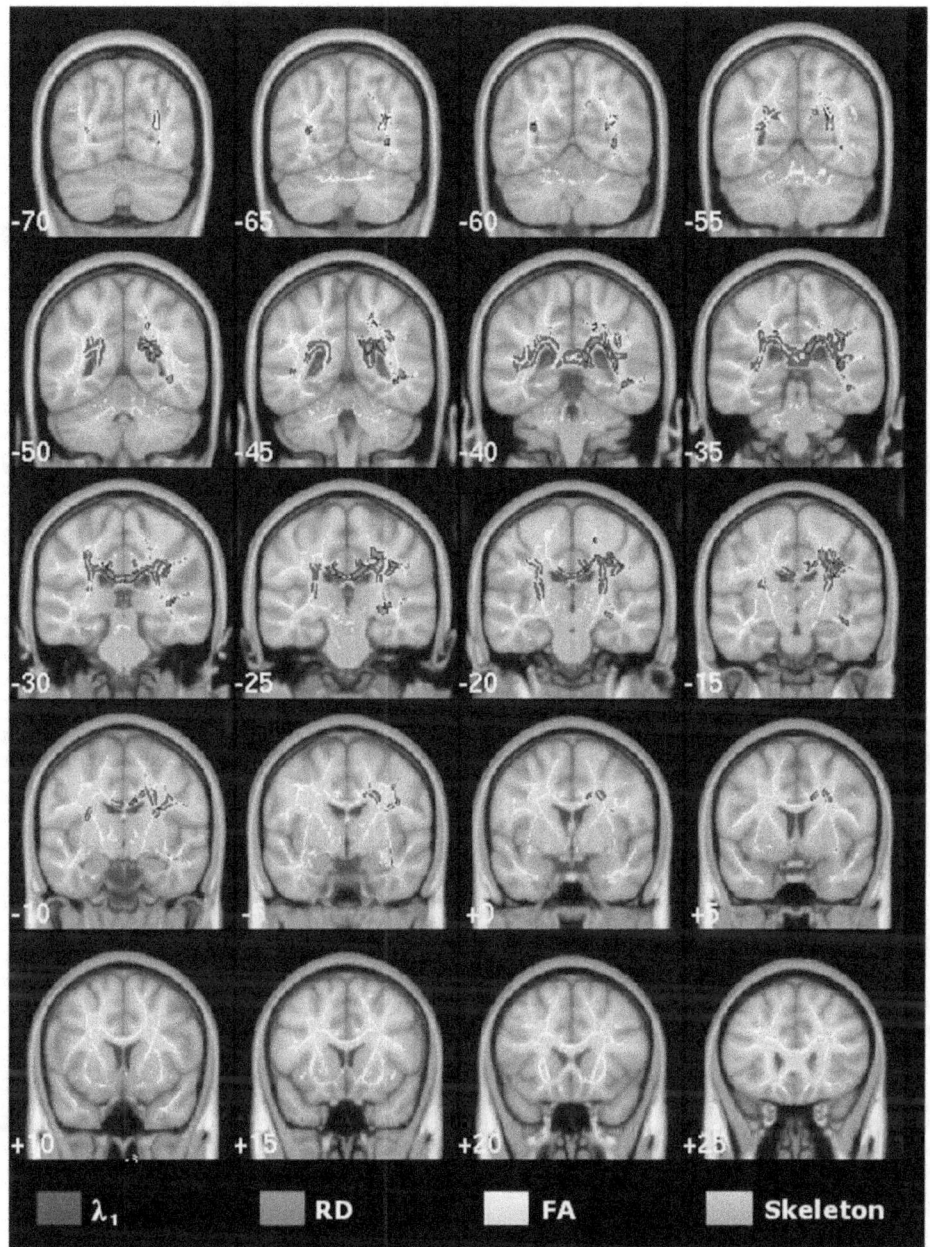

Figure 3. Cross-sectional study of very mild Alzheimer's disease. TBSS results for the very mild Alzheimer's disease group compared to controls. Statistical maps (thresholded at TFCE-P<0.05) for increased axial/radial diffusivity and reduced FA overlaid onto the mean FA skeleton and the MNI152 template. Coronal depths are given in millimetres.
doi:10.1371/journal.pone.0049072.g003

compute the diagonal elements (λ_1, λ_2 and λ_3) at each brain voxel, from which the derived metrics RD, MD and FA were also inferred. Note that negative primary eigenvalues were deemed unphysical and were set to 0–a visual inspection of the spatial distribution of negative eigenvalues revealed that they were located in the periphery of white matter bundles *i.e.* adjacent to other tissue types and far from tract centres.

Tract-based spatial statistics (TBSS) analysis. The TBSS approach [25] was used to perform whole-brain statistical analyses at white matter tract centres. Spatial normalisation was achieved by warping all FA images to the $1\times1\times1$ mm^3 FMRIB58_FA standard template (FMRIB, University of Oxford, UK) in MNI152 space (Montreal Neurological Institute, McGill University, Canada) using the FMRIB's non-linear image registration tool

(FNIRT v1.0). All–patients (N = 43) and controls (N = 26)–warped FA maps were averaged to create the mean FA template, from which the mean FA skeleton was derived (FA>0.2). Finally, all subjects' spatially normalised FA, λ_1, RD and MD data were projected onto the skeleton and fed into voxel-wise statistics, where 10,000 permutations of the data were generated using randomise v2.1 with threshold-free cluster enhancement (TFCE) enabled [26]. The following statistical comparisons were made: (i) cross-sectional: very mild (N = 21) and mild (N = 22) Alzheimer's disease patients versus controls (N = 26); and (ii) longitudinal: Alzheimer's disease (N = 16) at 12 months versus baseline data. Note that for subgroup comparisons–*i.e.* very mild and mild Alzheimer's disease against controls–and for the longitudinal assessment, we used the mean FA skeleton derived from all 69 subjects to compute the

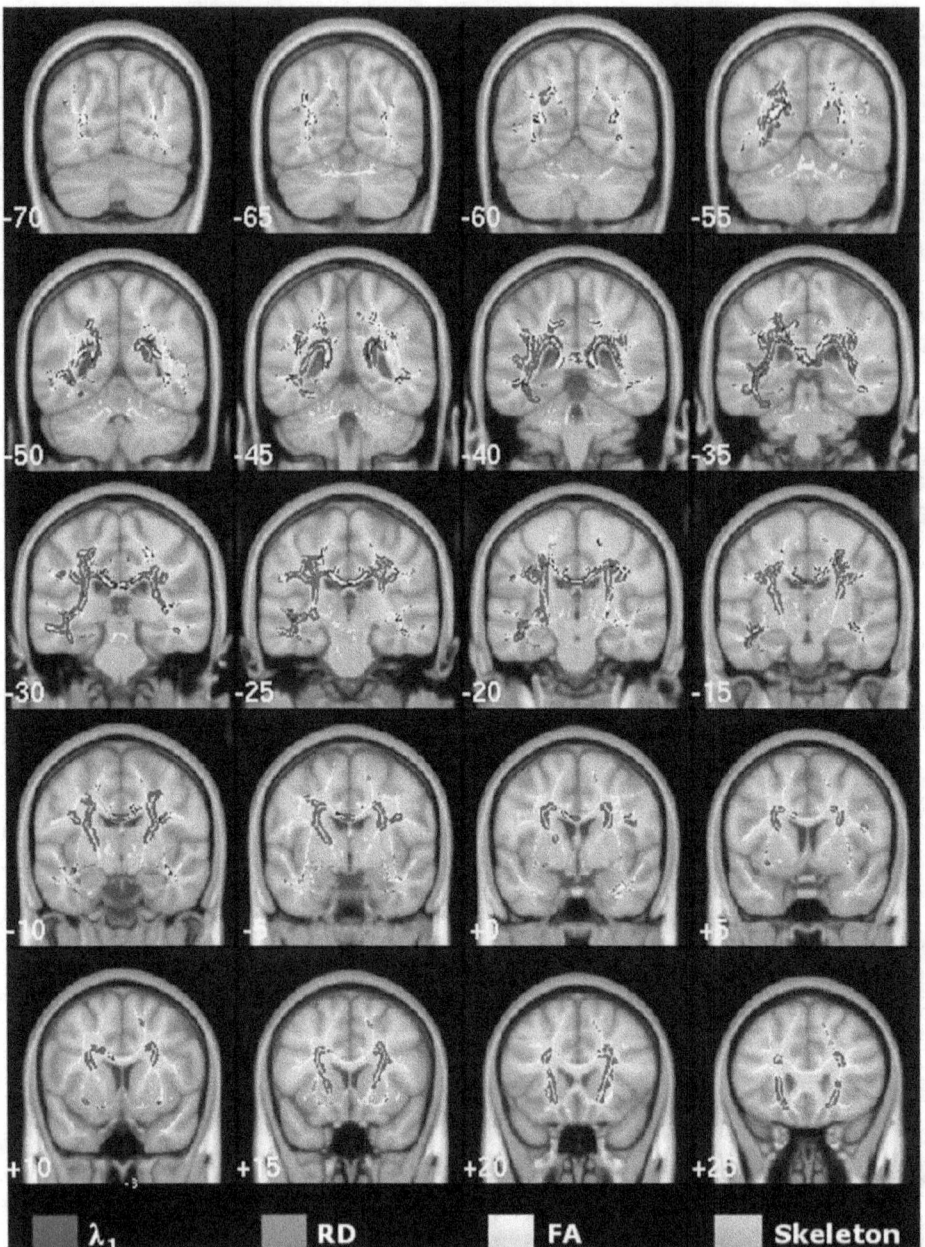

Figure 4. Cross-sectional study of mild Alzheimer's disease. TBSS results for the mild-stage Alzheimer's disease group compared to controls. Thresholded (TFCE-P<0.05) statistical maps for increased axial/radial diffusivity and reduced FA were overlaid onto the mean FA skeleton and the MNI152 template. Coronal depths are given in millimetres.
doi:10.1371/journal.pone.0049072.g004

skeletonisation vectors. All statistical maps were thresholded at a TFCE level of P<0.05 to help prevent the known issue of Type I errors in voxel-wise experiments.

Regional analysis. Region-of-interest analyses can be confounded in DTI studies where tracts are not directly visualised such as in the white matter of the cerebral hemispheres. For instance, the effect of atrophy in a patient group could mean that regions of interest are subtly–though systematically–misplaced with respect to tract anatomy, and this could cause spurious alterations in tensor metrics. Furthermore, the impact of crossing fibres can make changes in tensor behaviour difficult to interpret. For instance, increased λ_1 has been previously reported in Alzheimer's disease [5,7,8,11], which was a somewhat unanticipated finding as it implied that disease was associated with greater diffusivity along the preferential orientation of white matter tracts.

An alternate hypothesis to explain this phenomenon, however, was that it might relate to differential disease involvement in crossing tracts *e.g.* if tract A and B cross, but only tract B is affected by disease, then its degeneration will lead to an apparent increase in λ_1–and greater anisotropy–because the tensor is now being influenced more exclusively by tract A [13]. To avoid these confounds, the midline corpus callosum was studied because (i) it can be directly visualised with obvious boundary limits and (ii) it is devoid of crossing fibres. It has further advantages in that it is a large structure (*cf.* the fornix, which can also be directly visualised) hence minimising partial volume effects; finally, prior knowledge in Alzheimer's disease, indicates that one expects greater degenerative change in the splenium compared to the genu [7]; hence one can study differential disease effects in the same white matter bundle.

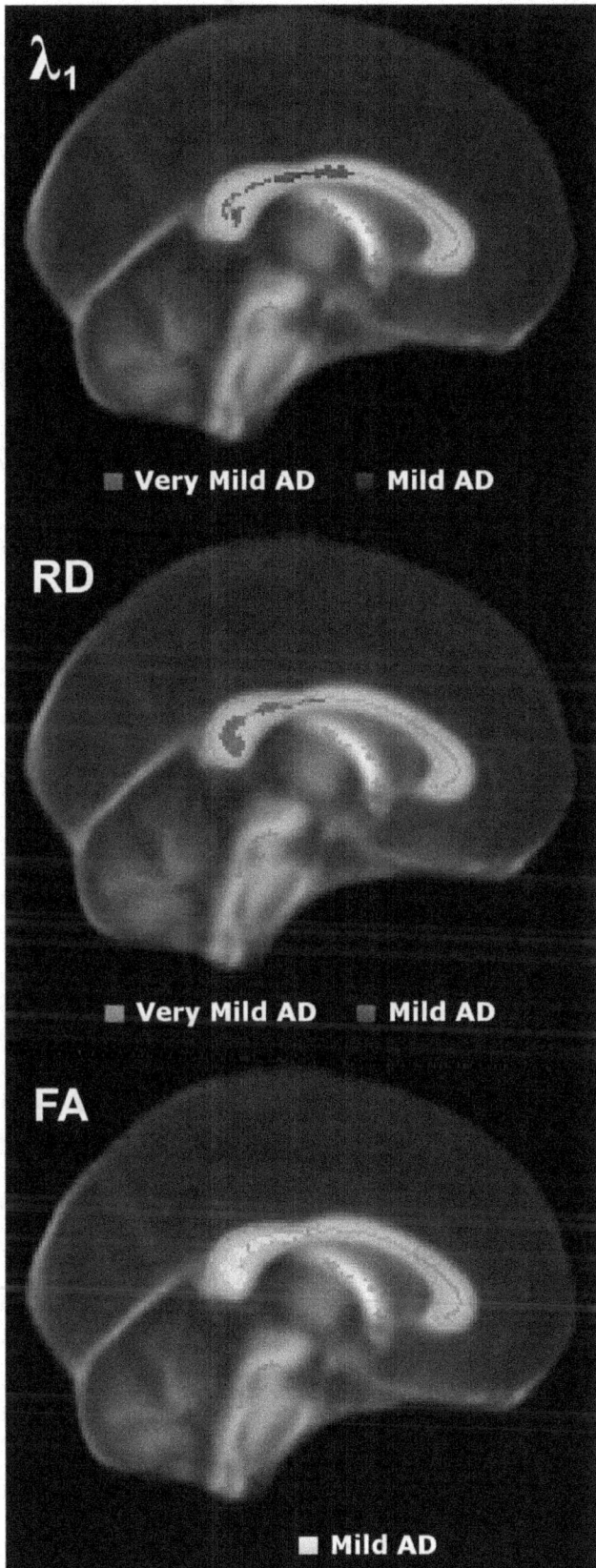

Figure 5. Cross-sectional results in the mid-sagittal corpus callosum. TBSS results across the sagittal midline for very mild and mild Alzheimer's disease groups compared to controls.
doi:10.1371/journal.pone.0049072.g005

Each T1-weighted structural volume was affine-registered to its corresponding *b*0 image, hence enabling the midline corpus callosum to be individually traced with Analyze v8.1 (Biomedical Imaging Resource, Mayo Foundation, Rochester, MN, USA), while minimising partial-volume contamination. Then in Matlab v2008a (The Mathworks Inc., Natick, MA, USA), we automated the subdivision of each corpus callosum mask into three regions–splenium, truncus and genu as illustrated in Figure 2 (top panel)–of equal length along the axis that connects the most distal–caudal and rostral–points from the mid-sagittal corpus callosum's centre-of-mass. Note that although rigorous, tractography-based strategies have been proposed to subdivide the corpus callosum [27], in this study we were ultimately interested in discerning overall tensor differences between caudal and rostral callosal tracts; thus, for simplicity, we followed a widely-used previous classification [28]– we collapsed the isthmus and splenium regions into a single splenial region of interest, and the truncus included both anterior and posterior sections of the callosal midbody. It should also be noted that although both schemes were highly concordant in the caudal third, they disagreed on the definition of genu, which only extended across the anterior sixth of the corpus callosum in the most-recently proposed classification [27].

We computed mean values for each region of interest in native space and for comparison, we also extracted mean values–directly in standard space–resulting from the intersection of each region of interest (segmented from the standard FMRIB58_FA template) with the mean FA skeleton mask (N = 69, FA>0.2) as depicted in Figure 2 (bottom panel). It is important to note that the latter method only required tracing the template corpus callosum mask once; whereas the former approach needed corpus callosum masks to be delineated for every individual. Although manual extraction is considered to be the "gold standard" method [14], it is a time-consuming process and in neurodegeneration, atrophy can lead to systematic misregistration to template of a patient group relative to controls [29]. In order to circumvent this problem, TBSS projects tract centres onto a skeleton containing all major white matter bundles; thereby minimising the effect of misregistration, but also excluding peripheral white matter tracts. In this study, we also tested the hypothesis that skeletonised mid-sagittal corpus callosum DTI data contains all the relevant information needed both to detect early white matter damage in Alzheimer's disease and to monitor disease progression.

To address the research questions posed in this study, we first collapsed all DTI measurements from all Alzheimer's disease subjects (N = 43), which, for each callosal subregion, were cross-sectionally compared against control data (N = 26) and regressed against a measure of global cognitive status (ACE-R scores). These tests aimed to find differential behaviours across regions. Subsequently, the patient group was subdivided–as proposed in the 'Subjects' subsection (very mild, N = 21; and mild Alzheimer's disease, N = 22)–, and further cross-sectional comparisons were performed to assess the overall trend of each DTI parameter across disease severity. The group study designs were as follows: both very mild and mild patient groups were contrasted against controls; additionally, mild patients were compared against the very mild cohort. Further confirmation of the observed tensor behaviour was sought by testing a smaller group of Alzheimer's patients (N = 16) longitudinally: 12 months versus baseline, and contrasting data from both time-points against controls.

In Matlab, we first applied a numerical Lilliefors test of the default null hypothesis that mean-subject values came from a distribution in the normal family [30], which revealed that they did not at $\alpha = 0.05$ for any DTI metric in any cohort. We therefore compared unpaired DTI-derived values from independent

Table 3. Alzheimer's disease skeletonised DTI parametric comparisons in different mid-sagittal callosal areas.

Alzheimer's disease (N = 43) vs. Control (N = 26)	Splenium	Truncus	Genu
λ_1	−2.24[§]	−1.39	−0.22
RD	−3.08**	−0.76	0.53
MD	−3.39**	−1.08	0.30
FA	2.45[§]	0.40	−1.18

Results are given as Wilcoxon rank-sum Z-statistic.
Significance levels: [§]0.01<P<0.05 (Alzheimer's disease worse than controls, two-tailed); **P<0.05 (Alzheimer's disease worse than controls, two-tailed, Bonferroni-corrected on n = 12).
doi:10.1371/journal.pone.0049072.t003

samples (*i.e.* patients versus controls or very mild versus mild patients) using nonparametric Wilcoxon rank-sum–*i.e.* Mann–Whitney *U*–tests [31,32], and paired longitudinal samples (*i.e.* same patient cohort at different time-points) were tested with the Wilcoxon signed-rank approach [32]. For consistency, all two-sample hypotheses on cognitive profiles were tested with the same relevant (*i.e.* rank-sum if cross-sectional; signed-rank if longitudinal) method. Linear dependence with ACE-R was tested using pairwise Pearson's correlations [33]. Note that statistical significances were computed combining both tails of the sampling distributions.

To assess for atrophy in the midline corpus callosum, we compared cross-sectional callosal areas in native space. Each measurement was normalised for differences in total intracranial volume using an analysis of covariance approach, where the measured areas were adjusted by an amount proportional to the difference between each individual's observed total intracranial volume and the global total intracranial volume mean for all control subjects [34]. Total brain volumes were also computed and normalised (by total intracranial volume) to compare (N = 43) mid-sagittal callosal areas with a measure of global atrophy. Total intracranial and brain volumes were determined using a previously validated method that involved summing grey matter, white matter and cerebrospinal-fluid tissue segments [35].

Simultaneous inference procedure. In order to correct for the statistical effect of simultaneous regional testing in the present study, we applied Bonferroni inequalities to each family of hypotheses with $\alpha = 0.05$. We corrected inferences separately if the hypotheses under evaluation were different. For instance, we performed 28 cross-sectional statistical tests to identify the nature of cognitive deficits across groups at differing disease stages relative to controls. This experiment was treated as a family (n = 28 tests); the family-wise error (FWE) rate associated with $\alpha = 0.05$ was therefore $P_{FWE} = 0.0018$. Analogously, statistical significance (corrected for multiple comparisons) on longitudinal comparisons of cognitive performance was established at $P < 0.0071$ (n = 7). The cross-sectional analyses (N = 43 patients versus controls)–performed to characterise the different imaging parameters in each callosal subdivision–were treated as a separate family (n = 12, $P_{FWE} = 0.0042$). Pearson's correlations were also treated as a family (n = 12, $P_{FWE} = 0.0042$). In addition, the cross-sectional assessments of each patient subgroup (*i.e.* very mild and mild Alzheimer's disease versus controls) were corrected together (n = 24, $P_{FWE} = 0.0021$). Note though that for each region of interest, longitudinal DTI data was corrected separately (n = 12, $P_{FWE} = 0.0042$).

Results

Cross-sectional TBSS Study of Very Mild Alzheimer's Disease

TBSS results for the voxel-wise group contrast of very mild Alzheimer's disease versus controls are shown in Figure 3. The λ_1 statistical map showed significant bilateral and confluent change that predominantly involved parietal white matter, with strongest abnormalities along the posterior cingulum and the inter-hemispheric tracts of the caudal corpus callosum. In contrast, there was relative sparing of caudal occipital, rostral temporal lobe and prefrontal white matter, and, the more rostral tracts of the corpus callosum. RD abnormalities spatially overlapped with those found for λ_1 in parietal and superior temporal white matter–though only

Table 4. DTI group comparisons across disease stages and linear dependence on global cognition for all patients in the splenium.

Splenium	Cross-sectional			ACE-R Linear Dependence (N = 43)
	Very mild Alzheimer's (N = 21) vs. Control (N = 26)	Mild Alzheimer's (N = 22) vs. Control (N = 26)	Mild Alzheimer's (N = 22) vs. Very mild Alzheimer's (N = 21)	
λ_1	2.62*	1.19	1.54	0.15
RD	2.13[§]	3.07**	−0.89	−0.40**
MD	3.01**	2.74*	0.21	−0.21
FA	−1.27	−2.85*	1.4	0.44**

Group results are given as Wilcoxon rank-sum Z-statistic; statistical dependencies are given as Pearson correlation coefficient with 41 degrees of freedom.
Significance levels: [§]0.01<P<0.05 (Alzheimer's disease worse than controls, two-tailed); *P<0.01 (Alzheimer's disease worse than controls, two-tailed); **P<0.05 (Alzheimer's disease worse than controls, two-tailed, Bonferroni-corrected on n = 24; or DTI measure correlated with Alzheimer's disease cognitive status, two-tailed, Bonferroni-corrected on n = 12).
doi:10.1371/journal.pone.0049072.t004

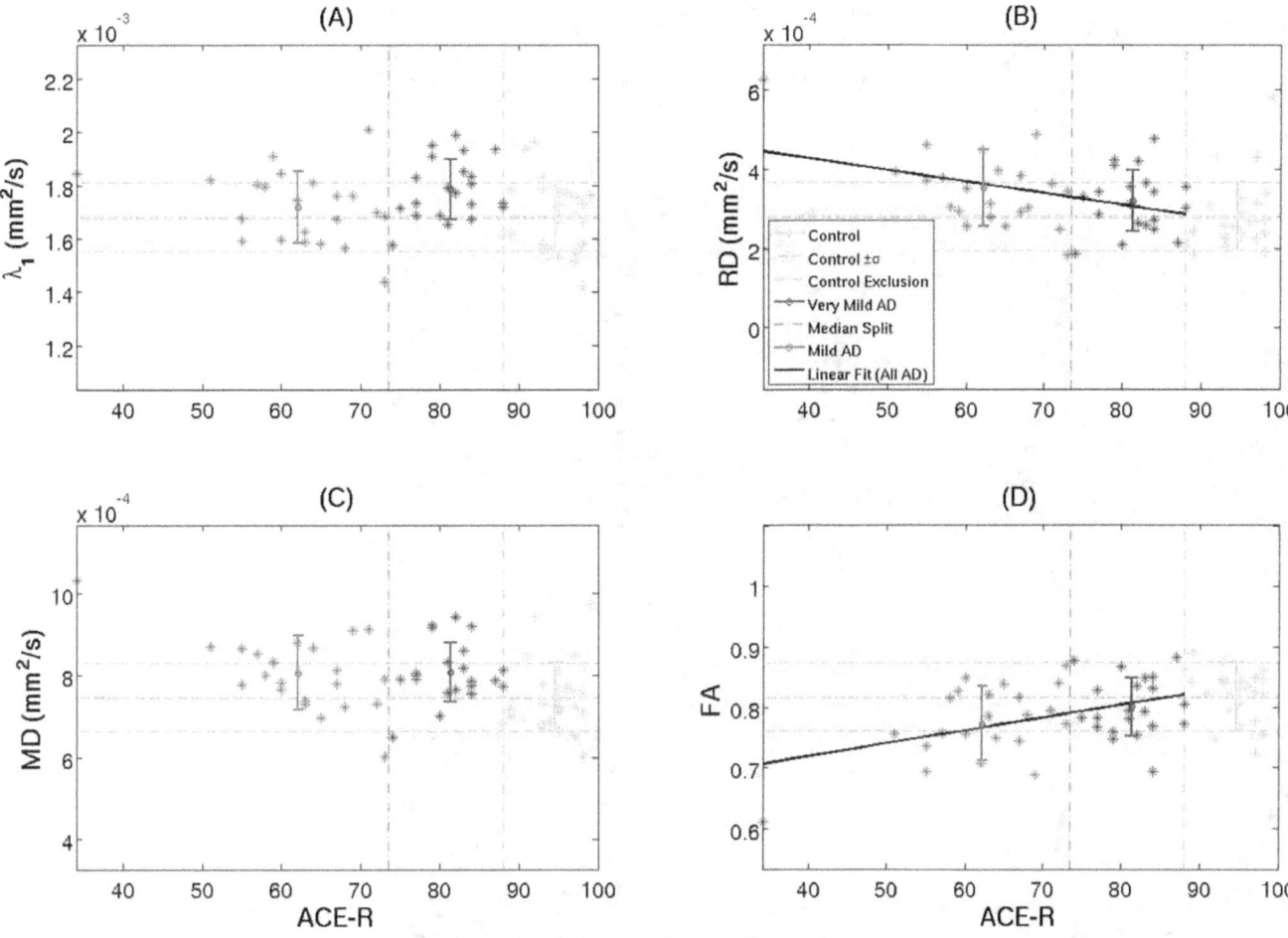

Figure 6. Cross-sectional diffusion tensor behaviour in the splenial region. Mean subject values for skeletonised DTI parameters in the splenium as a function of cognitive status (ACE-R scores) for controls (green), very mild Alzheimer's disease (blue) and mild Alzheimer's disease patients (red). The error bars represent ± one group standard deviation. The vertical axes were scaled to 10 control standard deviations. The vertical lines delimit the control exclusion criteria (ACE-R<88/100) and the median split (ACE-R = 74). A least-square linear fit was displayed if Pearson's correlation coefficient was deemed statistically significant (Table 4).
doi:10.1371/journal.pone.0049072.g006

across the right hemisphere. FA changes were similarly distributed, but overall were the least widespread.

Cross-sectional TBSS Study of Mild Alzheimer's Disease

Extensive, mostly bilateral distributions of DTI abnormalities for all metrics (increased diffusivities and reduced FA) were found in the mild Alzheimer's disease versus control group contrast using TBSS. As illustrated in Figure 4, λ_1 showed the most extensive and confluent clusters of significance. These were located in parietal white matter regions including the caudal corpus callosum and the posterior cingulum bundle; caudal temporal areas with a slightly greater predilection for the left side and bilateral frontal lobe involvement Although RD and FA abnormalities were highly concordant and largely overlapped with λ_1 clusters, overall they were less extensive; in particular, frontal lobe involvement of RD and FA was minimal. Note that all regions found to be abnormal in the very mild Alzheimer's disease group (Figure 3), were also clearly damaged in the mild group (Figure 4).

The cross-sectional MD results for both Alzheimer's disease groups were also extensive and unsurprisingly overlapped to a high degree with those of its components; more specifically with the spatial distribution of increased λ_1, but it did not reveal any additional involvement (see Figure S1).

Mid-sagittal Corpus Callosum

TBSS. Unlike total brain volume in Alzheimer's disease, which was significantly reduced compared to controls (standard score, Z = −0.80; P = 0.002), atrophy in the cross-sectional area of the corpus callosum did not reach statistical significance (Z = −0.43, P = 0.1).

Figure 5 shows DTI abnormalities across the mid-sagittal corpus callosum for both very mild and mild Alzheimer's disease stages. The caudal corpus callosum was heavily involved, whereas there was preservation of white matter tracts running across the mid-sagittal genu. λ_1 featured prominently in the very mild Alzheimer's disease cohort but it did not become more extensive in the more-impaired group; in contrast, RD/FA abnormalities were more extensive in mild-stage Alzheimer's disease. Note that the fornix was abnormal for all DTI metrics in both Alzheimer's disease groups (uncorrected-P<0.01, data not shown), but the clusters of significance did not survive our attempt to correct for multiple comparisons.

Regions of Interest

The regional analyses were consistent with the above TBSS observations. Table 3 highlights the preservation of the midline truncus and genu relative to the splenium when contrasting all Alzheimer's patients (N = 43) with the control group. Examining

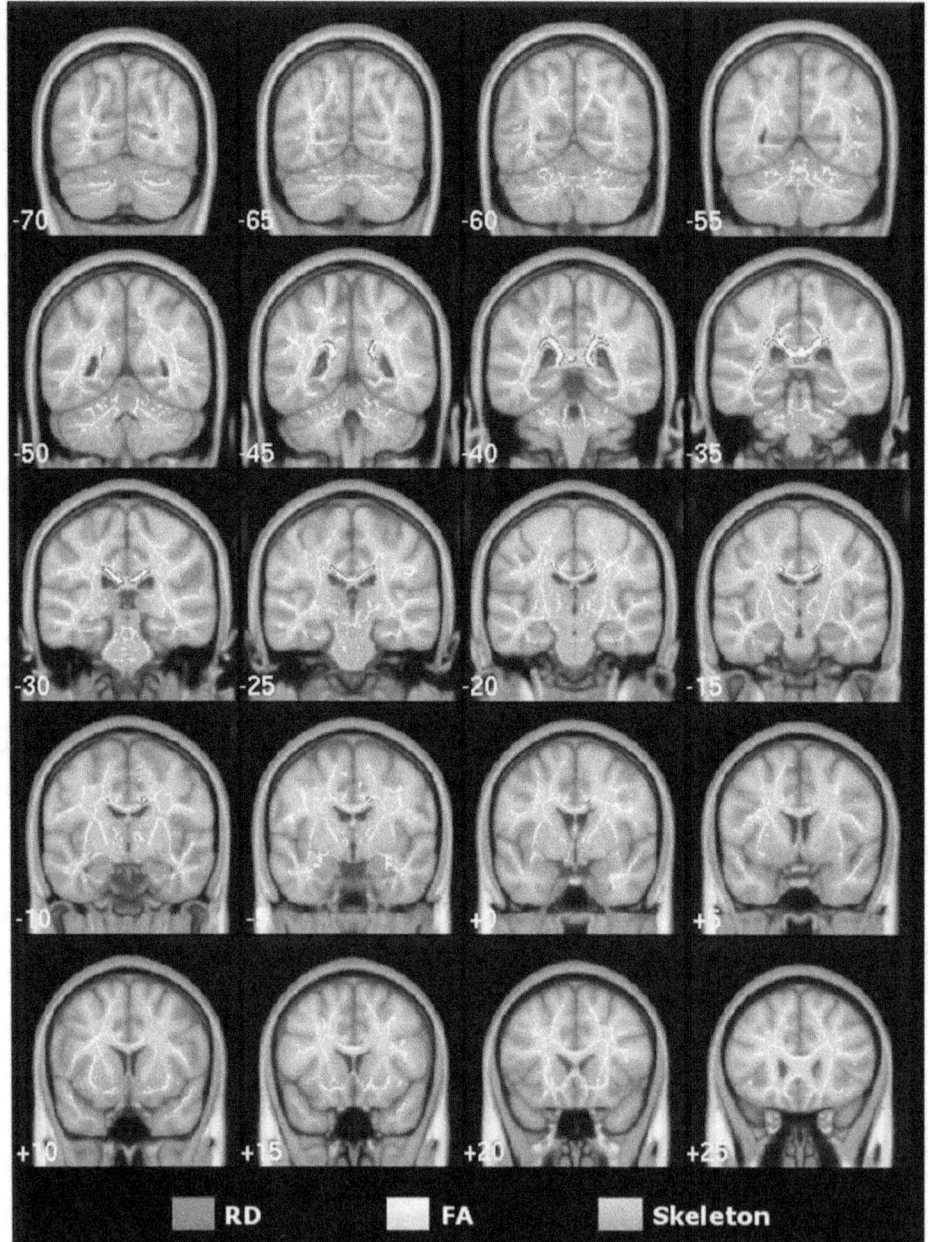

Figure 7. Longitudinal study of Alzheimer's disease. Whole-brain TBSS contrast on 12-month follow-up versus baseline in the longitudinal Alzheimer's disease cohort (TFCE-P<0.05) for increased radial diffusivity and reduced FA *n.b.* no significant results for λ_1 or MD were found.
doi:10.1371/journal.pone.0049072.g007

for differential behaviour of the diffusion tensor across varying disease stages reinforced the finding that in early disease, λ_1 is more prominently abnormal than RD indicating that a significant contributor to early MD increase is an increase in λ_1 (Table 4). RD and FA, however, showed the most prominent alterations in the more cognitively-impaired group of patients–where λ_1 remained relatively stable–, suggesting that MD abnormalities in later disease stages are primarily driven by increased RD (Table 4). The latter finding was supported by a statistically significant correlation between dementia severity (ACE-R score) and either FA or RD (Table 4). It should be noted that statistical tests for the truncus and genu–equivalent to those reported in Table 4 for the splenium–yielded, as expected, no significant results.

Focusing on the splenial lesion, this being the key pathological region, Figure 6 illustrates all mean patient DTI values relative to control data as a function of cognitive status. As shown in Table 4, splenial λ_1 appeared to increase significantly in very mild subjects, but it did not follow that more impaired patients were increasingly abnormal–if anything there was a trend to attenuation of abnormality with advancing dementia (Figure 6a). In stark contrast, RD and FA were essentially less sensitive in very mild disease but there was a linear progression observed for these behaviours with advancing severity (Figure 6b and 6d). Note that the behaviour of MD followed a similar pattern to that of λ_1 in early disease stages but appeared to be largely driven by RD in more advanced cases (Figure 6c).

It should be noted that the regional results reported in this section–using skeletonised DTI data–were replicated with data extracted from entire callosal regions of interest in native space (see plots in Figure S2).

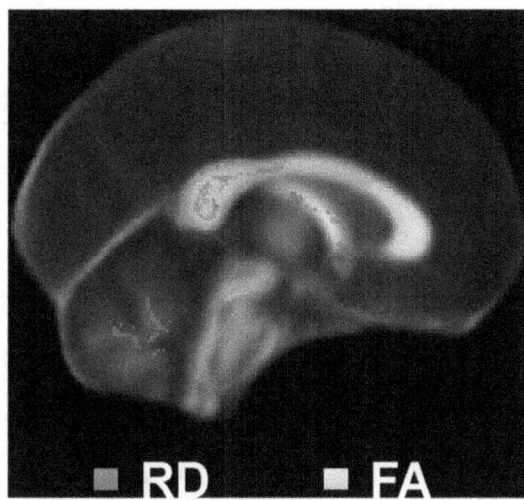

Figure 8. Longitudinal results in the mid-sagittal corpus callosum. Longitudinal TBSS results for radial diffusivity and fractional anisotropy across the midline.
doi:10.1371/journal.pone.0049072.g008

Longitudinal Study of Alzheimer's Disease

The contrast of 12-month follow-up scans with baseline in the longitudinal Alzheimer's disease cohort (N = 16) found that λ_1 remained unchanged in the whole brain's skeletonised white matter at TFCE-P<0.05. However, consistent with the cross-sectional analyses, RD/FA abnormalities progressed significantly in the caudal corpus callosum and posterior cingulum bilaterally, and in a left superior temporal region (Figure 7). The clusters of significance found in the longitudinal assessments were highly co-localised with the strongest DTI abnormalities found in the very mild Alzheimer's disease group relative to controls; this was also clearly illustrated in the mid-sagittal TBSS results (Figure 8).

The splenial results shown in Table 5 revealed a very consistent scenario. λ_1 was slightly abnormal at baseline but it did not progress. RD and FA differences, however, –above the statistical threshold at baseline–showed emphatic abnormalities at 12 months and during the longitudinal time-span. MD was found to be similarly abnormal at baseline and 12 months, thus resulting in no apparent progression.

When the extracted mean DTI values from each subject's skeletonised splenium were plotted against ACE-R scores (Figure 9), the findings were in remarkable agreement with those observed in the cross-sectional study. Overall, RD/FA longitudi-

nal pairs (Figure 9b and 9d, respectively) followed more coherently progressive evolutions than axial and mean diffusivities (Figure 9a and 9c).

Discussion

This study aimed to investigate the biomarker potential of DTI metrics in Alzheimer's disease through whole-brain analyses as well as by taking a reductionist approach in the corpus callosum to eliminate ambiguities generated by uncertain tract visualisation and crossing fibres. The evolution of DTI changes was examined in both cross-sectional and longitudinal datasets; the former by way of a median spilt in which 76% of the very mild patients were in the mild-cognitive impairment stage of Alzheimer's disease, and the latter by contrasting 12-month follow-up scans to baseline. Across the various analyses, a consistent picture emerged in which an increase in λ_1 is the first significant change in Alzheimer's disease, but then remains relatively steady. In contrast, RD–and therefore FA–become progressively more abnormal with disease evolution, making them the candidate metrics for stage-specific biomarkers. In other words, these markers could have value to track change over time. Given that FA reduction is a function of both RD and λ_1, and the early increase in λ_1 appeared to attenuate with disease progression, it may be that FA is the superior measure of decline compared to RD in longitudinal studies. It should be emphasized, however, that the attenuation of λ_1 was subtle and, unless replicated in similar studies, could simply represent random variability in the current dataset. A further caveat to this proposal is that the preference for FA would only apply to areas in which the λ_1 abnormality has already peaked– such as the splenium in the present analyses. For instance, in a repeated-measure longitudinal design, in areas that are initially spared in terms of λ_1, the first movement of this metric would be to increase, leading to a loss of sensitivity for FA to detect change. This was exemplified by the cross-sectional results, in which frontal and left temporal white matter was normal in the very mild group, but became abnormal (mostly in terms of λ_1) in the mild group. This problem would, of course, be avoided by studying RD, which–unlike FA–is independent of λ_1.

In contrast to RD and FA, the results indicated that λ_1 has no role at all as staging biomarker for a given region of interest. Although one could, in theory, propose it as a staging marker by looking at the differential spatial extent of λ_1 abnormalities over time, this would be difficult to implement as a marker of progression given that some degree of heterogeneity would be expected across subjects; furthermore, such an approach would also be confounded if it proved correct in future studies that the λ_1

Table 5. Longitudinal DTI assessment of Alzheimer's disease in the splenium.

Splenium				Longitudinal
	Baseline (N = 16) vs. Control (N = 26)	12 months (N = 16) vs. Control (N = 26)		12 months (N = 16) vs. Baseline (N = 16)
λ_1	2.37§	1.54		−0.52
RD	1.72	2.97**		−2.59*
MD	2.47§	2.71*		−1.76
FA	−0.87	−2.58*		−2.64*

Baseline and 12 months versus controls comparisons are reported as Wilcoxon rank-sum Z-statistic values; paired longitudinal results are given as Wilcoxon signed-rank Z-statistic.
Significance levels: §0.01<P<0.05 (Alzheimer's disease worse than controls, two-tailed); *P<0.01 (Alzheimer's disease worse than controls; or 12 months worse than baseline, two-tailed); **P<0.05 (Alzheimer's disease worse than controls, two-tailed, Bonferroni-corrected on n = 12).
doi:10.1371/journal.pone.0049072.t005

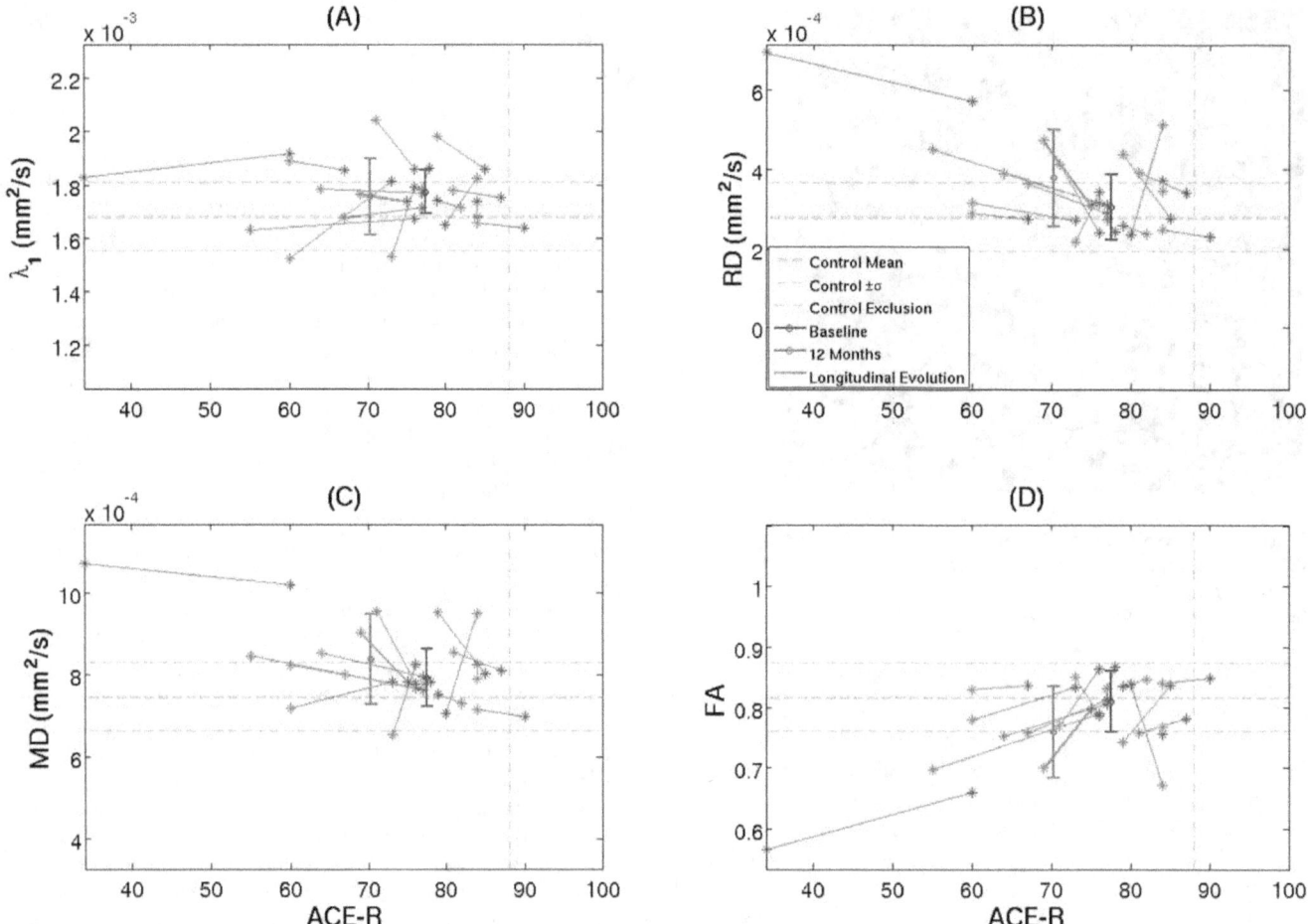

Figure 9. Longitudinal tensor behaviour in the splenium. Longitudinal pairs of mean subject skeletonised DTI parameters as a function of cognitive status (ACE-R) for Alzheimer's disease subjects at baseline (blue) and 12 months (red).
doi:10.1371/journal.pone.0049072.g009

effect attenuates in early affected regions. Nevertheless, the results of both cross-sectional and longitudinal studies clearly indicate that an increase in λ_1 is the first sign of change in Alzheimer's disease, suggesting therefore that it could have a role as an early state-specific marker. This was particular notable in the cross-sectional data, in which posterior temporo-parietal white matter including the splenium showed increased λ_1 in the very mild group with the same regions showing involvement of RD and FA in the mild group *i.e.* at a more advanced disease stage. In the more advanced group, however, new areas–notably frontal and left temporal white matter–showed increased λ_1, suggesting that as degeneration spreads to new areas, an increase in λ_1 is the first sign of this involvement. Similarly, the longitudinal data also showed that there was a prominent increase in λ_1 in posterior temporo-parietal white matter at baseline (cross-sectional comparison against the control population not shown), with RD and FA abnormalities emerging in the same spatial distribution with follow-up.

Increased λ_1 as found in this and other recent studies [5,7] was an unanticipated finding in Alzheimer's disease and its mechanism is uncertain. The finding that the λ_1 abnormalities were the most spatially extensive extends the results of our earlier study using the TBSS method [5], and are also consistent with a recent independent TBSS study in showing that this metric has the greatest sensitivity to change in early disease [36]. Using a similar TBSS-based approach, Huang et al. [7] also found that the most prominent features in less affected areas in Alzheimer's disease

were increased λ_1 and MD whereas, also consistent with our findings, in areas such as the cingulum and fornix that would be expected to have most advanced pathology, RD and FA were highly abnormal but λ_1 was not.

It was recently proposed that λ_1 increase might represent differential tract involvement in areas of crossing white matter tracts [13]–*i.e.* if two tracts cross then the tensor in such areas will be the average contribution of both; therefore, if one of these tracts degenerates, the tensor will be driven by the remaining tract and hence an increase in λ_1 could be predicted. While this seems a very plausible theory in crossing fibres, it cannot explain the λ_1 increase in very early Alzheimer's disease because the observation is equally apparent in areas such as the splenium [5,7] and fornix [5,37], in which crossing tracts are not present. One clue from the current study was the finding that increased λ_1 in the splenium showed no correlation with global dementia severity. This, in turn, implies that increased λ_1 might be completely independent of axonal loss. It must be stressed, nevertheless, that the failure of λ_1 to correlate with dementia severity is only demonstrated at a global level. It may still be the case that the phenomenon driving the early increase in λ_1 is associated with local dysfunction of specific cognitive processes. For instance, a recent study noted correlation between increased λ_1 and route-learning impairment in Alzheimer's disease [38]; the area of correlation was tightly co-incident with correlations between the same task and both metabolism and atrophy of adjacent grey matter suggesting that it was not an artefactual result.

Studies in Alzheimer's disease, to date, have mostly tended to conceptualise DTI abnormalities in terms of neuronal loss or damage, but it is important to keep in mind that although robust tensor changes can be found in Alzheimer's disease, their precise underlying mechanism is essentially unknown. Furthermore, studies often infer mechanisms by citing homology with animal models, but this can only ever be *consistent with* rather than *proof of* a given mechanism; for instance, if myelin loss in an animal model causes a particular tensor metric to change in a certain way, it does not follow that myelin loss is the *only* mechanism that could generate such a tensor behaviour. Returning to the present findings, RD, and therefore FA, correlated with dementia severity implying that whatever these metrics capture, it is likely to be related to neuronal loss. The fact that increased λ_1 was both independent of dementia severity and a precursor to RD/FA changes (*n.b.* areas where RD and FA changes emerged were characteristically those that had first seen an increase in λ_1), suggests that λ_1 may be capturing an upstream event to axonal degeneration. It is also noteworthy that the spread of λ_1 increase was not random but, rather, closely mirrored the expected progression of degeneration as would be measured by cerebral glucose metabolism–*i.e.* posterior (posterior cingulate/precuneus spreading out to lateral temporo-parietal association tracts), then later to anterior (prefrontal) areas [39,40].

Although a completely speculative hypothesis, one possible upstream event could be inflammation. The role of inflammatory change in Alzheimer's disease is presently of considerable interest [41] and it is at least conceivable, given that λ_1 increase appears to represent something other than axonal loss, that it could be driven by factors such as microglial activation. Whatever its mechanism, understanding the true sequence in the cascade of events leading to neuronal loss in Alzheimer's disease is arguably the most important question in understanding pathogenesis. As such, further work to understand what this early λ_1 increase might represent in areas that subsequently degenerate, seems to be, therefore, critically important.

The differing behaviour of tensor metrics identified in the course of Alzheimer's disease in this study goes some way to explain inconsistencies reported in previous studies. For instance, some studies in early disease have reported little abnormality in FA [5,6]. That said, it is difficult to identify a coherent picture from previous DTI results in Alzheimer's disease, even if one only considers the corpus callosum–for review see [42]. Factors contributing to this inconsistency likely include: differing levels of dementia severity; an almost universal lack of outcome data in cohorts labelled mild-cognitive impairment; variable region-of-interest placement; and variable acquisition protocols. In the present study, the cross-sectional and longitudinal data highlighted the critical effect of dementia severity, while clinical follow-up ensured that all cases scanned in the mild-cognitive impairment stage had incipient Alzheimer's disease. The issue of region-of-interest placement is critical to standardisation if DTI data is to be used as a biomarker. Because TBSS fits tract centres common to all subjects, this appears to be an appropriate method for whole-brain analyses. Meanwhile, the midline corpus callosum offers a cleaner target to study a tract in isolation; critically, however, as would be expected from prior knowledge, it is not homogenously affected but, rather, the splenium is the site of maximum damage. The current study offers an automated method for extracting corpus callosum regions that could go some way to optimising comparability across studies. Finally, the issue of acquisition is critical to consider. The present study used a 63-direction

acquisition with one b-value, and as already mentioned, yielded a spread of abnormalities with advancing severity that is highly consistent with the evolution of Alzheimer's disease from other imaging modalities. Recent methods work has validated the use of 30 directions with two b-values as an alternative, whereas fewer (than 30) directions may be less reliable for tensor modelling unless a large number of b-values are used [43]; to this end, it is important to note that most early DTI studies employed less than 10 directions with only one b-value, which may have contributed to noisy or inconsistent results. It should also be noted that at present, although RD, MD and FA are considered to be reliable DTI metrics, conflicting results have been reported with regard to the intra-scanner stability of λ_1 measurements at 3T [44,45]. In this study, λ_1 appeared to be robust in the corpus callosum, but further test-retest validations using the proposed experimental methodology are required to address this important question. A final technical point to note is that although it is discouraged to interpret primary diffusivities on the basis of the underlying neurobiological processes [46], the negligible effects of: (i) crossing fibres, (ii) partial volume–due to lack of atrophy–and (iii) eigenvector sorting bias–due to the large differences in signal-to-noise ratio between λ_1 and RD *e.g.* $\lambda_1 \approx 6 \cdot \text{RD}$ in the skeletonised splenium–, makes the mid-sagittal corpus callosum a suitable white matter structure to monitor early-stage Alzheimer's disease.

In conclusion, the cross-sectional and longitudinal data examined in the present study identified that RD and FA have utility as staging biomarkers in Alzheimer's disease. Both whole-brain TBSS and a skeletonised splenial region of interest appear to be good methods to standardise sampling in repeated-measures designs. The sensitivity of these measures compared to other biomarkers needs to be established, however, one final point argues for their potential added value in practical terms. Structural MRI is already a standard procedure in longitudinal studies; a diffusion sequence can be readily acquired in the same scanning session, meaning that this added value can be achieved with little extra cost or inconvenience compared to nuclear medicine imaging or cerebrospinal-fluid analysis. Axial diffusivity (λ_1) in a given region is a state-, rather than a stage-specific biomarker, that predates changes in RD/FA and appears to represent something other than axonal loss.

Supporting Information

Figure S1 Increased mean diffusivity results for very mild and mild Alzheimer's disease. TBSS results for very mild- and mild-stage Alzheimer's disease groups compared to controls. Thresholded (TFCE-P<0.05) statistical maps for increased mean diffusivity were overlaid onto the mean FA skeleton and the MNI152 template with coronal depths given in millimetres. Extensive, mostly bilateral distributions of DTI abnormalities for increased mean diffusion were found in the very mild and mild Alzheimer's disease group comparisons. Significant abnormalities were located in parietal white matter regions including the caudal corpus callosum and the posterior cingulum bundle, and in caudal temporal areas. All clusters of significance found in the very mild Alzheimer's disease group, were also found in the mild group. As expected, overall MD abnormalities were highly concordant and largely overlapped with the spatial distribution of λ_1 clusters of significance shown in Figure 3 and Figure 4 (main manuscript).
(TIF)

Figure S2 Regional analysis of the splenium in native space. Mean subject values for DTI parameters in the native splenial region as a function of cognitive status (ACE-R) for controls (green), very mild Alzheimer's disease (blue) and mild Alzheimer's disease patients (red). The error bars represent ± one group standard deviation, and the vertical axes were scaled to 10 control standard deviations. The vertical lines delimit the control exclusion criteria (ACE-R<88) and the median split (ACE-R = 74). A least-square linear fit was displayed if Pearson's correlation coefficient was deemed statistically significant for N = 43 patients. In agreement with the skeletonised data shown in Figure 6 (main manuscript), λ_1 appeared to increase most significantly in very mild subjects, whereas RD and FA followed a linear progression with advancing disease severity.

(TIF)

Acknowledgments

We are grateful for the support from our patients and healthy volunteers.

Author Contributions

Conceived and designed the experiments: JAC GBW PJN. Performed the experiments: JAC GP. Analyzed the data: JAC SA. Wrote the paper: JAC GBW GP PJN.

References

1. Jack CR, Jr., Petersen RC, Xu YC, O'Brien PC, Smith GE, et al. (1999) Prediction of AD with MRI-based hippocampal volume in mild cognitive impairment. Neurology 52: 1397–1403.
2. Fellgiebel A, Schermuly I, Gerhard A, Keller I, Albrecht J, et al. (2008) Functional relevant loss of long association fibre tracts integrity in early Alzheimer's disease. Neuropsychologia 46: 1698–1706.
3. Mielke MM, Kozauer NA, Chan KC, George M, Toroney J, et al. (2009) Regionally-specific diffusion tensor imaging in mild cognitive impairment and Alzheimer's disease. Neuroimage 46: 47–55.
4. Takahashi S, Yonezawa H, Takahashi J, Kudo M, Inoue T, et al. (2002) Selective reduction of diffusion anisotropy in white matter of Alzheimer disease brains measured by 3.0 Tesla magnetic resonance imaging. Neurosci Lett 332: 45–48.
5. Acosta-Cabronero J, Williams GB, Pengas G, Nestor PJ (2010) Absolute diffusivities define the landscape of white matter degeneration in Alzheimer's disease. Brain 133: 529–539.
6. Fellgiebel A, Wille P, Muller MJ, Winterer G, Scheurich A, et al. (2004) Ultrastructural hippocampal and white matter alterations in mild cognitive impairment: a diffusion tensor imaging study. Dement Geriatr Cogn Disord 18: 101–108.
7. Huang H, Fan X, Weiner M, Martin-Cook K, Xiao G, et al. (2012) Distinctive disruption patterns of white matter tracts in Alzheimer's disease with full diffusion tensor characterization. Neurobiol Aging 33: 2029–2045.
8. Shu N, Wang Z, Qi Z, Li K, He Y (2011) Multiple diffusion indices reveals white matter degeneration in Alzheimer's disease and mild cognitive impairment: a tract-based spatial statistics study. J Alzheimers Dis 26 Suppl 3: 275–285.
9. Zhang Y, Schuff N, Du AT, Rosen HJ, Kramer JH, et al. (2009) White matter damage in frontotemporal dementia and Alzheimer's disease measured by diffusion MRI. Brain 132: 2579–2592.
10. Huang J, Auchus AP (2007) Diffusion tensor imaging of normal appearing white matter and its correlation with cognitive functioning in mild cognitive impairment and Alzheimer's disease. Ann N Y Acad Sci 1097: 259–264.
11. Bosch B, Arenaza-Urquijo EM, Rami L, Sala-Llonch R, Junque C, et al. (2012) Multiple DTI index analysis in normal aging, amnestic MCI and AD. Relationship with neuropsychological performance. Neurobiol Aging 33: 61–74.
12. Zhang Y, Schuff N, Jahng GH, Bayne W, Mori S, et al. (2007) Diffusion tensor imaging of cingulum fibers in mild cognitive impairment and Alzheimer disease. Neurology 68: 13–19.
13. Douaud G, Jbabdi S, Behrens TE, Menke RA, Gass A, et al. (2011) DTI measures in crossing-fibre areas: increased diffusion anisotropy reveals early white matter alteration in MCI and mild Alzheimer's disease. Neuroimage 55: 880–890.
14. Fellgiebel A, Muller MJ, Wille P, Dellani PR, Scheurich A, et al. (2005) Color-coded diffusion-tensor-imaging of posterior cingulate fiber tracts in mild cognitive impairment. Neurobiol Aging 26: 1193–1198.
15. Zhang J, Jones M, DeBoy CA, Reich DS, Farrell JA, et al. (2009) Diffusion tensor magnetic resonance imaging of Wallerian degeneration in rat spinal cord after dorsal root axotomy. J Neurosci 29: 3160–3171.
16. Hanyu H, Asano T, Sakurai H, Imon Y, Iwamoto T, et al. (1999) Diffusion-weighted and magnetization transfer imaging of the corpus callosum in Alzheimer's disease. J Neurol Sci 167: 37–44.
17. McKhann G, Drachman D, Folstein M, Katzman R, Price D, et al. (1984) Clinical diagnosis of Alzheimer's disease: report of the NINCDS-ADRDA Work Group under the auspices of Department of Health and Human Services Task Force on Alzheimer's Disease. Neurology 34: 939–944.
18. Folstein MF, Folstein SE, McHugh PR (1975) "Mini-mental state". A practical method for grading the cognitive state of patients for the clinician. J Psychiatr Res 12: 189–198.
19. Mioshi E, Dawson K, Mitchell J, Arnold R, Hodges JR (2006) The Addenbrooke's Cognitive Examination Revised (ACE-R): a brief cognitive test battery for dementia screening. Int J Geriatr Psychiatry 21: 1078–1085.
20. Reese TG, Heid O, Weisskoff RM, Wedeen VJ (2003) Reduction of eddy-current-induced distortion in diffusion MRI using a twice-refocused spin echo. Magn Reson Med 49: 177–182.
21. Griswold MA, Jakob PM, Heidemann RM, Nittka M, Jellus V, et al. (2002) Generalized autocalibrating partially parallel acquisitions (GRAPPA). Magn Reson Med 47: 1202–1210.
22. Smith SM, Jenkinson M, Woolrich MW, Beckmann CF, Behrens TE, et al. (2004) Advances in functional and structural MR image analysis and implementation as FSL. Neuroimage 23 Suppl 1: S208–219.
23. Jenkinson M, Smith S (2001) A global optimisation method for robust affine registration of brain images. Med Image Anal 5: 143–156.
24. Smith SM (2002) Fast robust automated brain extraction. Hum Brain Mapp 17: 143–155.
25. Smith SM, Jenkinson M, Johansen-Berg H, Rueckert D, Nichols TE, et al. (2006) Tract-based spatial statistics: voxelwise analysis of multi-subject diffusion data. Neuroimage 31: 1487–1505.
26. Smith SM, Nichols TE (2009) Threshold-free cluster enhancement: addressing problems of smoothing, threshold dependence and localisation in cluster inference. Neuroimage 44: 83–98.
27. Hofer S, Frahm J (2006) Topography of the human corpus callosum revisited–comprehensive fiber tractography using diffusion tensor magnetic resonance imaging. Neuroimage 32: 989–994.
28. Witelson SF (1989) Hand and sex differences in the isthmus and genu of the human corpus callosum. A postmortem morphological study. Brain 112: 799–835.
29. Snook L, Plewes C, Beaulieu C (2007) Voxel based versus region of interest analysis in diffusion tensor imaging of neurodevelopment. Neuroimage 34: 243–252.
30. Lilliefors HW (1967) On the Kolmogorov-Smirnov test for normality with mean and variance unknown. Journal of the American Statistical Association 62: 399–402.
31. Mann HB, Whitney DR (1947) On a Test of Whether one of Two Random Variables is Stochastically Larger than the Other. Annals of Mathematical Statistics 18: 50–60.
32. Wilcoxon F (1946) Individual comparisons of grouped data by ranking methods. J Econ Entomol 39: 269.
33. Pearson K (1896) Mathematical Contributions to the Theory of Evolution. III. Regression, Heredity and Panmixia. Philosophical Transactions of the Royal Society A 187: 253–318.
34. Jack CR, Jr., Twomey CK, Zinsmeister AR, Sharbrough FW, Petersen RC, et al. (1989) Anterior temporal lobes and hippocampal formations: normative volumetric measurements from MR images in young adults. Radiology 172: 549–554.
35. Pengas G, Pereira JM, Williams GB, Nestor PJ (2009) Comparative reliability of total intracranial volume estimation methods and the influence of atrophy in a longitudinal semantic dementia cohort. J Neuroimaging 19: 37–46.
36. O'Dwyer L, Lamberton F, Bokde AL, Ewers M, Faluyi YO, et al. (2011) Multiple indices of diffusion identifies white matter damage in mild cognitive impairment and Alzheimer's disease. PLoS One 6: e21745.
37. Oishi K, Akhter K, Mielke M, Ceritoglu C, Zhang J, et al. (2011) Multi-modal MRI analysis with disease-specific spatial filtering: initial testing to predict mild cognitive impairment patients who convert to Alzheimer's disease. Front Neurol 2: 54.
38. Pengas G, Williams GB, Acosta-Cabronero J, Ash TWJ, Hong YT, et al. (2012) The relationship of topographical memory performance to regional neurodegeneration in Alzheimer's disease. Front Ag Neurosci 4: 17.
39. Chase TN, Foster NL, Fedio P, Brooks R, Mansi L, et al. (1984) Regional cortical dysfunction in Alzheimer's disease as determined by positron emission tomography. Ann Neurol 15 Suppl: S170–174.
40. Nestor PJ, Fryer TD, Smielewski P, Hodges JR (2003) Limbic hypometabolism in Alzheimer's disease and mild cognitive impairment. Ann Neurol 54: 343–351.
41. Wyss-Coray T, Rogers J (2012) Inflammation in Alzheimer disease-a brief review of the basic science and clinical literature. Cold Spring Harb Perspect Med 2: a006346.
42. Di Paola M, Spalletta G, Caltagirone C (2010) In vivo structural neuroanatomy of corpus callosum in Alzheimer's disease and mild cognitive impairment using different MRI techniques: a review. J Alzheimers Dis 20: 67–95.

43. Correia MM, Carpenter TA, Williams GB (2009) Looking for the optimal DTI acquisition scheme given a maximum scan time: are more b-values a waste of time? Magn Reson Imaging 27: 163–175.

44. Danielian LE, Iwata NK, Thomasson DM, Floeter MK (2010) Reliability of fiber tracking measurements in diffusion tensor imaging for longitudinal study. Neuroimage 49: 1572–1580.

45. Takao H, Hayashi N, Kabasawa H, Ohtomo K (2012) Effect of scanner in longitudinal diffusion tensor imaging studies. Hum Brain Mapp 33: 466–477.

46. Wheeler-Kingshott CA, Cercignani M (2009) About "axial" and "radial" diffusivities. Magn Reson Med 61: 1255–1260.

Cost-Effectiveness of Magnetic Resonance Imaging with a New Contrast Agent for the Early Diagnosis of Alzheimer's Disease

Maria Biasutti[1,2], Natacha Dufour[1,2], Clotilde Ferroud[3], William Dab[1], Laura Temime[1]*

1 Laboratoire Modélisation et Surveillance des risques sanitaires – Conservatoire national des Arts et Métiers – 75003, Paris, France, **2** Ecole des Ponts ParisTech – 77700, Marne la Vallée, France, **3** Laboratoire Transformations Chimiques et Pharmaceutiques – Conservatoire national des Arts et Métiers – 75003, Paris, France

Abstract

Background: Used as contrast agents for brain magnetic resonance imaging (MRI), markers for beta-amyloid deposits might allow early diagnosis of Alzheimer's disease (AD). We evaluated the cost-effectiveness of such a diagnostic test, MRI+CLP (contrastophore-linker-pharmacophore), should it become clinically available.

Methodology/Principal Findings: We compared the cost-effectiveness of MRI+CLP to that of standard diagnosis using currently available cognition tests and of standard MRI, and investigated the impact of a hypothetical treatment efficient in early AD. The primary analysis was based on the current French context for 70-year-old patients with Mild Cognitive Impairment (MCI). In alternative "screen and treat" scenarios, we analyzed the consequences of systematic screenings of over-60 individuals (either population-wide or restricted to the ApoE4 genotype population). We used a Markov model of AD progression; model parameters, as well as incurred costs and quality-of-life weights in France were taken from the literature. We performed univariate and probabilistic multivariate sensitivity analyses. The base-case preferred strategy was the standard MRI diagnosis strategy. In the primary analysis however, MRI+CLP could become the preferred strategy under a wide array of scenarios involving lower cost and/or higher sensitivity or specificity. By contrast, in the "screen and treat" analyses, the probability of MRI+CLP becoming the preferred strategy remained lower than 5%.

Conclusions/Significance: It is thought that anti-beta-amyloid compounds might halt the development of dementia in early stage patients. This study suggests that, even should such treatments become available, systematically screening the over-60 population for AD would only become cost-effective with highly specific tests able to diagnose early stages of the disease. However, offering a new diagnostic test based on beta-amyloid markers to elderly patients with MCI might prove cost-effective.

Citation: Biasutti M, Dufour N, Ferroud C, Dab W, Temime L (2012) Cost-Effectiveness of Magnetic Resonance Imaging with a New Contrast Agent for the Early Diagnosis of Alzheimer's Disease. PLoS ONE 7(4): e35559. doi:10.1371/journal.pone.0035559

Editor: David W. Dowdy, Johns Hopkins Bloomberg School of Public Health, United States of America

Received July 22, 2011; **Accepted** March 20, 2012; **Published** April 20, 2012

Funding: This research was financed by a grant from the Cnam, a public higher education establishment by which all authors were employed at the time. The funders had no role in study design, data collection and analysis, decision to publish, or preparation of the manuscript.

Competing Interests: The authors have declared that no competing interests exist.

* E-mail: laura.temime@cnam.fr

Introduction

Alzheimer's disease (AD) is the main cause of dementia in older people, with approximately 26 million cases worldwide [1,2,3]. What is more, a major increase in this prevalence is expected in years to come [3]. In France, while 850.000 people were diagnosed with AD in 2004, 2.1 million may be affected by 2040 [4].

There are currently no treatments that may cure AD or halt the course of the disease. However, in recent years, drugs such as acetylcholinesterase inhibitors have demonstrated efficacy at reducing the intensity of certain symptoms. Moreover, new avenues for research are being investigated. Many scientists believe that one of the main causes of the AD has to do with beta-amyloid, microscopic protein which accumulate throughout the cortex of Alzheimer patients. This is called the "amyloid hypothesis" [2]. They believe that the destruction of brain cells seen in AD is caused by defects in the way beta-amyloid is produced, how it accumulates and how it is eliminated. Animal studies in mice have suggested that anti-beta-amyloid drugs can reduce brain amyloid level and improve memory problems in diseases similar to AD. At the present time, there is no clear evidence that these drugs can improve Alzheimer symptoms or protect brain cells but it is thought that they could halt the development of dementia in patients with early stage AD [5].

With these prospects of further therapeutic developments, attention has now focused on improving the sensitivity and specificity of diagnostic tools, and in developing tools that would allow early diagnosis.

The current standard diagnostic strategy of AD generally comprises a detailed history, a standardized assessment of cognition and functional status and laboratory testing. Brain imaging examinations such as nonenhanced computed tomography imaging, positron emission tomography imaging, or magnetic resonance imaging (MRI) are also sometimes used in order to exclude other conditions or to measure brain atrophy.

Finding more accurate diagnostic tools implies discovering non-invasive sensitive and specific biomarkers for AD. One avenue of research lies in the detection of β-amyloid plaques [6,7]. This detection could be achieved through the use of new contrast agents for MRI which bind to β-amyloid plaques, thus allowing a valid diagnosis of AD at a very early stage [6,8].

A few studies have attempted to assess the cost-effectiveness of imaging diagnosis tools for AD [9,10,11], or to evaluate the impact of screening the general population [12]. However, none has focused on combinations of MRI and new contrast agents.

In this study, we evaluate the cost-effectiveness of a diagnostic strategy based on MRI with a new contrast agent detecting β-amyloid plaques (contrastophore-linker-pharmacophore or CLP). We compare this strategy with other current standard diagnostic strategies. In the primary analysis, the new strategy is simply introduced as an alternative to current diagnostic tools and made available to the same population. In this setting, we investigate the consequences of the introduction of a new AD treatment with significant efficacy at an early stage of the disease.

In alternative scenarios, we assume that the availability of this new treatment would naturally raise the issue of the opportunity of screening for AD. We thus evaluate the cost-effectiveness of diagnostic strategies in the context of hypothetical national screening programs.

Methods

1. Framework of the cost-effectiveness analyses

We performed cost-effectiveness analyses in order to compare the costs and benefits of several alternative diagnostic strategies in the French context. Costs were measured in Euros (€) and benefits were measured in quality-adjusted life-years (QALYs), which assign to each year of life a weight between 0 (dead) and 1 (perfect health).

A strategy was considered dominated if another strategy had a better or similar efficacy at a lower cost; conversely, a strategy was considered strongly dominant when it was both more effective and cheaper than all other strategies. We computed incremental cost-effectiveness ratios (ICERs), in which changes in resource use, compared with the next best strategy, were included in the numerator, while additional health effects, compared with the next best strategy, were included in the denominator. Finally, we compared ICERs to the willingness-to-pay (WTP) for an additional QALY, which was assumed equal to three times the gross national product per capita in France, as recommended by the World Health Organization Choice working group [13,14], that is, 76.171€ per QALY in 2009. If no strategy was strongly dominant, the preferred strategy was that with the highest ICER under the willingness-to-pay threshold.

The study was conducted from a societal perspective, meaning it included all costs and benefits, no matter who incurred them. Future costs and QALYs were discounted at 5% annually.

The cost-effectiveness analyses were conducted using the TreeAge software [15]. We performed expected value analyses, based on the computation over simulated cycles of percentages of a hypothetical cohort in each modeled AD stage. For the multivariate sensitivity analyses, we also performed Monte Carlo simulations with 10.000 trials, in order to derive the distribution of incremental cost-effectiveness ratios for the MRI+CLP strategies, as well as acceptability curves for all strategies.

Table 1 details the compared strategies.

1.1. Primary analysis. In the primary analysis, three diagnostic strategies were compared over a three year period for a cohort of 70 year-old individuals consulting for the first time following mild cognitive impairment (MCI) symptoms:

- the standard diagnosis strategy based on an interview with an AD specialist, cognition tests such as mini-mental state evaluation (MMSE) and laboratory tests (standard diagnosis strategy)
- a strategy combining the standard strategy with standard MRI (standard MRI strategy)
- and a strategy combining the standard strategy with MRI used with a new contrast agent detecting β-amyloid plaques (MRI+CLP strategy)

Figure 1A depicts the tree showing the possible outcomes of using one of the investigated diagnostic tests in this scenario. The choice of a 3-year horizon for this analysis was motivated by data on the duration of efficacy of currently available AD treatments and mortality rates of over-70 dementia patients.

As part of the sensitivity analysis, we assumed that a new treatment had been developed which delayed significantly the course of AD at an early stage and that this treatment was offered to MCI patients diagnosed with AD but with high MMSE scores (who were either false positives or early AD patients).

1.2. "Screen and treat" analyses. In the "screen and treat" analyses, it was assumed that a new treatment had been developed which delayed significantly the course of AD at an early stage, and that a national screening campaign targeted at individuals over 60 years-old took place. Screening could either be population-wide or limited to individuals carrying the ε4 allele of the apolipoprotein E gene (ApoE4), in whom the risk of AD has been shown to be significantly higher [16].

In this context, three diagnostic strategies were compared over a fifteen year period for a cohort of 60 year-old individuals taking part in the screening campaign:

- the standard diagnosis strategy,
- the standard MRI,
- and the MRI+CLP strategy

Figure 1B depicts the tree showing the possible outcomes of the screening procedure with one of the investigated diagnostic tests in this scenario.

Following the initial screening, individuals who were not diagnosed as AD patients were screened again every 5 years, unless they developed dementia symptoms between these scheduled screenings, in which case they were immediately tested.

The choice of a 15 year horizon for this second analysis was motivated by the need to follow 60 year-old mostly healthy individuals through several screening campaigns.

2. Models of disease progression

We used a Markov model of the evolution of AD based on previous work [17] in which the disease evolved in 5 stages: no AD, mild AD, moderate AD, severe AD and death. For the screen and treat analyses, a 6th stage was added for asymptomatic patients with early AD. We also distinguished patients that were taken care of at home from institutionalized patients, at each stage of AD. Initially, all patients in the cohort began in the community setting and had a probability in each cycle, conditional on disease state (and, for the 2d analysis, on age), of making a transition to nursing home care. File S1 and Figure S1 present the models we used in more detail.

Table 1. Compared strategies.

Strategy	Tests	Imaging
Standard diagnosis	Laboratory tests, clinical examination, cognition test	None
Standard MRI	Laboratory tests, clinical examination, cognition test	Non-enhanced MRI
MRI+CLP	Laboratory tests, clinical examination, cognition test	MRI with a new contrast agent detecting β-amyloid plaques

doi:10.1371/journal.pone.0035559.t001

Considering the natural history of AD, we chose to model disease progression using 6 month cycles. Transition probabilities over 6 months were obtained from the square root of the matrix of annual transition probabilities which were based on the literature [17,18,19] and available data on age-specific mortality rates [20] and age-specific AD incidence [4] in France.

Table S1 lists all model parameters, with their base-case values.

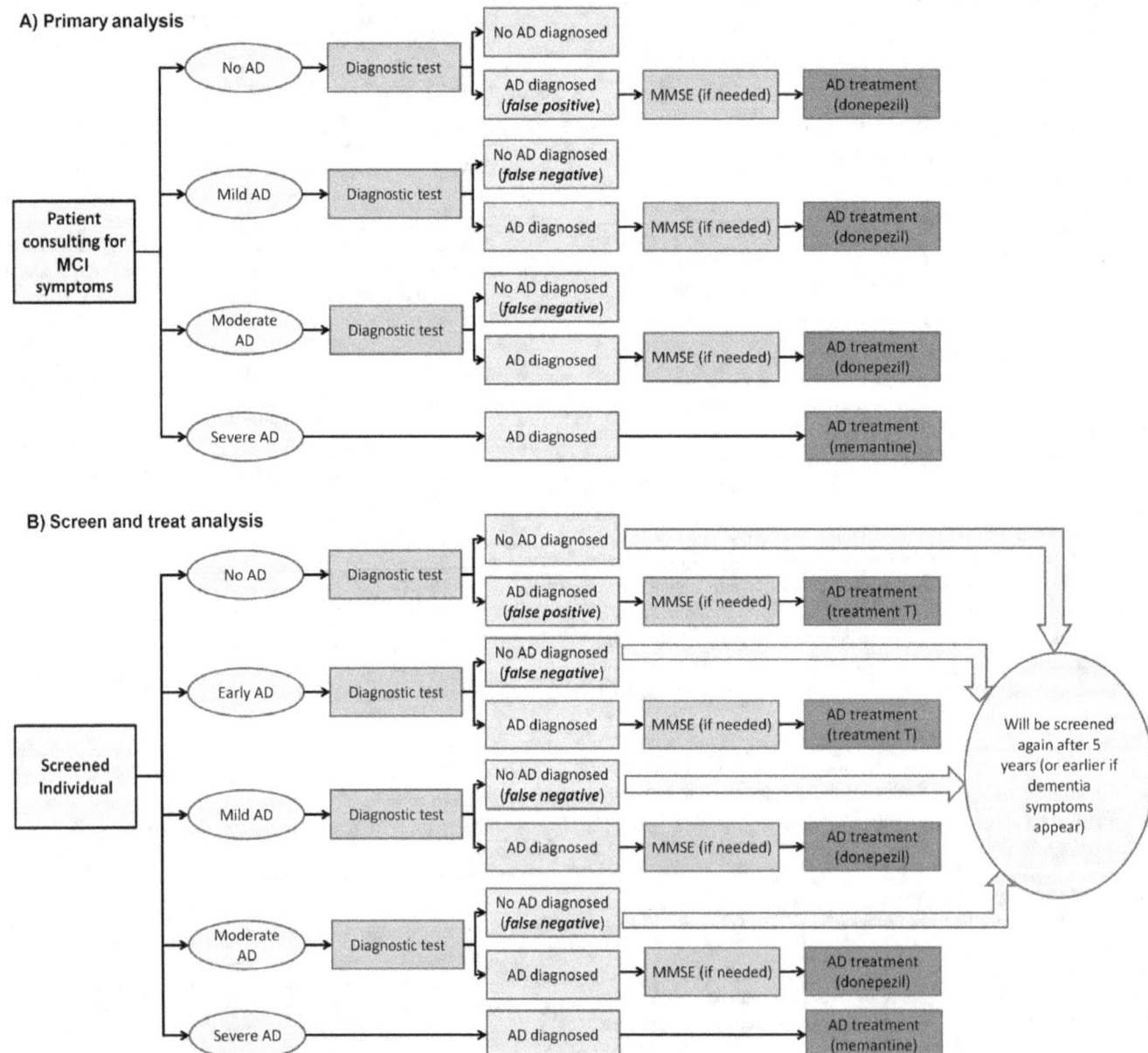

Figure 1. Decision tree for an individual tested for Alzheimer's disease (AD). Possible outcomes of the testing procedure are depicted as a function of the individual's health status for: (a) The primary scenario (testing of over-70 patients consulting for dementia symptoms). (b) The "screen and treat" scenario (systematic screening of the over-60 population). Depending on the investigated strategy, the generic "diagnostic test" mentioned in the trees may be standard diagnosis, standard MRI or MRI+CLP. When AD is diagnosed, the imaging procedures are followed by a cognition test (MMSE) in order to determine the disease stage. No test is performed in severe AD patients, who are assumed to be diagnosed directly.
doi:10.1371/journal.pone.0035559.g001

3. Available treatments

The model assumes that all patients who receive a diagnosis of probable Alzheimer disease receive treatment with donepezil, memantine or a hypothetical higher-efficacy drug.

If the patient is diagnosed at a mild or moderate stage, donepezil is prescribed, to be replaced by memantine when the patient has evolved to a severe stage of AD. If the patient is diagnosed when the disease is already severe, memantine is prescribed.

In addition, a hypothetical treatment T which is efficient at early stages of AD may be prescribed to patients who are diagnosed with AD but have high MMSE scores in the primary analysis, or to patients who are diagnosed with early AD in the "screen and treat" analyses.

Donepezil treatment has been shown to improve significantly memory and other cognitive functions in patients with mild to moderate AD [21], and to reduce the annual decline in cognition in these patients when compared with patients in a placebo group [22]; similarly, memantine treatment has been shown to cause a clinically noticeable reduction in deterioration over 28 weeks, compared with placebo, in patients with moderate-to-severe AD [23,24]. It is to be noted that actually, donepezil or memantine help treat the symptoms of AD although there is no evidence that they modify the underlying pathology of the disease. On the basis of these data, we assumed that treatment modified transition probabilities between disease stages, both reducing the speed of AD progression and increasing the chance of symptom lessening (Table S1). For treatment T, we only assumed a decrease in the progression from early to mild and moderate stage AD, as we supposed that reversal to asymptomatic AD of mild stage patients was not possible. In the base-case analysis, these effects were assumed to be constant throughout the duration of treatment; long-term clinical studies suggest that treatment efficacy may last for up to 3 years [21,25].

4. AD prevalence and incidence

In the primary analysis, the simulated cohort comprised 70 year old individuals who consulted for cognitive impairment symptoms. There is evidence that older persons with Mild Cognitive Impairment (MCI) feature neurobiological AD in 50% to 70% of the cases [26]. Based on this evidence and on data from a study at Massachusetts General Hospital [10], we estimated that 56% of the cohort patients had AD initially. The distribution between disease stages at this first consultation was estimated, based on a French study [27], at 55.9% mild stage AD, 39.9% moderate stage AD and 4.2% severe stage AD.

MCI is often a precursor to Alzheimer's dementia and the annual rate of development of AD for patients with MCI is 10 to 15% [26,28]. Here, we assumed a 10%/year AD incidence in untreated patients of the cohort.

In the first "screen and treat" analysis, the cohort was representative from the French population of individuals over 60 years old, as it was assumed that a national screening was underway. Therefore the initial prevalence of AD (including early asymptomatic stage AD) in the cohort was assumed to be 1% [3]. We further assumed that there was an 8/7 ratio between the prevalences of early stage and mild stage AD [Personal communication, Pr. Verny, AP-HP, Paris, 2009]. The distribution between mild, moderate and severe stages was the same as in the primary analysis.

Age-specific AD incidence rates for individuals between 60 and 75 years old were chosen to be consistent with data from recent cohort studies [29,30].

In the second "screen and treat" analysis, screening was restricted to individuals carrying the ε4 allele of the apolipoprotein E gene (ApoE4). Based on earlier studies showing significantly higher risk of AD occurrence in ApoE4 individuals [16], we assumed that age-specific incidence rates were doubled.

5. Diagnostic tests

The standard diagnostic strategy of AD was assumed to comprise a detailed history of the patient, an assessment of cognition and functional status using a questionnaire test such as the MMSE, and laboratory testing. Other strategies combined MRI (with or without a new contrast agent) for AD diagnosis with a questionnaire test such as the MMSE aimed at determining the stage of the disease.

In the case of severe AD, it was assumed that dementia symptoms allowed direct diagnosis over a consultation (without need for a diagnostic test). Hence, all severe stage AD patients were assumed to be diagnosed and to receive treatment.

As in [10], we estimated the sensitivity of the standard diagnostic tests at 75% and their specificity at 90%; in early stage AD, we assumed that patients were asymptomatic and that the standard diagnostic therefore performed as it did in non-AD patients, declaring only 10% ($=1-0.9$) of them as having AD. Based on data from a clinical study, we also hypothesized a sensitivity of 50% in early stage, 88% in mild stage and 95% in moderate stage AD, as well as a 96% specificity, for standard MRI diagnosis [31].

Regarding the hypothetical diagnostic test using MRI with the new contrast agent (MRI+CLP), we based our assumptions on available data on PET-scan amyloid imaging. As studies on amyloid plaques suggest that amyloid deposition reaches a plateau by the early clinical stages of Alzheimer's disease (amyloid cascade hypothesis), we assumed the sensitivity of the MRI+CLP diagnostic test to be independent of the disease stage. In one study on PET tracers, the sensitivity and specificity were estimated at 90% [32]; in another, a 95% sensitivity and 83% specificity were found [33]. Here, we assumed a 96% sensitivity and 87% specificity for MRI+CLP.

6. Costs and effectiveness

All costs were measured at their 2009 level.

6.1. Costs of diagnostic tests. The cost of the standard diagnosis was computed as the sum of the cost of a specialist consultation in France, estimated at 55€ [34], that of mental state evaluation tests, estimated at 69€ [35], and that of standard laboratory tests, estimated at 50€ [36]. The cost of MRI was obtained from the "Classification Commune des Actes Médicaux", a fixed-costs scale of medical procedures based on practitioners' fees, fixed costs for the medical procedures themselves, and fixed costs for operating the equipment [35]. Finally, we estimated the cost of the new contrast product for MRI at 250€ [Personal Communication, Guerbet company, Paris, 2009].

6.2. Costs of AD follow-up. Diagnosed AD patients were assumed to have a follow-up consultation every 6 month with an AD specialist. These specialist consultations were estimated at 41€ [34].

6.3. Costs of treatment. We used prices for generic AD drugs, that is, 572€ per 6-month period for generic donepezil (Aricept) and 286€ per 6-month period for generic memantine (Ebixa) [37]. We further assumed that the hypothetical new drug that would be efficient in early stage AD would have a cost similar to that of generic donepezil.

6.4. Costs of care. We took into account both living and care costs. For institutionalized patients, living costs included hostel costs, based on a French study of AD patients [18], and costs of care included caregiver wages. In an earlier study, caregivers were estimated to spend 517 hours over a 3 month period caring for moderate-to-severe AD patients [38]. Here, we therefore computed costs associated with caregivers over 6 months by multiplying hourly wages (estimated at 13 €/h for professional caregivers) with 1034 hours.

For patients living at home, "basic" costs included living and medical expenditures [39], based on a French study of home-cared AD patients and controls; the cost of care by unprofessional caregivers was also estimated as an opportunity cost. In order to do this, we valued informal care at a conservative value of 8.4 €/h, and we assumed that these unpaid caregivers spent the same amount of time caring for AD patients than professional caregivers, that is, 1034 hours over a 6 month cycle.

6.5. Indirect costs. In this study, we took into account several indirect costs of AD. First, we assigned an opportunity cost to unprofessional caregivers who took care of AD patients leaving at home, as described before.

Second, we took into account the burden of AD care on the health state of unprofessional caregivers. Based on an earlier study [38], 35% of AD caregivers take medication related to their activity; they have high rates of depression and anxiety, as well as high overall morbidity and mortality rates, compared to non-AD caregiver controls [40]. We estimated the cost of this health impact as that as of a weekly psychiatrist consultation, plus that of an antidepressant treatment, for 35% of unprofessional caregivers.

Finally, we also evaluated the cost associated with the loss of productivity of AD patients. This is generally not done in cost-effectiveness studies of AD, since AD patients are for the most part retired. However, recent data shows that pensioners are becoming more and more involved in volunteer activities within nonprofit organizations (NPOs), as well as performing informal volunteer activities [41].

Here, based on French data [42], we estimated that 60 to 75 year-old individuals performed on average 63.8 hours of informal volunteering activities over a 6 month period – mostly within the family sphere, such as childcare for instance. This was valued at 7.7€/hour, which was the minimum wage in France in 2009, and multiplied by an "efficiency coefficient" of 0.7 to arbitrarily take into account the reduced productivity in older individuals.

Similarly, we estimated that 50% of 60 to 75 year-old individuals are involved in NPOs, with a mean of 12 hours of volunteer activities per month. On average, we hence estimated that 60 to 75 year-old individuals performed a total of 36 hours of volunteer activities within NPOs over a 6 month period [43], which were valued at 7.9€/hour and multiplied by the aforementioned 0.7 efficiency coefficient.

We added the resulting estimated productivity benefit of a French pensioner to our analyses as a cost associated to AD, in full for moderate-to-severe patients and multiplied by 0.6 for mild AD patients (assuming that mild AD only reduces productivity by 40%).

6.6. Effectiveness. We estimated quality-of-life weights (QALYs) for over-60 patients without Alzheimer disease at 0.826 on a scale of 0 to 1, on the basis of the mean of time trade-off scores for men and women aged 65–84 years old published in a study of health outcomes in the general population [44].

Quality-of-life weights for patients with Alzheimer disease at each disease stage and care setting (institution or community) were based on previously published Health Utilities Index Mark 2 (HUI:2) scores [17].

7. Sensitivity analysis

The ranges investigated in the Sensitivity Analysis are summarized in Table S1, along with the data sources. We performed both univariate and multivariate sensitivity analyses. For the multivariate analyses, we performed a Monte-Carlo simulation with 10.000 trials, using *a priori* triangular distributions for model parameters. We then identified the most influential parameters in the cost-effectiveness of the MRI+CLP strategy by calculating the partial rank correlation coefficient (PRCC) between each input parameter and the ICER of this strategy and assessing their statistical significance.

7.1. Drug effects and prices. We investigated the impact of the introduction of new drugs, which would have the same costs and indications as donepezil and memantine, respectively, but with varying efficacy: the probabilities of transitions under treatment from mild to moderate or moderate to severe stage were further reduced by a factor (f_{mM} or f_{MS}) ranging from 0.5 to 1, and the probabilities of transitions under treatment from moderate to mild or severe to moderate stage were further increased by a factor (f_{Mm} or f_{SM}) ranging from 1 to 2 [17]. For simplicity reasons, we also summarized these four avenues for improvement of current AD treatment through a single parameter f, assuming a linear relationship between the multiplying factors:
$$f = f_{ML} = f_{SM} = -2 \times f_{LM} + 3$$

Regarding the hypothetical drug efficient for early stage AD (treatment T), we investigated both more and less efficient drugs, with probabilities of progression from early to mild and moderate stage AD under treatment T ranging from 0 to their values without treatment T; f_T was the reduction factor applied to these transition probabilities due to treatment T (in [0–1]).

The assumed cost for a 6-month cure with treatment T was also varied, between 0 and 1000€.

7.2. Diagnostic tests characteristics. We investigated sensitivities from 0.9 to 1 and specificities from 0.7 to 1 in early to moderate stage AD patients for the hypothetical diagnostic test using MRI with the CLP contrast product. We also investigated sensitivities ranging from 0.75 to 0.90 for the standard diagnosis in moderate stage AD.

In the "screen and treat" analyses, we investigated sensitivities of standard MRI between 0.1 and 0.5 for early stage AD.

7.3. Disease progression. To model faster or slower progression of AD, we investigated state transition probabilities in our Markov model ranging from 10% lower to 10% higher than their base-case values.

7.4. Initial distribution of patients and prevalence. In the primary analysis, we investigated AD prevalences among consulting individuals ranging from 50 to 70%. For each fixed prevalence, we varied the proportion of patients with mild AD between 50 and 75% of all AD patients; the ratio between moderate and severe AD prevalence remained the same, that is, 10 moderate stage patients for 1 severe stage patient.

In the "screen and treat" analyses, we investigated initial AD prevalences among screened individuals ranging from 1 to 10%. For each fixed prevalence, we varied the proportion of patients with early asymptomatic AD from 30 to 75% of all AD patients; the distribution of mild to severe stages remained the same.

7.5. Discount rate. As the "screen and treat" analyses spanned a 15 year period, we assessed the impact of variations in the assumed discount rate for costs and QALYs, from 0 to 10% per year.

7.6. Frequency of screenings. In the "screen and treat" analyses, we investigated the impact of varying durations between screening campaigns, ranging from one to ten years.

Table 2. Results of the primary analysis (base-case hypothesis): computed cost, efficacy and cost-effectiveness (C/E) ratio of the standard diagnosis, standard MRI and MRI+CLP strategies, and incremental cost-effectiveness ratios (ICER) of the MRI+CLP strategy as compared with the standard MRI strategy.

Strategy	Cost (in €)	Efficacy (in QALYs)	C/E	ICER
In the current context				
Standard diagnosis	36 294	1.7663	20 548	Dominated
Standard MRI	36 131	1.7710	20 401	
MRI+CLP	36 313	1.7731	20 480	88 439 €/QALY
Assuming hypothetical treatment T has been made available				
Standard diagnosis	36 260	1.7668	20 523	Dominated
Standard MRI	36 117	1.7712	20 391	
MRI+CLP	36 268	1.7737	20 447	60 923 €/QALY

doi:10.1371/journal.pone.0035559.t002

Results

1. Primary analysis

1.1. Base Case. The first part of Table 2 summarizes the results of the primary cost-effectiveness analysis in the base case; in the second part of Table 2, hypothetical treatment T is offered to all MCI patients diagnosed with AD but with high MMSE scores. In both cases, the standard diagnosis strategy was dominated by the standard MRI strategy (more costly and less effective).

Cost and effectiveness increased from standard MRI to MRI+CLP strategies. In the base-case, the ICER of the MRI+CLP strategy was higher than the French willingness-to-pay threshold (estimated at 76 171 €/QALY). Hence, standard MRI was found to be the preferred strategy. However, assuming that treatment T had been made available led to a lower ICER for MRI+CLP, making it the preferred strategy.

1.2. Sensitivity analysis. Detailed results of the univariate sensitivity analysis are presented in Table S2 (without treatment T). Assuming either more effective AD treatments, higher speed of AD progression, a larger initial AD prevalence in 70 year-old MCI individuals, a larger initial portion of mild AD, higher sensitivity or specificity of MRI+CLP diagnosis or a lower cost of the CLP product could lead to MRI+CLP becoming the preferred strategy, with an ICER lower than the willingness-to-pay threshold.

Table 3 (columns 1 and 2) provides partial rank correlation coefficients (PRCC) between input values and the ICER of the MRI+CLP strategy (compared with the standard MRI strategy, without treatment T). Only parameters whose PRCC with this ICER is statistically significant at the confidence level of 5% or lower are shown, namely: the speed of disease progression; the initial AD prevalence in the studied population; the initial portion of mild stage AD; the discount rate; the sensitivity and specificity of the MRI+CLP diagnostic test; and the cost of the CLP contrast agent.

In Figure 2, the sensitivity of our conclusions on the MRI+CLP diagnostic test characteristics (sensitivity, specificity and cost) is assessed. MRI+CLP is the preferred strategy in a wide array of scenarios, including some assuming lower sensitivity or specificity or higher cost than in the base-case.

Figure S2 provides the distribution of incremental cost-effectiveness ratios for the MRI+CLP strategy, compared with standard diagnosis, as well as an acceptability curve depicting the probability for each of the three investigated strategies to be preferred as a function of the willingness-to-pay threshold. For willingness-to-pay thresholds larger than 90 000€/QALY, MRI+CLP becomes the preferred strategy.

With the assumed WTP threshold at 76 171€/QALY, the probability that MRI+CLP was the preferred strategy increased from 43% to 64% when treatment T was assumed to be available (data not shown). Figure S3 investigates the impact of the efficacy and cost of treatment T on these results.

2. "Screen and treat" analyses

2.1. Base Case. Table 4 summarizes the results of the "screen and treat" cost-effectiveness analyses in the base case; in the first part, the whole over-60 population is screened, while in the second part, the screening is targeted at ApoE4 individuals. In both cases, the standard diagnosis strategy was dominated by the standard MRI strategy.

Table 3. Partial rank correlation coefficients (PRCC) between input values and the ICER of the MRI+CLP strategy (compared with the preferred strategy).

Primary cost-effectiveness analysis		"Screen and treat" cost-effectiveness analysis (population-wide screening)	
Parameter	PRCC	Parameter	PRCC
Speed of disease progression	−0,41	Initial prevalence of AD	−0,86
Initial prevalence of AD	−0,51	Initial portion of early AD	−0,15
Initial portion of mild AD	−0,26	Sensitivity of MRI+CLP test	−0,17
Sensitivity of MRI+CLP test	−0,92	Specificity of MRI+CLP test	−0,64
Specificity of MRI+CLP test	−0,73	Discount rate	0,29
Discount rate	0,19	Cost of the CLP contrast agent	0,41
Cost of the CLP contrast agent	0,79	Cost of treatment T	0,78
		Impact of treatment T (from high to low)	0,41
		Speed of disease progression	−0,23
		Sensitivity of standard MRI in early AD	0,51

All PRCCs are statistically significant at the confidence level of 5%. A higher absolute value of PRCC indicates a strong relationship between that parameter and the ICER; a positive (resp. negative) value of PRCC implies that the value of the ICER increases (resp. decreases) when the value of the input increases.
doi:10.1371/journal.pone.0035559.t003

A) Cost of CLP = 50€/injection

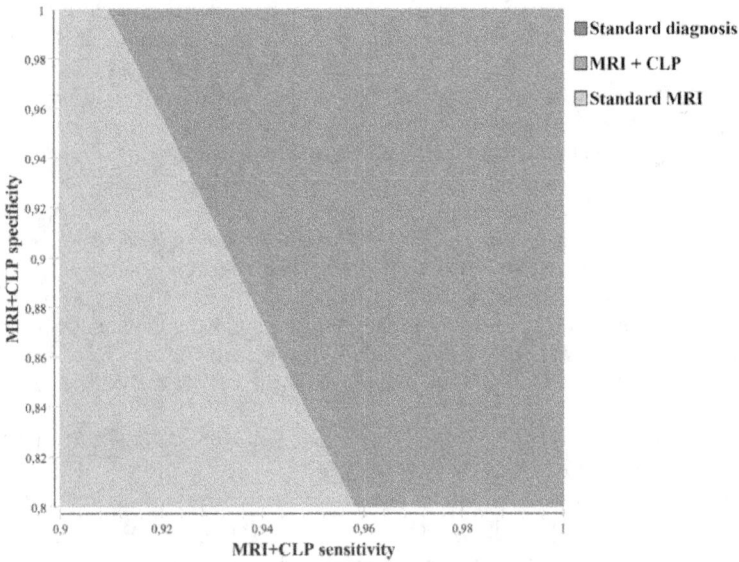

B) Cost of CLP = 250€/injection

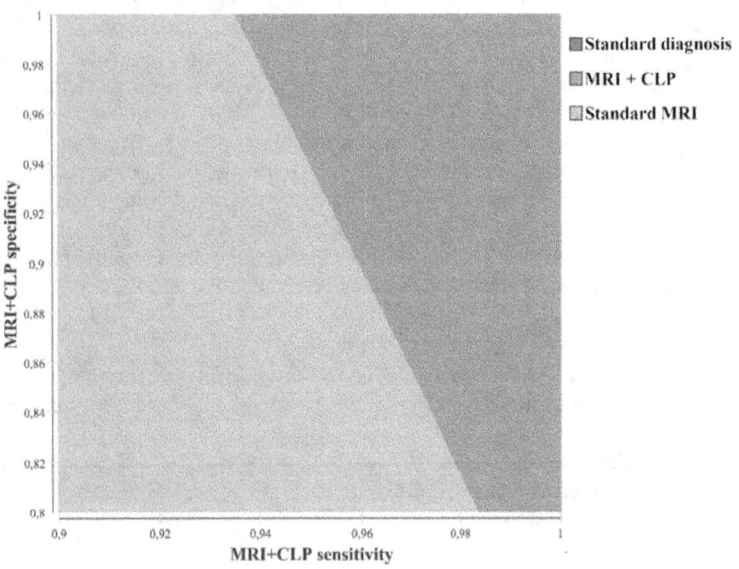

C) Cost of CLP = 450€/injection

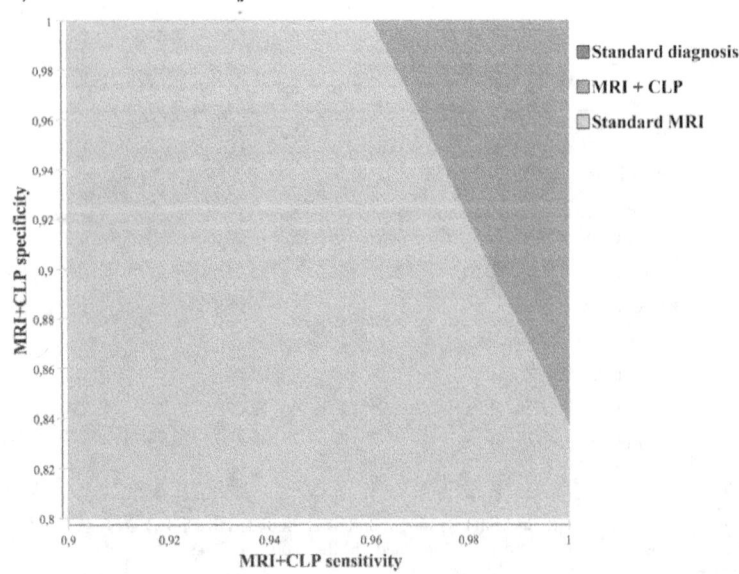

Figure 2. Results of the primary analysis: multivariate sensitivity analysis. The strategy with maximum net monetary benefit is depicted as a function of the assumed sensitivity and specificity of the MRI+CLP diagnostic test, for assumed costs of the CLP contrast agent between 0 and 500€ per injection (in the absence of treatment T): (a) Cost of the CLP contrast agent at 50 €/injection. (b) Cost of the CLP contrast agent at 250 €/injection. (c) Cost of the CLP contrast agent over 450 €/injection.
doi:10.1371/journal.pone.0035559.g002

Although overall computed costs and QALYs were lower when assuming a screening targeted at the ApoE4 population, the main base-case results were similar in both our screening analyses. The MRI+CLP strategy was both more costly and more efficient than the standard MRI strategy. Its ICER, compared with the standard MRI strategy, was much higher than the French willingness-to-pay estimated at 76 171 €/QALY. Therefore, standard MRI was the preferred strategy in the base case.

2.2. Sensitivity analysis. Detailed results of the univariate sensitivity analysis are presented in Table S3 for the population-wide screening scenario. For an assumed specificity of MRI+CLP higher than 98%, MRI+CLP became the preferred strategy; it was strongly dominant for specificities over 99%. No other individual model parameter had enough impact on our results to make MRI+CLP the preferred strategy.

Table 3 (columns 3 and 4) provides partial rank correlation coefficients (PRCC) between inputs values and the ICER of the MRI+CLP strategy (compared with the standard MRI strategy), for the population-wide screening scenario. Only parameters whose PRCC with this ICER is statistically significant at the confidence level of 5% or lower are shown, namely: the initial AD prevalence in the studied population; the specificity of the MRI+CLP diagnostic test; and the efficacy and cost of new treatment T.

Figure 3 depicts results from a multivariate analysis performed on the efficacy and cost of the hypothetical new treatment and MRI+CLP specificity, while Figure 4 depicts results from a multivariate analysis performed on the initial prevalence of AD in the general over-60 population, the specificity of MRI+CLP diagnosis and the assumed cost of the CLP contrast agent. Several combinations of these parameters allow for MRI+CLP strategy dominance, but all include high specificity of MRI+CLP diagnosis. For instance:

- assuming 98% specificity for MRI+CLP diagnosis and that treatment T reduces AD progression from the early stage by

half, MRI+CLP is the preferred strategy for the base-case cost of treatment T (500€/6 months of treatment)

- assuming an initial AD prevalence of 4% and the base-case cost of 250€ per injection for the CLP contrast agent, MRI+CLP is the preferred strategy as long as MRI+CLP diagnosis is more than 97% specific.

Figure S4 provides the distribution of incremental cost-effectiveness ratios for the MRI+CLP strategy, compared with standard MRI, as well as an acceptability curve depicting the probability for the MRI+CLP strategy to be the preferred strategy as a function of the willingness-to-pay threshold. This probability remains lower than 4% even assuming a willingness-to-pay at 200 000€/QALY.

When assuming a screening targeted at the ApoE4 population, the probability that MRI+CLP was the preferred strategy increased slightly, reaching 5% for a 200 000 €/QALY willingness-to-pay threshold (data not shown).

Discussion

Here, we investigated the cost-effectiveness of a new diagnostic tool for AD allowing early diagnosis in two different contexts. First, we assumed that this new diagnostic tool would be made available to the same individuals who are currently offered other diagnostic tests. Second, we hypothesized that a treatment with significant efficacy in early stage AD was developed, and that, as a consequence, a national screening campaign was put into place, using either the currently available diagnostic tests or the new diagnostic test.

We found that in both analyses, the preferred base-case strategy was the standard MRI strategy. However, multivariate sensitivity analyses showed that, while in the primary analysis combining MRI with a new contrast product could prove the preferred strategy under a wide array of realistic scenarios, the probability of this happening was inferior to 5% in the hypothesis of a national screening campaign. Even assuming the availability of a low-cost highly efficient treatment in early AD, novel contrast agents would need to have very high specificity to be cost-effective when used for systematic screening of the entire population.

1. Models of disease progression

We used Markov models of AD progression. Although widely used in similar cost-effectiveness analyses [10,11,17,18,45,46], this approach presents several limitations. First, it has been shown that using time-independent transition probabilities may lead to either overestimate or underestimate disease progression, depending on the AD stage [47]. Second, in order for the model complexity to remain manageable, we were led to limit the number of states. In order to take into account indirect consequences of AD, such as the loss of productivity of AD patients in their volunteer activities, we incorporated them as aggregate factors in the computation of costs.

Using other modeling approaches, such as discrete events simulation, would allow a more detailed and realistic description of AD progression and, in turn, derive more reliable conclusions [12,48].

Table 4. Results of the "screen and treat" analyses (base-case hypothesis): computed cost, efficacy and cost-effectiveness (C/E) ratio of the standard diagnosis, standard MRI and MRI+CLP strategies, and incremental cost-effectiveness ratio (ICER) of the MRI+CLP strategy as compared with the standard MRI strategy.

Strategy	Cost (in €)	Efficacy (in QALYs)	C/E	ICER
Population-wide screening				
Standard diagnosis	43 559	8.0722	5 396	Dominated
Standard MRI	43 009	8.0732	5 327	
MRI+CLP	44 945	8.0752	5 566	991 972 €/QALY
Screening targeted at ApoE4 individuals				
Standard diagnosis	44 711	8.0377	5 563	Dominated
Standard MRI	44 180	8.0386	5 496	
MRI+CLP	46 075	8.0415	5 730	641 326 €/QALY

doi:10.1371/journal.pone.0035559.t004

A) Specificity inferior to 0.97

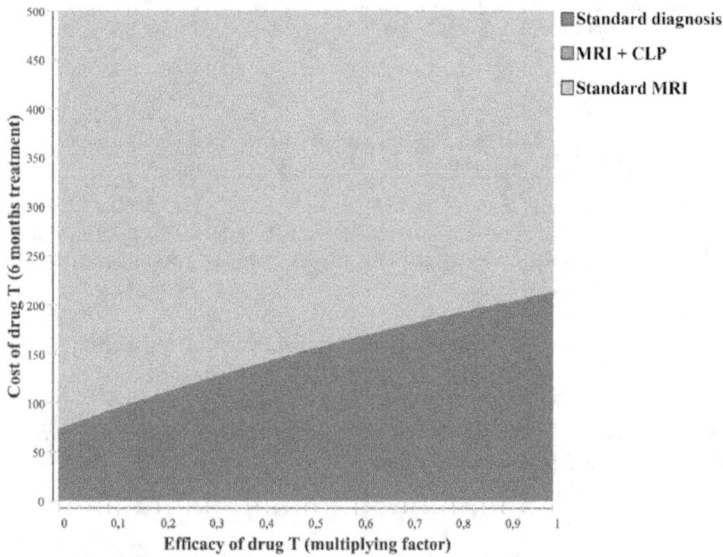

B) 0.98 specificity

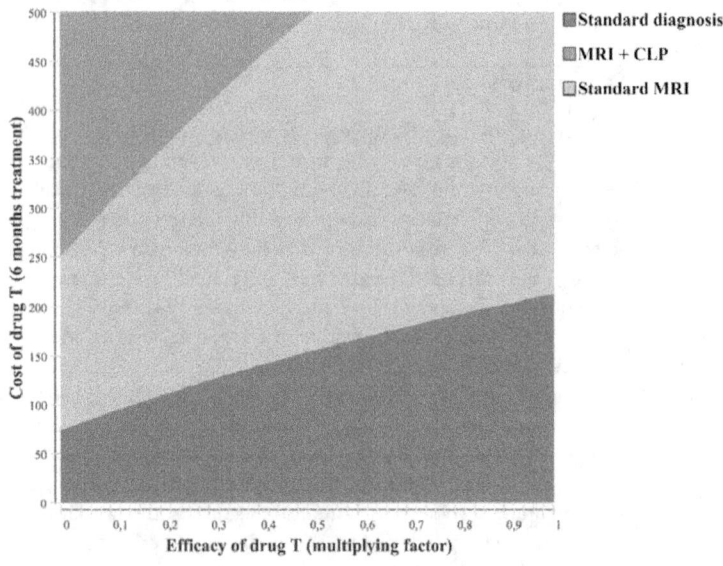

C) 0.99 specificity

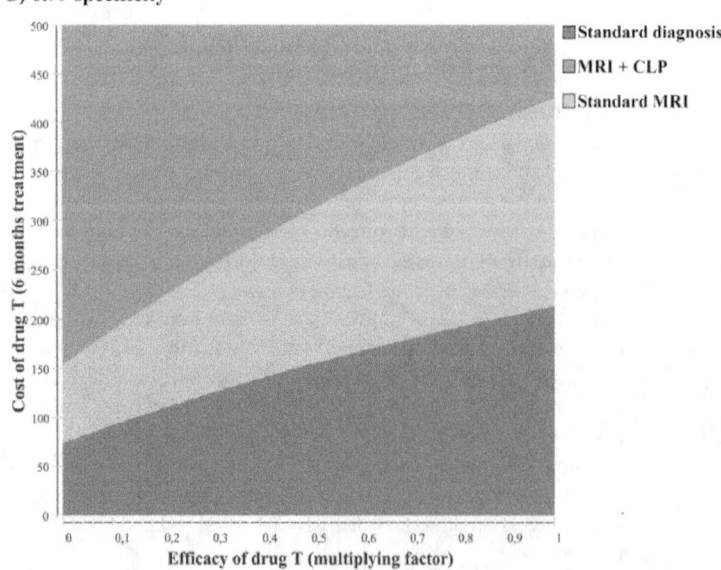

Figure 3. Results of the "screen and treat" (population-wide screening) analysis: multivariate sensitivity analysis. The strategy with maximum net monetary benefit is depicted as a function of the assumed efficacy and cost of the hypothetical new drug T, for assumed specificities of the MRI+CLP diagnosis test between 0.80 and 0.99. The efficacy of treatment T is expressed as a 0-to-1 ratio between assumed probabilities of transition from early stage AD with and without treatment T; 0 corresponds to maximum efficacy and 1 to no efficacy (in the base case, $f_T = 0.5$: 50% reduction). Only costs lower than the base-case cost of 500€ per 6-month treatment are investigated here. (a) specificity for MRI+CLP inferior to 0.97 (including base case). (b) 0.98 specificity for MRI+CLP. (c) 0.99 specificity for MRI+CLP.
doi:10.1371/journal.pone.0035559.g003

2. Assumed properties of the MRI+CLP diagnostic test

Because the new CLP contrast agent for MRI is still under development, assumptions had to be made regarding its sensitivity and specificity for diagnosing AD. As mentioned in the Methods, we based these assumptions in part on available data on PET-scan used with amyloid markers [32,33]. We also investigated relatively wide ranges for these characteristics in our sensitivity analyses.

Regarding the specificity, it should be noted that amyloid plaques have been detected in 10 to 30% of otherwise apparently normal elderly subjects. This may limit the capacity of MRI+CLP to correctly identify healthy subjects, which is why we investigated specificities as low as 0.70 in our sensitivity analyses. However, several studies also suggest that the presence of amyloid plaques is associated with declining cognitive test scores and with structural and functional brain changes suggestive of early AD [49]. In two recent follow-up studies, about one third of patients with mild cognitive impairment in whom amyloid plaques were detected converted to AD over the following 2 years [50,51]. It could therefore be argued that at least part of these 10–30% amyloid-positive individuals may not be "false positive", but very early stage AD patients.

Figure S5 illustrates the influence of false positives and false negatives associated with the MRI+CLP diagnosis in terms of additional cost per QALY in both our primary analysis and our "screen and treat" analysis.

3. Included costs

In this study, we chose to include indirect costs in addition to direct costs. The importance of these indirect costs, which include costs associated with the loss of productivity of AD patients and costs associated with informal caregiving at the homes of AD patients, has indeed been underlined in several recent studies, which showed that they may dominate direct costs of care in early stages of the disease [52]. As a consequence, it has been suggested in recent reviews that future cost-effectiveness studies should take into account such indirect costs [48,53].

4. Results and limits of the primary analysis

The results we obtained in our primary analysis are similar to those from previously published cost-efficacy studies, in the sense that in the base-case, adding a new marker to MRI was not cost-effective [10,11]. However, in our multivariate sensitivity analysis, there was a high probability of MRI+CLP becoming the preferred strategy.

In addition, it is to be noted that we found the standard MRI strategy to dominate the standard diagnosis strategy, whereas earlier studies found very high ICERs for similar imaging strategies [10,11]. This may be due to the fact that in these earlier studies, MRI was supposed to come as an addition to the standard diagnosis procedure, which included a detailed history, a questionnaire test such as the MMSE, laboratory testing and nonenhanced CT imaging. In our study, the standard MRI strategy only comprised the initial specialist consultation, the MMSE and MRI itself.

Because of the high level of uncertainty surrounding the assumed sensitivity and specificity of both standard diagnosis and standard MRI, we also explored how our results changed when assuming higher sensitivity and specificity for the standard diagnosis, or lower sensitivity and specificity for standard MRI. Irrespective of the assumed specificity, the standard diagnosis strategy remained dominated by the standard MRI strategy. However, as shown in Figure S6, standard diagnosis could become preferable to standard MRI under a wide array of combinations of lower sensitivity for standard MRI and higher sensitivity for standard diagnosis in moderate AD.

All in all, it should be underlined here that comparing standard MRI to the current standard diagnosis strategy for AD was not the focus of this study and that our results should not be taken as evidence that large-scale screening using standard MRI should be undertaken.

Several limitations of this analysis lie with the assumptions we made on AD treatment.

First, we neglected all adverse effects from the treatments. Including a cost associated with such adverse effects in treated individuals would lead to reduced ICERs for all strategies. As costs would be expected to increase while QALYs remained unchanged, the ICER of the MRI+CLP strategy should only increase.

Second, we assumed that all diagnosed individuals were treated. This is in reality probably false, as AD patients may end up rejecting treatment or not taking it properly.

Finally, another limitation of this analysis is that we did not take into account the psychological impact of early diagnosis of AD in the absence of efficient treatment at this stage. Including this factor would increase the cost associated to the MRI+CLP strategy, and in turn its ICER.

5. Results and limits of the "screen and treat" analyses

In our "screen and treat" analyses, we investigated a hypothetical future in which new treatments effective in early stage AD were available. To our knowledge, ours is the first study to do so, although earlier works investigated improvements in currently available treatments for mild to severe stage AD [10,11]. Innovatively, this second analysis also included a community-wide screening program and repeated rounds of testing. Indeed, if such treatments were to become available, population screening programs – which are not currently recommended by any health Agency – would have to be discussed.

Because the investigated context was hypothetical, we had to make several assumptions which influenced our results. First, we had to estimate the prevalence of AD in the general over-60 population, including asymptomatic cases. There is obviously no data to document this prevalence, and we chose a rather conservative value of 1%; the actual figure may be well over this value and we investigated prevalences up to 10% in our sensitivity analysis. Our base-case analysis was a worst-case scenario for the MRI+CLP strategy, which included the only diagnosis tool adapted to early AD.

Second, as both the new treatment and the new diagnosis test were hypothetical, we chose values for their base-case characteristics based on personal communications with AD specialists and teams currently working on the development of CLP tracers [Personal Communication, Guerbet company, Paris, 2009], and

A) Cost of CLP = 50€/injection

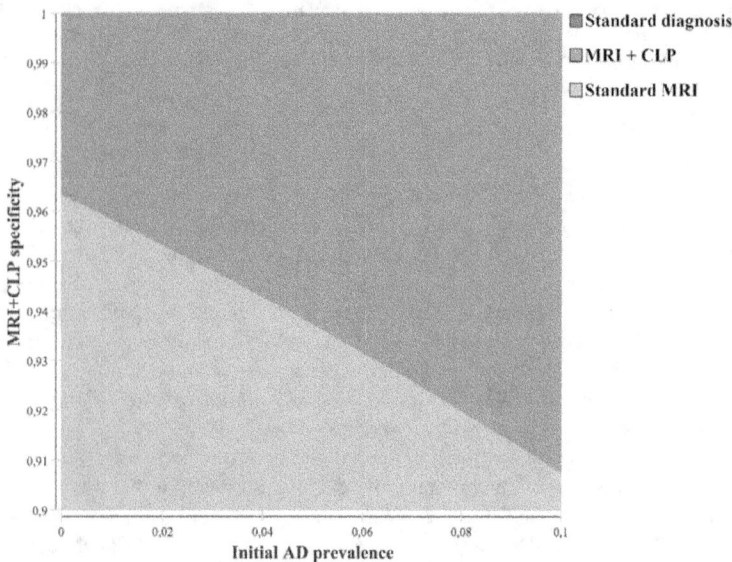

B) Cost of CLP = 250€/injection

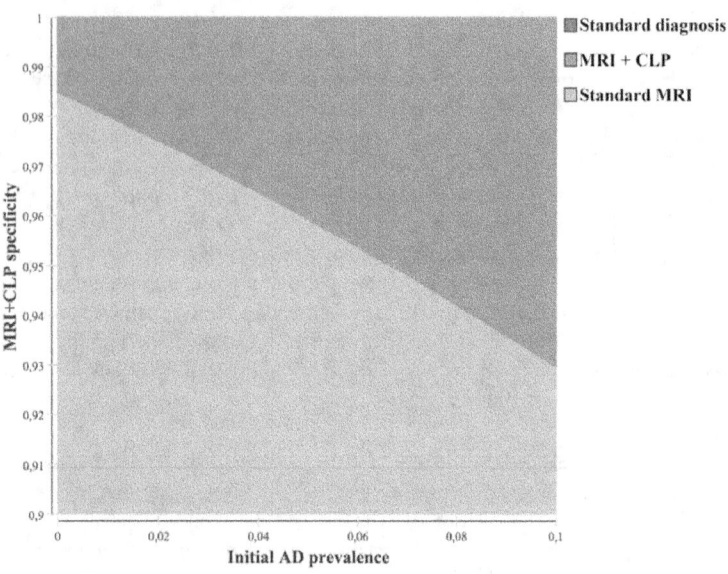

C) Cost of CLP = 500€/injection

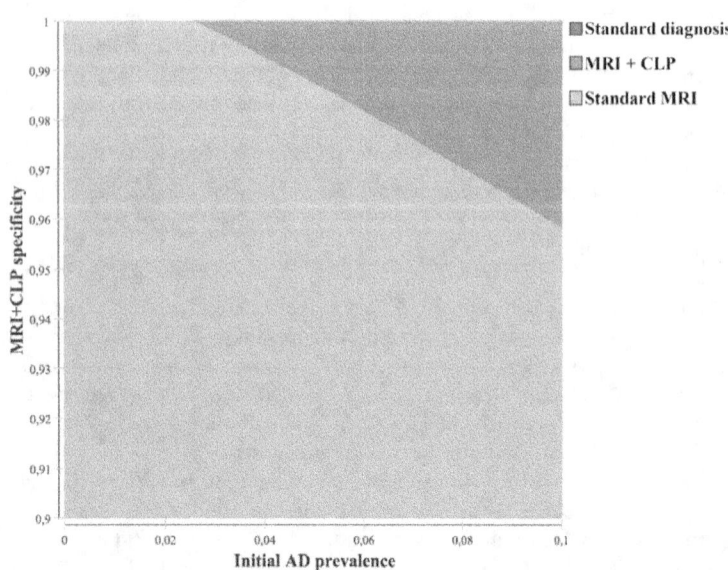

Figure 4. Results of the "screen and treat" (population-wide screening) analysis: multivariate sensitivity analysis. The strategy with maximum net monetary benefit is depicted as a function of the assumed prevalence of AD in the general over-60 population (between 0 and 10%) and specificity of the MRI+CLP diagnostic test between 0.90 and 1, for assumed costs of the CLP contrast agent between 0 and 500€ per injection: (a) Cost of the CLP contrast agent at 50 €/injection. (b) Cost of the CLP contrast agent at 250 €/injection (base-case). (c) Cost of the CLP contrast agent at 500 €/injection.
doi:10.1371/journal.pone.0035559.g004

investigated wide ranges of variation for these values in our sensitivity analysis. It is to be noted that the new treatment T may well be more expensive than 1000€, the top limit of our investigated range; however, as shown by our results, MRI+CLP would then systematically not prove cost-effective, irrespective of other characteristics.

Third, the participation rate to the screening campaign was unknown, and assumed to be 100%. Based on observed data from similar screening campaigns, actual rates are more around 60% at best, meaning that the screened population may not be representative of the general over-60 population. Also, being screened positive for AD may have a psychological impact, especially in asymptomatic patients. We chose not to take into account this impact in our analysis, considering that it should be reduced by the availability of a treatment efficient from early AD. Future studies should model screening participation and impact more realistically and investigate the potential repercussions.

Finally, this second analysis suffered from the same limitations related to AD treatment as the first. Including adverse effects of treatments in this analysis would increase the cost of the MRI+CLP strategy. Moreover, as the time horizon for this analysis was 15 years, it would have been interesting to investigate the impact of varying durations of treatment efficacy. This will be made easier in future years when more data on the long-term impact of AD treatment becomes available.

Because there is evidence that individuals carrying the ApoE4 gene are at increased risk for AD, we felt it was pertinent to investigate a scenario under which screening was targeted at these individuals. It should be noted however, that, in order to fully investigate such a scenario, other factors may have to be taken into account. Indeed, some epidemiological studies suggest that the ApoE4 genotype increases mortality rates, in particular cardio-vascular mortality in older individuals [54], hence age-specific mortality rates would need to be obtained for ApoE4 individuals. In addition, amyloid plaque density in cognitively healthy adults has been shown to be higher in ApoE4 carriers [55]. Depending on the interpretation of this finding, this may have different implications for a diagnostic tool based on the detection of amyloid plaques. On the one hand, it could be assumed that ApoE4 carriage increases the speed of amyloid plaque accumulation in AD patients; in that case, MRI+CLP would have better sensitivity in early stage AD in ApoE4 carriers. On the other hand, it could also be assumed that the ApoE4 genotype increases the density of amyloid plaques irrespective of AD; in that case, MRI+CLP would be expected to have lower specificity in ApoE4 carriers.

6. Conclusions

Assuming that a treatment with proven efficacy in early AD becomes available, as well as a diagnostic test allowing early detection of the disease, the issue of screening the population will arise. Our study suggests that, in order for this screening to be cost-effective, key parameters are the specificity of the new diagnostic test and the cost and effectiveness of the new treatment. These preliminary results ought to be taken into account in the currently underway research on early detection and treatment of AD, including work on β-amyloid plaques detection and elimination.

When this research yields results, a new cost-effectiveness analysis should be performed in order to evaluate the available tools with observed data.

Supporting Information

Figure S1 Markov models of Alzheimer's disease progression. All states are further subdivided in two, for individuals living at home vs. inside an institution (retirement or nursing home). A) Model for the primary analysis. B) Model for the "screen and treat" analyses.
(TIF)

Figure S2 Multivariate sensitivity analysis of the primary cost-effectiveness study. A) Distribution of incremental cost-effectiveness ratios (ICER) of the MRI+CLP strategy, compared to the standard diagnosis strategy. B) Acceptability curve: probability that each strategy either is dominant or has an ICER inferior to the willingness-to-pay, as a function of the willingness-to-pay threshold.
(TIF)

Figure S3 Multivariate sensitivity analysis of the primary cost-effectiveness study with treatment T. The strategy with maximum net monetary benefit is depicted as a function of the assumed efficacy and cost of the hypothetical new drug T. The efficacy of treatment T is expressed as a 0-to-1 ratio between assumed probabilities of transition from early stage AD with and without treatment T; 0 corresponds to maximum efficacy and 1 to no efficacy (in the base case, $f_T = 0.5$: 50% reduction).
(TIF)

Figure S4 Multivariate sensitivity analysis of the "screen and treat" (population-wide screening) cost-effectiveness study. A) Distribution of incremental cost-effectiveness ratios (ICER) of the MRI+CLP strategy, compared to the standard MRI strategy. B) Acceptability curve: probability that the MRI+CLP strategy either is dominant or has an ICER inferior to the willingness-to-pay, as a function of the willingness-to-pay threshold.
(TIF)

Figure S5 Analysis of the influence of MRI+CLP false positives and false negatives on the cost-effectiveness of the MRI+CLP strategies (tornado diagram). The range of incremental cost-effectiveness ratios (ICER) of the MRI+CLP strategy (compared to the standard MRI strategy) in A) the primary analysis and B) the "screen and treat" analysis is depicted for MRI+CLP sensitivities ranging from 0.9 to 1 and specificities ranging from 0.7 to 1. A sensitivity lower than 0.96 (base-case value) implies a higher risk of false negatives (FN, dotted green bars) than in the base-case. A specificity lower than 0.87 (base-case value) implies a higher risk of false positives (FP, dotted yellow bars) than in the base-case.
(TIF)

Figure S6 Multivariate sensitivity analysis of the results of the primary cost-effectiveness study on standard MRI vs. standard diagnosis. The strategy with maximum net monetary benefit among these two strategies is depicted as a

function of the assumed sensitivity of the standard MRI diagnostic test in mild and moderate AD, for an assumed sensitivity of the standard diagnosis strategy in moderate AD between 0.75 and 0.85 (in the absence of CLP and treatment T). A) 0.75 sensitivity in moderate AD for standard diagnosis (base-case value). B) 0.85 sensitivity in moderate AD for standard diagnosis.
(TIF)

File S1 Models of disease progression.
(DOCX)

Table S1 Model parameters: base-case values and ranges investigated in the sensitivity analyses.
(DOCX)

Table S2 Univariate sensitivity analysis: incremental cost-effectiveness ratio (ICER) of the MRI+CLP strategy, compared to the reference strategy, in the primary cost-effectiveness analysis, depending on the values of model parameters.
(DOCX)

Table S3 Univariate sensitivity analysis: ICER of the MRI+CLP strategy compared with the reference strategy, in the universal "screen and treat" cost-effectiveness analysis, depending on the values of model parameters.
(DOCX)

Author Contributions

Conceived and designed the experiments: CF WD LT. Performed the experiments: MB ND LT. Analyzed the data: MB ND LT. Wrote the paper: WD LT. Helped formulate realistic assumptions: CF WD.

References

1. Alzheimer's Association (2009) 2009 Alzheimer's disease facts and figures. Alzheimers Dement 5: 234–270.
2. Ballard C, Gauthier S, Corbett A, Brayne C, Aarsland D, et al. (2011) Alzheimer's disease. Lancet 377: 1019–1031.
3. Ferri CP, Prince M, Brayne C, Brodaty H, Fratiglioni L, et al. (2005) Global prevalence of dementia: a Delphi consensus study. Lancet 366: 2112–2117.
4. Helmer C, Pasquier F, Dartigues JF (2006) [Epidemiology of Alzheimer disease and related disorders]. Med Sci (Paris) 22: 288–296.
5. Hampel H, Broich K, Hoessler Y, Pantel J (2009) Biological markers for early detection and pharmacological treatment of Alzheimer's disease. Dialogues Clin Neurosci 11: 141–157.
6. Forlenza OV, Diniz BS, Gattaz WF (2010) Diagnosis and biomarkers of predementia in Alzheimer's disease. BMC Med 8: 89.
7. McKhann GM (2011) Changing concepts of Alzheimer disease. JAMA 305: 2458–2459.
8. Weiner MW, Aisen PS, Jack CR, Jr., Jagust WJ, Trojanowski JQ, et al. (2010) The Alzheimer's disease neuroimaging initiative: progress report and future plans. Alzheimers Dement 6: 202–211 e207.
9. Kulasingam SL, Samsa GP, Zarin DA, Rutschmann OT, Patwardhan MB, et al. (2003) When should functional neuroimaging techniques be used in the diagnosis and management of Alzheimer's dementia? A decision analysis. Value Health 6: 542–550.
10. McMahon PM, Araki SS, Neumann PJ, Harris GJ, Gazelle GS (2000) Cost-effectiveness of functional imaging tests in the diagnosis of Alzheimer disease. Radiology 217: 58–68.
11. McMahon PM, Araki SS, Sandberg EA, Neumann PJ, Gazelle GS (2003) Cost-effectiveness of PET in the diagnosis of Alzheimer disease. Radiology 228: 515–522.
12. Furiak NM, Klein RW, Kahle-Wrobleski K, Siemers ER, Sarpong E, et al. (2010) Modeling screening, prevention, and delaying of Alzheimer's disease: an early-stage decision analytic model. BMC Med Inform Decis Mak 10: 24.
13. Moatti JP, Le Corroller Soriano AG, Protiere C (2003) The "Plan Cancer" in France: an economists' point of view. Bull Cancer 90: 1010–1015.
14. Tan-Torres Edjerer T, Baltussen R, Adam T, Hutubessy R, Acharya A, et al. (2003) WHO guide to cost-effectiveness analysis. Geneva: World Health Organization.
15. TreeAge Software I (2009) TreeAge Pro Healthcare. Williamstown, USA.
16. Genin E, Hannequin D, Wallon D, Sleegers K, Hiltunen M, et al. (2011) APOE and Alzheimer disease: a major gene with semi-dominant inheritance. Mol Psychiatry 16: 903–907.
17. Neumann PJ, Hermann RC, Kuntz KM, Araki SS, Duff SB, et al. (1999) Cost-effectiveness of donepezil in the treatment of mild or moderate Alzheimer's disease. Neurology 52: 1138–1145.
18. Fagnani F, Lafuma A, Pechevis M, Rigaud AS, Traykov L, et al. (2004) Donepezil for the treatment of mild to moderate Alzheimer's disease in France: the economic implications. Dement Geriatr Cogn Disord 17: 5–13.
19. Himes CL, Wagner GG, Wolf DA, Aykan H, Dougherty DD (2000) Nursing home entry in Germany and the United States. J Cross Cult Gerontol 15: 99–118.
20. INED (2008) Age- and sex-specific mortality rates, France, 2008. Paris, .
21. Winblad B, Engedal K, Soininen H, Verhey F, Waldemar G, et al. (2001) A 1-year, randomized, placebo-controlled study of donepezil in patients with mild to moderate AD. Neurology 57: 489–495.
22. Rogers SL, Farlow MR, Doody RS, Mohs R, Friedhoff LT (1998) A 24-week, double-blind, placebo-controlled trial of donepezil in patients with Alzheimer's disease. Donepezil Study Group. Neurology 50: 136–145.
23. McShane R, Areosa Sastre A, Minakaran N (2006) Memantine for dementia. Cochrane Database Syst Rev. CD003154 p.
24. Reisberg B, Doody R, Stoffler A, Schmitt F, Ferris S, et al. (2003) Memantine in moderate-to-severe Alzheimer's disease. N Engl J Med 348: 1333–1341.
25. Atri A, Shaughnessy LW, Locascio JJ, Growdon JH (2008) Long-term course and effectiveness of combination therapy in Alzheimer disease. Alzheimer Dis Assoc Disord 22: 209–221.
26. Drago V, Babiloni C, Bartres-Faz D, Caroli A, Bosch B, et al. (2011) Disease tracking markers for Alzheimer's disease at the prodromal (MCI) stage. J Alzheimers Dis 26 Suppl 3: 159–199.
27. Blum-Boisgard C, Ulmann P (2007) Médicaments spécifiques de la maladie d'Alzheimer. Régime Social des Indépandants. pp 1–130.
28. Bowen J, Teri L, Kukull W, McCormick W, McCurry SM, et al. (1997) Progression to dementia in patients with isolated memory loss. Lancet 349: 763–765.
29. Commenges D, Joly P, Letenneur L, Dartigues JF (2004) Incidence and mortality of Alzheimer's disease or dementia using an illness-death model. Stat Med 23: 199–210.
30. Katz MJ, Lipton RB, Hall CB, Zimmerman ME, Sanders AE, et al. (2011) Age-specific and Sex-specific Prevalence and Incidence of Mild Cognitive Impairment, Dementia, and Alzheimer Dementia in Blacks and Whites: A Report From the Einstein Aging Study. Alzheimer Dis Assoc Disord.
31. Harris GJ, Lewis RF, Satlin A, English CD, Scott TM, et al. (1998) Dynamic susceptibility contrast MR imaging of regional cerebral blood volume in Alzheimer disease: a promising alternative to nuclear medicine. AJNR Am J Neuroradiol 19: 1727–1732.
32. Mormino EC, Kluth JT, Madison CM, Rabinovici GD, Baker SL, et al. (2009) Episodic memory loss is related to hippocampal-mediated beta-amyloid deposition in elderly subjects. Brain 132: 1310–1323.
33. Hansson O, Zetterberg H, Buchhave P, Londos E, Blennow K, et al. (2006) Association between CSF biomarkers and incipient Alzheimer's disease in patients with mild cognitive impairment: a follow-up study. Lancet Neurol 5: 228–234.
34. Ministère de la Santé (2009) Tarifs conventionnels des consultations de médecins spécialistes. In: Santé Mdl, ed. Paris: Assurance Maladie, Ministère de la Santé.
35. Ministère de la Santé (2009) Classification Commune des Actes Médicaux. In: Santé Mdl, ed. Paris: Assurance Maladie, Ministère de la Santé.
36. Ministère de la Santé (2009) Nomenclature des actes de biologie médicale. In: Santé Mdl, ed. Paris: Assurance Maladie, Ministère de la Santé.
37. Dictionnaire VIDAL. Paris: Editions du Vidal.
38. Feldman H, Gauthier S, Hecker J, Vellas B, Hux M, et al. (2004) Economic evaluation of donepezil in moderate to severe Alzheimer disease. Neurology 63: 644–650.
39. Rigaud AS, Fagnani F, Bayle C, Latour F, Traykov L, et al. (2003) Patients with Alzheimer's disease living at home in France: costs and consequences of the disease. J Geriatr Psychiatry Neurol 16: 140–145.
40. Elliott AF, Burgio LD, Decoster J (2010) Enhancing caregiver health: findings from the resources for enhancing Alzheimer's caregiver health II intervention. J Am Geriatr Soc 58: 30–37.
41. Reimat A (2002) Production associative et bénévolat informel : quelle signification économique pour les activités de production des retraités ? Innovations 15: 73–98.
42. Marbot C (2008) Travailler pour des particuliers : souvent une activité d'appoint. Insee Références, Les salaires en France.
43. France Bénévolat (2010) La situation du bénévolat en France en 2010. IFOP – France Bénévolat.
44. Fryback DG, Dasbach EJ, Klein R, Klein BE, Dorn N, et al. (1993) The Beaver Dam Health Outcomes Study: initial catalog of health-state quality factors. Med Decis Making 13: 89–102.
45. Gagnon M, Rive B, Hux M, Guilhaume C (2007) Cost-effectiveness of memantine compared with standard care in moderate-to-severe Alzheimer disease in Canada. Can J Psychiatry 52: 519–526.
46. Lejeune C, Bismuth MJ, Conroy T, Zanni C, Bey P, et al. (2005) Use of a decision analysis model to assess the cost-effectiveness of 18F-FDG PET in the

management of metachronous liver metastases of colorectal cancer. J Nucl Med 46: 2020–2028.

47. Faissol DM, Griffin PM, Swann JL (2009) Bias in Markov models of disease. Math Biosci 220: 143–156.

48. Cohen JT, Neumann PJ (2008) Decision analytic models for Alzheimer's disease: state of the art and future directions. Alzheimers Dement 4: 212–222.

49. Villemagne VL, Pike KE, Darby D, Maruff P, Savage G, et al. (2008) Abeta deposits in older non-demented individuals with cognitive decline are indicative of preclinical Alzheimer's disease. Neuropsychologia 46: 1688–1697.

50. Forsberg A, Engler H, Almkvist O, Blomquist G, Hagman G, et al. (2008) PET imaging of amyloid deposition in patients with mild cognitive impairment. Neurobiol Aging 29: 1456–1465.

51. Wolk DA, Price JC, Saxton JA, Snitz BE, James JA, et al. (2009) Amyloid imaging in mild cognitive impairment subtypes. Ann Neurol 65: 557–568.

52. Reese JP, Hessmann P, Seeberg G, Henkel D, Hirzmann P, et al. (2011) Cost and Care of Patients with Alzheimer's Disease: Clinical Predictors in German Health Care Settings. J Alzheimers Dis.

53. Mauskopf J, Mucha L (2011) A review of the methods used to estimate the cost of Alzheimer's disease in the United States. Am J Alzheimers Dis Other Demen 26: 298–309.

54. Schachter F, Faure-Delanef L, Guenot F, Rouger H, Froguel P, et al. (1994) Genetic associations with human longevity at the APOE and ACE loci. Nat Genet 6: 29–32.

55. Caselli RJ, Walker D, Sue L, Sabbagh M, Beach T (2010) Amyloid load in nondemented brains correlates with APOE e4. Neurosci Lett 473: 168–171.

Multi-Method Analysis of MRI Images in Early Diagnostics of Alzheimer's Disease

Robin Wolz[1][9], Valtteri Julkunen[2][9], Juha Koikkalainen[3], Eini Niskanen[2,4], Dong Ping Zhang[1], Daniel Rueckert[1], Hilkka Soininen[2,5], Jyrki Lötjönen[3]*, the Alzheimer's Disease Neuroimaging Initiative[¶]

1 Biomedical Image Analysis Group, Department of Computing, Imperial College London, London, United Kingdom, 2 Department of Neurology, Kuopio University Hospital, Kuopio, Finland, 3 Knowledge Intensive Services, VTT Technical Research Centre of Finland, Tampere, Finland, 4 Department of Applied Physics, University of Eastern Finland, Kuopio, Finland, 5 Institute of Clinical Medicine, Neurology, University of Eastern Finland, Kuopio, Finland

Abstract

The role of structural brain magnetic resonance imaging (MRI) is becoming more and more emphasized in the early diagnostics of Alzheimer's disease (AD). This study aimed to assess the improvement in classification accuracy that can be achieved by combining features from different structural MRI analysis techniques. Automatically estimated MR features used are hippocampal volume, tensor-based morphometry, cortical thickness and a novel technique based on manifold learning. Baseline MRIs acquired from all 834 subjects (231 healthy controls (HC), 238 stable mild cognitive impairment (S-MCI), 167 MCI to AD progressors (P-MCI), 198 AD) from the Alzheimer's Disease Neuroimaging Initiative (ADNI) database were used for evaluation. We compared the classification accuracy achieved with linear discriminant analysis (LDA) and support vector machines (SVM). The best results achieved with individual features are 90% sensitivity and 84% specificity (HC/AD classification), 64%/66% (S-MCI/P-MCI) and 82%/76% (HC/P-MCI) with the LDA classifier. The combination of all features improved these results to 93% sensitivity and 85% specificity (HC/AD), 67%/69% (S-MCI/P-MCI) and 86%/82% (HC/P-MCI). Compared with previously published results in the ADNI database using individual MR-based features, the presented results show that a comprehensive analysis of MRI images combining multiple features improves classification accuracy and predictive power in detecting early AD. The most stable and reliable classification was achieved when combining all available features.

Citation: Wolz R, Julkunen V, Koikkalainen J, Niskanen E, Zhang DP, et al. (2011) Multi-Method Analysis of MRI Images in Early Diagnostics of Alzheimer's Disease. PLoS ONE 6(10): e25446. doi:10.1371/journal.pone.0025446

Editor: Celia Oreja-Guevara, University Hospital La Paz, Spain

Received July 12, 2011; Accepted September 5, 2011; Published October 13, 2011

Funding: This project is partially funded under the 7th Framework Programme by the European Commission (http://cordis.europa.eu/ist/). Data collection and sharing for this project was funded by the Alzheimer's Disease Neuroimaging Initiative (ADNI; Principal Investigator: Michael Weiner; NIH grant U01 AG024904). ADNI is funded by the National Institute on Aging, the National Institute of Biomedical Imaging and Bioengineering (NIBIB), and through generous contributions from the following: Pzer Inc., Wyeth Research, Bristol-Myers Squibb, Eli Lilly and Company, GlaxoSmithKline, Merck & Co. Inc., AstraZeneca AB, Novartis Pharmaceuticals Corporation, Alzheimer's Association, Eisai Global Clinical Development, Elan Corporation, plc, Forest Laboratories, and the Institute for the Study of Aging, with participation from the U.S. Food and Drug Administration. Industry partnerships are coordinated through the Foundation for the National Institutes of Health. The grantee organization is the Northern California Institute for Research and Education, and the study is coordinated by the Alzheimer's Disease Cooperative Study at the University of California San Diego. ADNI data are disseminated by the Laboratory of Neuro Imaging at the University of California Los Angeles. Data used in the preparation of this article were obtained from the ADNI database (www.loni.ucla.edu/ADNI). As such, the investigators within the ADNI contributed to the design and implementation of ADNI and/or provided data but did not participate in analysis or writing of this report. ADNI investigators include (complete listing available at http://adni.loni.ucla.edu/wp-content/uploads/how_to_apply/ADNI_Authorship_List.pdf).

Competing Interests: The authors have declared that no competing interests exist.

* E-mail: jyrki.lotjonen@vtt.fi

[9] These authors contributed equally to this work.

[¶] For information on the Alzheimer's Disease Neuroimaging Initiative please see the Acknowledgments section.

Introduction

Alzheimer's disease (AD) is the most common cause of dementia globally and one of the major healthcare issues of the future. It has been estimated that during the next four decades the prevalence of AD will quadruple from 27 to 106 million by which time 1 in 85 persons worldwide will be living with the disease [1]. Even a modest delay of one year in disease onset and progression could reduce the number of cases by 9 million [1]. Interventions are postulated to be most effective when directed at patients at the earliest stages of the disease, which underlines the importance of early diagnosis of AD [2]. Mild cognitive impairment (MCI) is a heterogeneous syndrome that increases the risk of developing AD markedly [3]. However, not all MCI subjects convert to AD and some may even return to normal cognition [4].

The search for reliable biomarkers of AD-type pathology and predictors of disease progression among MCI subjects is ongoing. AD is characterized by neurofibrillary tangles and amyloid plaques in the brain [5]. Degenerative changes in the human neurotransmitter system lead to atrophy in selected brain regions [6]. The most promising candidate biomarkers are the ones derived from structural and functional neuroimaging as well as those measured in cerebrospinal fluid (CSF) and plasma [7]. Amyloid-based measures like the CSF-peptide $A\beta_{42}$ and the uptake of the PiB tracer on positron emission imaging (PET) show the earliest AD-type changes [7]. However, there is evidence that the number of amyloid plaques reach their saturation levels already by the time patients have clinically apparent symptoms of cognitive impairment [8,9], whereas atrophy, neuronal loss, synaptic loss, and the number of tangles increase with severity of illness [10]. These findings suggest that, although amyloid-based biomarkers may be used as longitudinal markers of AD type pathology, they seem to offer only limited insight into which MCI subjects will most likely convert to AD in the near future. In a recently published dynamic model of biomarker behavior in the AD spectrum, biomarkers based on structural magnetic resonance imaging (MRI) have been shown to be correlated with a progression from MCI to AD [11]. Such biomarkers could therefore improve the accuracy of early AD diagnostics and reduce especially the amount of false positive diagnoses. Besides providing chance for a more focused and earlier intervention, structural MRI biomarkers of AD could also aid the development of new disease-modifying drugs by acting as surrogate markers of disease progression, reduce the number of subjects needed to detect significant drug effect and provide quantitative measures of treatment benefits [12].

It has been shown that the early diagnostics of AD can be improved by using multiple different biomarkers simultaneously. Usually these studies have combined MRI-based markers with biomarkers based on positron emission tomography (PET) [13,14], cerebrospinal fluid (CSF) [15,16] or both [17–19]. Achieved results vary from no additional benefit [15,17] to significant improvement [13,14,16,20]. However, availability of all three biomarkers (CSF, PET, MRI) is not very common in clinical practice since obtaining all measures is laborious for the patient and clinician, induces delays and increases the costs of the diagnosis significantly. Furthermore, measurements obtained from CSF and PET are considered invasive. Recent studies focusing on only structural MRI have reached correct classification accuracys (CCR) of 76–94% in identifying healthy controls (HC) from patients with AD and 64–82% in predicting which MCI subjects will convert to AD in the imminent future [21–27]. The high variation in these results can be attributed to differences in study populations as well as evaluation designs. With the Alzheimer's Disease Neuroimaging Study (ADNI) [28], a large multi-center study on MR imaging in AD has been established that is available to the wider research community. Based on a large sub-group of ADNI subjects, Cuingnet et al. [29] presented a comparison of ten MRI-based feature extraction methods and their ability to discriminate between clinically relevant subject groups. The ten methods evaluated comprise five voxel-based methods, three methods based on cortical thickness and two methods based on the hippocampus. Best sensitivity/specificity values reported are 81%/95% for AD vs HC, 70%/61% for S-MCI vs P-MCI and 73%/85% for HC vs P-MCI.

In this paper we use the ADNI database to evaluate the ability of the combination of different MR-based features to increase classification accuracy. We evaluate the power of hippocampal volume (HV), cortical thickness (CTH), tensor-based morphometry (TBM) and features extracted from a recently proposed manifold-based learning (MBL) framework to discriminate healthy controls from subjects with AD and to predict conversion from MCI to AD. For evaluation we used all 834 ADNI baseline images that were available from the ADNI webpage. Compared to previous work this paper aims at establishing the improvement in accuracy and stability that can be achieved by combining more than one MR-based feature. To the best of our knowledge it is the first comprehensive study that analyzes MRI-derived features for the full ADNI dataset. For direct comparison with the work by Cuingnet et al. [29] we also evaluated all results on the subset used in their work.

To test the influence of the classification method used, we utilized both support vector machines (SVMs) and a linear discriminant analys (LDA) to evaluate classification accuracy (CCR), sensitivity (SEN) and specificity (SPE) in each experiment.

Materials and Methods

Subjects

In the ADNI study, brain MR images were acquired at regular intervals after an initial baseline scan from approximately 200 cognitively normal older subjects (HC), 400 subjects with mild cognitive impairment (MCI), and 200 subjects with early AD. Detailed inclusion/exclusion criteria used for the different subject groups in ADNI are defined in [30]. The AD group has scores between 20–26 (inclusive) on the Mini-Mental State Examination (MMSE) [31], and a Clinical Dementia Rating (CDR) [32] of 0.5 or 1.0. Furthermore, these subjects fulfil the NINCDS/ADRDA criteria for probable AD [33]. MCI subjects included have MMSE scores between 24–30 (inclusive), a memory complaint, have objective memory loss measured by education adjusted scores on Wechsler Memory Scale Logical Memory II, a CDR of 0.5, absence of significant levels of impairment in other cognitive domains, essentially preserved activities of daily living, and an absence of dementia [30]. Healthy subjects have MMSE scores between 24–30 (inclusive), a CDR of 0, are non-depressed, non MCI, and nondemented. A more detailed description of the ADNI study is given in Appendix S1.

All 834 ADNI subjects (231 HC, 238 S-MCI, 167 P-MCI, 198 AD) for which a 1.5T T1-weighted MRI scan at baseline was available were included in this study. 167 subjects in the MCI group converted to AD as of July 2011. We therefore independently analysed progressive MCI (P-MCI) subjects and subjects with a stable diagnosis of MCI (S-MCI).

Table 1 shows the demographics for the 834 study subjects. Statistically significant differences in the demographics and clinical variables between the study groups were assessed using Student's unpaired t-test. In this work, the difference was considered statistically significant if $p < 0.05$ if not stated otherwise. There were more men than women in all other groups besides the AD group. MMSE scores were significantly different in the pairwise comparisons between all study groups. CDR scores of the HC and AD groups are significantly different to the ones of the two MCI groups. Healthy subjects had a significantly lower Geriatric Depression Scale (GDS) compared to all other groups. Compared to all other groups, AD subjects had significantly shorter education.

MRI Acquisition

Standard 1.5T screening/baseline T1-weighted images obtained using volumetric 3D MPRAGE protocol with resolutions

Table 1. Subjects.

Group	HC	S-MCI	P-MCI	AD
N	231	238	167	198
Men	52%	66%	62%	52%
Age	76.02 (5.0)	74.85 (7.8)	74.6 (7.0)	75.68 (7.7)
MMSE	29.1* (1.0)	27.3* (1.8)	26.6* (1.7)	23.3* (2.0)
CDR	0 (0)	0.49 (0.05)	0.50 (0)	0.75 (0.25)
GDS	0.83* (1.14)	1.60 (1.42)	1.53 (1.30)	1.67 (1.42)
Education	16.0 (2.8)	15.6 (3.1)	15.7 (2.9)	14.7* (3.1)
APOE4 status ($\varepsilon 3\varepsilon 4/\varepsilon 4\varepsilon 4$)	23%/2%	31%/8%	50%/16%	42%/18%
Months to conversion			18.2 (10.1)	

*means statistically significant different from all other groups.
doi:10.1371/journal.pone.0025446.t001

ranging from 0.9 mm × 0.9 mm × 1.20 mm to 1.3 mm × 1.3 mm × 1.20 mm were included from the ADNI database. For detailed information of the MRI protocols and preprocessing steps see [34].

Feature extraction

All fully automated feature extraction methods described below were applied to images that were preprocessed by the ADNI pipeline.

Hippocampal volume. Baseline hippocampal volumes were measured using an approach based on fast and robust multi-atlas segmentation [35,36]. In this approach, multi-atlas label propagation is applied in combination with atlas selection to obtain the hippocampus segmentation. A set of hippocampus atlases is selected from a pool of atlas images according to image similarity with the query image. After registering all atlases to the query image, a spatial prior is generated from the multiple label maps. This spatial prior is then used to obtain a final segmentation based on an expectation maximization (EM) segmentation algorithm [37].

Cortical thickness. CTH is measured in the baseline T1-weighted structural MR images by using an automated computational surface-based method developed at the McConnell Brain Imaging Centre, Montreal Neurological Institute, McGill University, Montreal, Canada (http://www2.bic.mni.mcgill.ca/) [38]. Individual MRI volumes were registered to standard space using the ICBM152 template [39]. Intensity non-uniformities were corrected [40] before the final brain mask was calculated [41]. Tissues were segmented into white matter (WM), grey matter (GM) and cerebrospinal fluid (CSF) using the INSECT-algorithm [42] and the magnitude of PVE was estimated by using the trimmed minimum covariance determinant (TMCD) method [43]. The brains were divided automatically into two separate hemispheres and the inner and outer surfaces of the cortex were extracted according to intersections between WM and GM (white matter surface, WMS) as well as GM and CSF (grey matter surface, GMS) using the Constrained Laplacian-Based Automated Segmentation with Proximities (CLASP) algorithm [44]. The inner surface was first formed by deforming an ellipsoid polygon mesh to the shape of the WMS. GMS was obtained by further expanding the inner surface. Each polygon mesh surface consisted of 81,920 polygons and 40,962 nodes per hemisphere. The thickness of the cortex was defined at each linked node as the distance between the two concentrically linked polygon meshes on the WMS and the GMS. This t-link metric has been proven to be the simplest yet most precise way to determine cortical thickness [38]. Although MR images were transformed to standard space to allow for group analysis, thickness calculations were performed in each subject's native space. Finally, cortical thickness maps were smoothed with a 20 mm FWHM diffusion smoothing kernel to improve the signal-to-noise ratio and statistical power [45]. The described toolbox did not achieve satisfactory results on some study subjects because of i) failure in tissue segmentation and brain masking (48 subjects) and ii) failure in partial volume effect estimation (59 subjects). As a result the pipeline crashed and CTH measures were not obtained for 76 subjects (24 control, 35 MCI, 17 AD). Also the cortical model of 31 subjects (10 control, 13 MCI, 8 AD) was completely deformed and thus unusable. For these 107 subjects the CTH features were considered as missing values. CTH features used in the classification experiments are introduced below.

Tensor-based morphometry. The TBM analysis was performed using a multi-template approach [46,47]. In TBM, a template image is non-rigidly registered to a study image, and, typically, the determinant of the Jacobian matrix ('the Jacobian') of the deformation is used to measure the voxel-level morphometry.

Instead of using just one template image, we used 30 randomly selected images (10 controls, 10 MCIs, and 10 ADs) from the ADNI database as template images. The template images were used also in the classification analysis to maximize the number of subjects. Each template image was registered to a study image, and Jacobian maps were computed for each template image. To combine the results of multiple templates, all template images were registered to the mean anatomical template generated from the 30 images, and all the results were normalized to this reference space [47]. The combination of the results was performed by averaging the ROI-wise feature values of all the templates as described in detail below.

Manifold-based learning. In this machine learning approach, non-linear dimensionality reduction with Laplacian eigenmaps [48] is used to learn features to discriminate between different subject groups. Laplacian eigenmaps estimates the low-dimensional representation of a set of input images based on a similarity graph that is defined with pairwise image similarities [48]. The hypothesis is that such a low-dimensional representation captures the variability in the dataset in a more compact way than pairwise image similarities directly. We estimate pairwise image similarities from the intensity appearance in a region around hippocampus and amygdala since both structures are known to be affected by AD in an early stage. All images are aligned in a template space using a coarse non-rigid registration (10 mm B-spline control-point spacing, [49]). Such a coarse non-rigid alignment ensures that corresponding brain structures are aligned but still allows to measure subject-specific differences. After performing dimensionality reduction, the first 20 dimensions of the resulting manifold are used as features to perform classification with the different methods used. More details on the theory and application of this manifold learning approach can be found in [20,50]. Figure 1 exemplarily shows a 2D embedding of a set of ADNI images acquired from healthy controls and subjects with AD. It can be seen that even two embedding dimensions give a relatively good separation between both groups. In our experiments we used a higher dimensional space allowing better discrimination.

ROI-wise features for CTH and TBM

Both CTH and TBM analyses produce local (point-wise) information, either on cortical thickness or the volume. Thus, the number of original features is enormous, and to make the classification more efficient and robust, the number of features has to be reduced. We evaluated both features in a statistical region of interest (ROI) defined as detailed in Appendix S2. Figures 2 and 3 show t-values for statistically significant differences between study groups for TBM and CTH respectively. A detailed description of the definition of these statistical ROIs is given in Appendix S2.

Study design

Table 2 presents an overview on the features calculated for all 834 available ADNI baseline images. All feature values were corrected for age and gender using a linear regression model where control subjects were used as the training set, i.e., the normal, not disease-related, age and gender related differences in the classification features were removed. Feature selection was then carried out on the corrected feature sets using stepwise regression [51].

We used two subsets to perform classification:

I. All 834 available baseline images described in the subjects section

II. 509 baseline images used by Cuingnet et al. [29] and detailed in their publication.

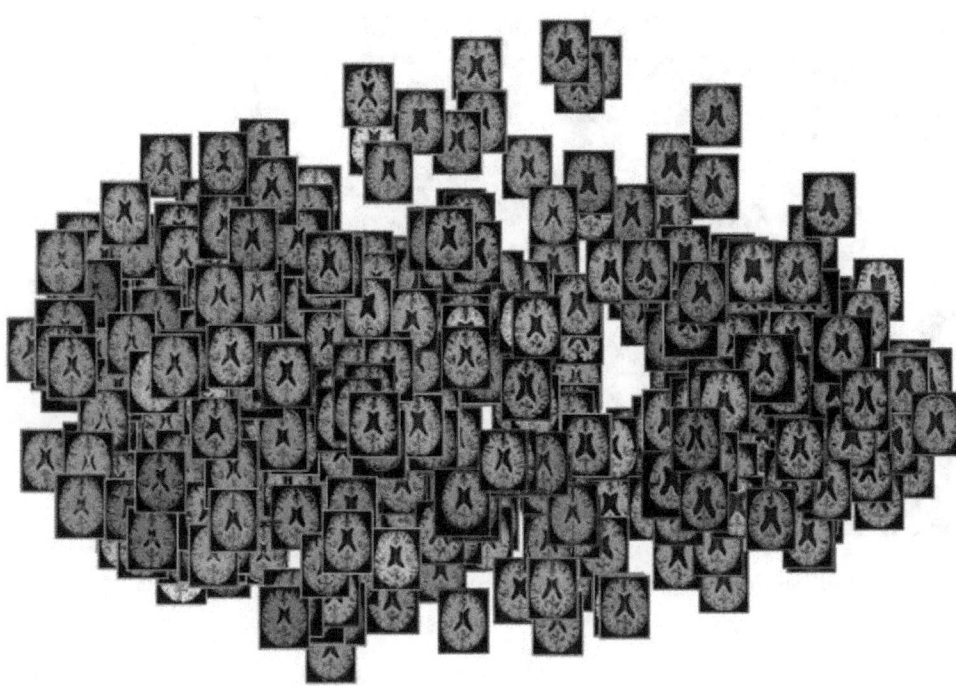

Figure 1. 2D manifold embedding of a set of images acquired from healthy controls (red) and subjects with AD (blue).
doi:10.1371/journal.pone.0025446.g001

The following sections describe the definition of the statistical ROIs and evaluation strategy used for the two datasets respectively.

Dataset I. In order to perform the study using cross-validation in the full dataset, it was divided into three equally sized parts. One part was used to perform the statistical tests for the CTH and TBM features, and the remaining two parts were used to evaluate the classification accuracy. This was repeated three times so that each part was once used to perform the statistical tests. Afterwards, the results of the three repetitions were averaged. The classification accuracy was evaluated using leave-N-out cross validation on those subjects not included in the statistical tests. Five percent of the evaluation subjects were regarded as the test set, and the remaining 95% of the subjects were used to train a classifier which was then applied to the test set. This was repeated table-1-caption100 times, each time selecting randomly the test set subjects. Finally, the results of the 100 repetitions were averaged.

Consequently, in overall, the classification evaluation was performed using 300 (3×100) repetitions, and the results presented in this paper are the average values of all these classifications.

Dataset II. Statistical ROIs for CTH and TBM feature extraction were calculated from the 325 baseline images that are not part of dataset II. In order to allow direct comparison of classification accuracy with the work by Cuingnet et al. [29], separate training and testing sets for the different comparisons were defined using the exact sub-groups reported in their manuscript. Around 50% of all subjects are used to train the different types of classifiers and the reported results are based on classifying the remaining subjects.

Classification methods

We used two different widely used methods to perform classification based on individual features and their combination:

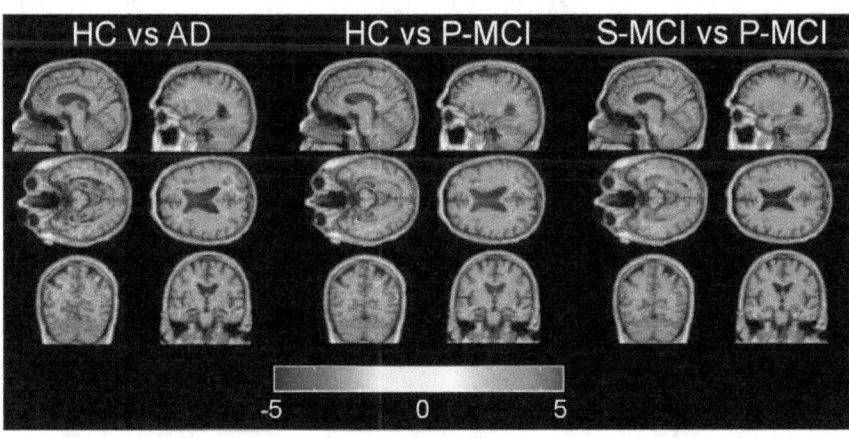

Figure 2. Results for voxelwise t-tests for statistically significant group differences with features extracted from TBM.
doi:10.1371/journal.pone.0025446.g002

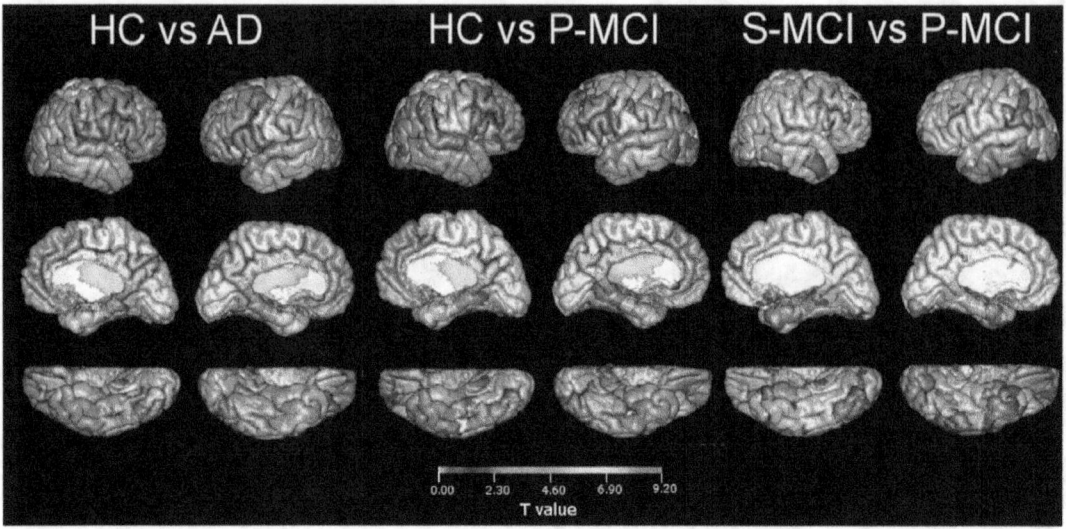

Figure 3. Results for t-tests for statistically significant group differences based on cortical thickness measurements.
doi:10.1371/journal.pone.0025446.g003

Linear discriminant analysis (LDA). Linear discriminant analysis (LDA) is a widely used technique to find a linear combination of features to best separate several classes [52]. In this work we used LDA as implemented in the *classify* function in Matlab with a multivariate normal density model with uninformative priors (p = 0.5).

Support vector machines (SVM). Support vector machines use training data to find a separating hyperplane in the n-dimensional training space that best separates two subject groups [53]. Test subjects are then classified according to their position relative to the defined hyperplane in the n-dimensional feature space. We used the libSVM library to perform the analysis. The radial basis function kernel was selected based on the guidelines provided by the libSVM library (Software available 2.3.2011 at http://www.csie.ntu.edu.tw/cjlin/libsvm).

Results

We used both classification methods to measure classification accuracy based on individual features as well as the combination of all features. The results for the comparisons HC vs AD, HC vs P-MCI and S-MCI vs P-MCI in the full ADNI database are presented in Tables 3, 4 and 5 respectively. Presented are classification accuracy (CCR), sensitivity (SEN) and specificity (SPE). Furthermore, the 95% confidence interval for the classification accuracy is estimated based on the multiple classification runs. Statistically

significant improvements achieved when combining all features are marked with † (p < 0.0001). To test for significance, unpaired t-tests were carried out between distribution estimates for the corresponding classification rates based on the multiple runs. All estimated distributions passed a normality test using a Kolmogorov-Smirnov test at α = 0.05.

For direct comparison with work presented by Cuingnet et al. [29], we performed classification based on the training- and testing sets defined in their manuscript as described above. S-MCI and P-MCI groups are defined in the same way as in the original publication. Sensitivity and specificity values for the classification in all three clinical pairings are reported in Table 6. Following the clear advantage for LDA in the performance on the full dataset, we only report results with this classifier for dataset II.

Discussion

In this study we assessed the automatic diagnostic capabilities of 4 structural MRI features (MBL, HC, CTH, TBM) separately and combined in 834 baseline images acquired in the ADNI study. When applied separately, TBM provided the overall best results, closely followed by MBL. Combining all features improved the results in all study experiments. Our results show how a combination of different MRI-based features can improve results based on only one measurement, resulting in a more powerful and stable classifier. The most significant improvement of the combination

Table 2. Features used in the study.

Method	No of features	Description
Hippocampal volume (HV)	1	total volume of left and right hippopcampus
Cortical thickness	9 (HC vs AD)	average cortical thickness within a ROI defined based on group-level statistical analysis
(CTH)	7 (HC vs P-MCI)	
	8 (S-MCI vs P-MCI)	
Tensor-based morphometry (TBM)	84	average Jacobian of atrophic voxels within a ROI, weighted based on voxel-wise p-values
Manifold-based learning (MBL)	20	coordinates of a subject in a low-dimensional manifold space learned from pairwise image similarities

doi:10.1371/journal.pone.0025446.t002

Table 3. Classification results for HC vs AD.

Feature	LDA			SVM		
	CCR [95% CI]	SEN	SPE	CCR [95% CI]	SEN	SPE
MBL	85† [64 100]	87	83	85 [64 100]	87	83
HV	81† [57 100]	81	79	81† [57 100]	84	77
CTH	81† [64 100]	89	71	82† [57 100]	90	73
TBM	87† [71 100]	90	84	87 [71 100]	89	84
All	89 [71 100]	93	85	86 [71 100]	94	78

†means statistically significant different from the combined results with $p < 0.0001$. CCR = Correct classification rate, SEN = Sensitivity, SPE = Specificity.
doi:10.1371/journal.pone.0025446.t003

Table 5. Classification results for S-MCI vs P-MCI.

Feature	LDA			SVM		
	CCR [95% CI]	SEN	SPE	CCR [95% CI]	SEN	SPE
MBL	65† [36 86]	64	66	65† [43 86]	77	48
HV	65† [36 86]	63	67	62 [36 86]	83	33
CTH	56† [29 86]	63	45	59 [36 79]	96	03
TBM	64† [36 86]	65	62	64† [36 86]	77	44
All	68 [43 93]	67	69	60 [36 86]	92	14

†means statistically significant different from the combined results with $p < 0.0001$.
doi:10.1371/journal.pone.0025446.t005

over the best individual feature can be observed for HC vs P-MCI with 5% units followed by 3 and 2% units for S-MCI vs P-MCI and HC vs AD, respectively. These improvements lead to 20, 12 and 9 subjects more being correctly classified respectively when using the combined feature set as compared to the best single feature for every comparison. Comparing two classification approaches based on LDA and SVMs resulted in a clear advantage of the former.

Several studies reported classification results using single MRI methods for the HC/AD classification (Table 7). Liu et al. [24] reported SEN/SPE of 92/90 in the classification of HC/AD subjects using regional cortical volumes in the AddNeuroMed dataset. McEvoy et al. [26] report a CCR of 89 on images from the ADNI database using features from cortical thickness and structural volumes. Vemuri et al. [54] present a SEN/SPE of 86/86 on 380 subjects using the STAND score. In our study the results obtained with single methods are lower (71–90) but almost identical when the methods were combined. It should be noted, however, that Liu and colleagues did not use cross-validation or separate training/testing sets when producing the results which could lead to overestimation of the results in a dataset outside the study cohort. Gerardin et al. [23] acquired a high SEN/SPE of 96/92 by using hippocampal shape analysis, but the number of subjects (25 HC, 23 AD) was quite low in order to produce results with good generalizability. Westman et al. [55] reported a CCR of 82 for HC vs AD classification and 73 for HC vs P-MCI classification by using various regional brain volumes. Our results are substantially more accurate, the group sizes are larger and clinical follow-up time is one year longer. Chupin et al. [21] reported SEN/SPE of 75/77 (hippocampal volume) and Querbes et al. [27] a CCR of 85 (cortical thickness), both lower than the

results acquired with the combination of features or TBM features independently in our study.

Varying results concerning AD prediction (S-MCI/P-MCI classification using baseline measurements) have been published (Table 7): Querbes et al. [27] reported a CCR of 73, Liu et al. [25] a SEN/SPE of 76/68, Chupin et al. [21] reported a SEN/SPE of 60/65 and Davatzikos et al. [15] SEN/SPE of 95/38. Our results with separate and combined baseline features lie in the range of these results (SEN/SPE 63/67, 64/66 and 67/69 when using HV, MBL and the combined features, respectively).

There can be several explanations for the variation in the reported results. A majority of the studies in this field have used different statistical methods and MRI feature extraction strategies on different datasets, which makes a comparison of the results complicated. Also the variation in the size of the study samples and the use (or ignoring) of cross-validation or separate training/testing sets are important factors, which both have crucial impact on the reliability and generalizability of the results. In Lötjönen et al. [36], we demonstrated that choosing from a population of 350 cases several times 2/3 for the training set and 1/3 for the test set and using hippocampus volume as a classification feature can lead to any classification accuracy between 53% and 77%. This observation is also confirmed by the high confidence intervals for the classification accuracies reported in Tables 3, 4 and 5. This shows that a fair comparison of methods based on the classification accuracy is difficult if not exactly the same data and classification approaches are used. Furthermore, since the ADNI study is still ongoing, several subjects labeled as S-MCI will progress in the future to the P-MCI group.

A recent study with a subset of ADNI subjects assessed the classification performance of several structural MRI methods in experiments comparable to our investigation [29]. Reported

Table 4. Classification results for HC vs P-MCI.

Feature	LDA			SVM		
	CCR [95% CI]	SEN	SPE	CCR [95% CI]	SEN	SPE
MBL	78† [54 100]	81	75	77† [54 92]	84	69
HV	76† [54 92]	77	76	78 [54 92]	83	71
CTH	77† [54 100]	85	65	77 [54 100]	89	62
TBM	79† [62 100]	82	76	80† [62 100]	85	74
All	84 [62 100]	86	82	82 [62 100]	93	67

†means statistically significant different from the combined results with $p < 0.0001$.
doi:10.1371/journal.pone.0025446.t004

Table 6. Classification results based on a subset of ADNI that was previously used for classification by Cuingnet et al. [29].

Feature	HC vs AD		HC vs P-MCI		S-MCI vs P-MCI	
	SEN	SPE	SEN	SPE	SEN	SPE
MBL	90	74	84	92	55	76
HV	80	69	75	76	63	70
CTH	85	75	86	59	72	35
TBM	93	76	90	84	63	59
All	94	76	94	89	69	54

doi:10.1371/journal.pone.0025446.t006

Table 7. Classification results of healthy control (HC), mild cognitive impairment (MCI) and Alzheimer's disease subjects reported in the recent literature.

Study	N	Features	HC vs AD			HC vs P-MCI			S-MCI vs P-MCI		
			CCR	SEN	SPE	CCR	SEN	SPE	CCR	SEN	SPE
Liu et al. [24]	333	Cortical volumes	91	92	90	-	-	-	-	-	-
Gerardin et al. [23]*	70	Hippocampus shape	94	96	92	-	-	-	-	-	-
Chupin et al. [21]*	605	Hippocampus volume	76	75	77	-	-	-	64	60	65
Querbes et al. [27]*	382	Cortical thickness	85	-	-	-	-	-	73	75	68
Liu et al. [25]	312	Amygdala/caudate volumes	-	-	-	-	-	-	69	76	68
Davatzikos et al. [15]*	356	SPARE-AD index	-	-	-	-	-	-	56	95	38
Cuingnet et al. [29]*	509	Various	-	81	95	-	73	85	-	62	69
Hinrichs et al. [14]*	159	MRI & PET	81	-	-	60	92	14	-	-	-
Westman et al. [55]	351	Various volumes	82	-	-	73	-	-	-	-	-
McEvoy et al. [26]*	398	Cortical thickness/various volumes	89	83	93	-	-	-	-	-	-
Vemuri et al. [54]	380	STAND score	-	86	86	-	-	-	-	-	-

N = Number of study subjects,
* = ADNI dataset.
doi:10.1371/journal.pone.0025446.t007

SEN/SPE lie in the ranges 59/81–81/95 (HC vs AD) and 70/73–73/85 (HC vs P-MCI). While most methods tested did not exceed the accuracy of a random classifier for the discrimination between S-MCI and P-MCI, the best results reported for this task were a SEN/SPE of 62/69 when using hippocampal volume. To allow a direct comparison of the results reported by Cuingnet et al. [29], we evaluated our features on the exact same training- and testing sets used in their paper. This direct comparison shows that our results compare favourably to other, established methods in neuroimaging. For HC vs AD classification, individual features in our study give more sensitive but less specific results than most methods in the previous publication. Combining all features gives an overall better classification accuracy than the majority of previously tested methods. Our results on the combined feature set furthermore outperform the majority of methods tested by Cuingnet et al. [29] when predicting MCI conversion as well as all methods for the classification between HC and P-MCI. A significant difference in classification accuracy can be observed between the full ADNI dataset and this smaller subset used for comparison with previous work. Reasons may include a strict separation into trainin- and testing sets which may result in less generalisability as well as the shorter follow-up period that was considered to define progression to AD.

Some studies have also combined different biomarkers (CSF, MRI, PET) with the idea of measuring different aspects of AD pathology and thus improve the classification accuracy. Hinrichs et al. [14] improved their HC/AD classification CCR by a few % units to 81 by combining MRI and PET. Eckerström et al. [16] studied the separation of a unified HC/S-MCI group from P-MCI group with CSF proteins and manual hippocampal volumes. They found CSF to be superior to MRI (SEN/SPE of 95/79 vs 86/66) while the combination performed best (SEN/SPE 90/91). However, it should be noted that the study sample in that particular study was small (a total of 68 subjects) and neither cross-validation or separate training/testing sets were used in order to ensure good generalizability of the results. In Kohannim et al. [17], the improvement from using multiple biomarkers was not significant and Davatzikos et al. [15] reported marginal improvements which, however, may be related to the fact that results with only one biomarker were not very good to begin with.

Considering solely the classification accuracies of the present study and those reported in literature, it seems questionable if the collection of several biomarkers is worth the effort and resource. A combination of different features extracted from a single MRI seems to provide results that are comparable or better than those obtained with other or multiple biomarkers. In a clinical point of view, this is interesting since it means that a single MRI scan provides not only aid to differential diagnostics of cognitive impairment, but also reliably describes a persons phase in the HC/AD continuum. MRI is also widely available, non-invasive and often useful in the differential diagnostics of memory problems thus making it a compelling option as the first biomarker that would be obtained from a patient with mild memory problems. However, a comprehensive differential diagnostics between AD and non-AD cognitive impairments will still require assessment of various different biomarkers. Also, it should be noted that the computational techniques used in this paper are not widely available in the clinical environment and thus limit their usage in the clinical work at present.

Strengths of the presented study are i) the use of multiple features extracted from one imaging modality, ii) large groups, iii) rigorous validation process of the results using cross-validation, and iv) results comparable or better than the ones published so far.

Our study has also some limitations that should be mentioned. The results are obtained from a single (although collected from multiple sites) cohort and should be also validated in other cohorts. A longer clinical follow-up time would be needed to see if the classification results of S-MCI/P-MCI experiment changed when more of the MCI subjects converted to AD. Furthermore, the ADNI study does not provide postmortem pathological confirmation of the clinical status. With this limitation, individual subjects might be wrongly categorized. Although a rigorous validation process was used, optimally we need to establish standardized cut-offs that would be well generalizable to other cohorts outside ADNI. That is, however, beyond the possibilities of this study and will require vast standardization and validation procedures. Also, the CTH pipeline had problems especially with severely atrophied brains or MRI scans with poor image quality. A more robust pipeline would be desirable in order to guarantee a more reliable feature extraction.

Supporting Information

Appendix S1   The Alzheimer's Disease Neuroimaging Initiative. (DOCX)

Appendix S2   ROI-wise features for CTH and TBM. (DOCX)

Acknowledgments

Data used in the preparation of this article were obtained from the ADNI database (www.loni.ucla.edu/ADNI). As such, the investigators within the ADNI contributed to the design and implementation of ADNI and/or provided data but did not participate in analysis or writing of this report. ADNI investigators include (complete listing available at http://adni.loni. ucla.edu/wp-content/uploads/how_to_apply/ADNI_Authorship_List. pdf).

Author Contributions

Conceived and designed the experiments: RW VJ JK DR HS JL. Performed the experiments: RW VJ JK EN DPZ. Analyzed the data: RW VJ JK. Contributed reagents/materials/analysis tools: RW JK DR JL. Wrote the paper: RW VJ.

References

1. Brookmeyer R, Johnson E, Ziegler-Graham K, Arrighi HM (2007) Forecasting the global burden of Alzheimer's disease. Alzheimer's and Dementia 3: 186–191.
2. Cummings J, Doody R, Clark C (2007) Disease-modifying therapies for alzheimer disease: challenges to early intervention. Neurology 69: 1622–1634.
3. Petersen R (2001) Practice parameter: early detection of dementia: mild cognitive impairment (an evidence-based review). Neurology 56: 1133.
4. Gauthier S, Reisberg B, Zaudig M, Petersen R, Ritchie K, et al. (2006) Mild cognitive impairment. Lancet 367: 1262–1270.
5. Braak H, Braak E (1991) Neuropathological stageing of Alzheimer-related changes. Acta Neuropathologica 82: 239–259.
6. Wenk G (2003) Neuropathologic changes in alzheimer's disease. Journal of Clinical Psychiatry 64 Suppl 9.
7. Hampel H, Brger K, Teipel SJ, Bokde AL, Zetterberg H, et al. (2008) Core candidate neurochemical and imaging biomarkers of alzheimer's disease. Alzheimer's and Dementia 4: 38–48.
8. Hyman BT, Marzloff K, Arriagada PV (1993) The lack of accumulation of senile plaques or amyloid burden in Alzheimer's disease suggests a dynamic balance between amyloid deposition and resolution. J Neuropathol Exp Neurol 52: 594–600.
9. Gmez-Isla T, Hollister R, West H, Mui S, Growdon J, et al. (1997) Neuronal loss correlates with but exceeds neurofibrillary tangles in alzheimer's disease. Ann Neurol 41: 17–24.
10. Ingelsson M, Fukumoto H, Newell KL, Growdon JH, Hedley-Whyte ET, et al. (2004) Early abeta accumulation and progressive synaptic loss, gliosis, and tangle formation in ad brain. Neurology 62: 925–31.
11. Jack C, Jr., Knopman D, Jagust W, Shaw L, Aisen P, et al. (2010) Hypothetical model of dynamic biomarkers of the alzheimer's pathological cascade. Lancet Neurology 27: 685–691.
12. Hampel H, Frank R, Broich K, Teipel S, Katz J, abd Hardy RG, et al. (2010) Biomarkers for alzheimer's disease: academic, industry and regulatory perspectives. NatRevDrug Discov 9: 560–574.
13. Fan Y, Resnick SM, Wu X, Davatzikos C (2008) Structural and functional biomarkers of prodromal alzheimer's disease: A high-dimensional pattern classification study. NeuroImage 41: 277–285.
14. Hinrichs C, Singh V, Xu G, Johnson S (2009) Mkl for robust multi-modality ad classification. In: MICCAI (II) Springer, volume 5762 of Lecture Notes in Computer Science. pp 786–794.
15. Davatzikos C, Bhatt P, Shaw LM, Batmanghelich KN, Trojanowski JQ (2010) Prediction of MCI to AD conversion, via MRI, CSF biomarkers, and pattern classification. Neurobiology of Aging In Press, Corrected Proof: -.
16. Eckerstrom C, Andreasson U, Olsson E, Rolstad S, Blennow K, et al. (2010) Combination of hippocampal volume and cerebrospinal uid biomarkers improves predictive value in mild cognitive impairment. Dement Geriatr Cogn Disord 29: 294–300.
17. Kohannim O, Hua X, Hibar DP, Lee S, Chou YY, et al. (2010) Boosting power for clinical trials using classifiers based on multiple biomarkers. Neurobiology of Aging 31: 1429–1442.
18. Landau S, Harvey D, Madison C, Reiman E, Foster N, et al. (2010) Comparing predictors of conversion and decline in mild cognitive impairment. Neurology 75: 230–8.
19. Walhovd KB, Fjell AM, Brewer J, McEvoy LK, Fennema-Notestine C, et al. (2010) Combining MR Imaging, Positron-Emission Tomography, and CSF Biomarkers in the Diagnosis and Prognosis of Alzheimer Disease. American Journal of Neuroradiology 31: 347–354+.
20. Wolz R, Aljabar P, Hajnal JV, Lotjonen J, Rueckert D (2011) Manifold learning combining imaging with non-imaging information. In: IEEE International Symposium on Biomedical Imaging. pp 960–963.
21. Chupin M, Hammers A, Liu R, Colliot O, Burdett J, et al. (2009) Automatic segmentation of the hippocampus and the amygdala driven by hybrid constraints: Method and validation. NeuroImage 46: 749–761.
22. Devanand DP, Pradhaban G, Liu X, Khandji A, De Santi S, et al. (2007) Hippocampal and entorhinal atrophy in mild cognitive impairment - Prediction of Alzheimer disease. Neurology 68: 828–836+.
23. Gerardin E, Chetelat G, Chupin M, Cuingnet R, Desgranges B, et al. (2009) Multidimensional classification of hippocampal shape features discriminates Alzheimer's disease and mild cognitive impairment from normal aging. NeuroImage 47: 1476–1486.
24. Liu Y, Paajanen T, Zhang Y, Westman E, Wahlund LO, et al. (2009) Combination analysis of neuropsychological tests and structural MRI measures in differentiating AD, MCI and control groups–The AddNeuroMed study. Neurobiology of Aging In Press, Corrected Proof: -.
25. Liu Y, Paajanen T, Zhang Y, Westman E, Wahlund LO, et al. (2010) Analysis of regional MRI volumes and thicknesses as predictors of conversion from mild cognitive impairment to Alzheimer's disease. Neurobiology of Aging 31: 1375–1385.
26. McEvoy L, Fennema-Notestine C, JC R, Hagler D, Holland D, et al. (2009) Alzheimer disease: quantitative structural neuroimaging for detection and prediction of clinical and structural changes in mild cognitive impairment. Radiology 251: 1950–205.
27. Querbes O, Aubry F, Pariente J, Lotterie JA, Dmonet JF, et al. (2009) Early diagnosis of alzheimer's disease using cortical thickness: impact of cognitive reserve. Brain 132: 2036–2047.
28. Mueller SG, Weiner MW, Thal LJ, Petersen RC, Jack C, et al. (2005) The Alzheimer's Disease Neuroimaging Initiative. Neuroimaging Clinics of North America 15: 869–877.
29. Cuingnet R, Gerardin E, Tessieras J, Auzias G, Lehricy S, et al. (2010) Automatic classification of patients with Alzheimer's disease from structural MRI: A comparison of ten methods using the ADNI database. NeuroImage In Press, Corrected Proof: -.
30. Petersen RC, Aisen PS, Beckett LA, Donohue MC, Gamst AC, et al. (2010) Alzheimer's Disease Neuroimaging Initiative (ADNI): clinical characterization. Neurology 74: 201–209.
31. Folstein MF, Folstein SE, McHugh PR (1975) Mini-mental state: A practical method for grading the cognitive state of patients for the clinician. Journal of Psychiatric Research 12(3): 189–198.
32. Morris J (1993) The Clinical Dementia Rating (CDR): current version and scoring rules. Neurology 43: 2412–2414.
33. McKhann G, Drachman D, Folstein M, Katzman R, Price D, et al. (1984) Clinical diagnosis of alzheimer's disease: report of the nincds-adrda work group under the auspices of department of health and human services task force on alzheimer's disease. Neurology 34: 939–944.
34. Jack CR, Jr., Bernstein M, Fox NC, Thompson P, Alexander G, et al. (2008) The Alzheimer's disease neuroimaging initiative (ADNI): MRI methods. Journal of Magnetic Resonance Imaging 27: 685–691.
35. Lotjonen JM, Wolz R, Koikkalainen JR, Thurfjell L, Waldemar G, et al. (2010) Fast and robust multi-atlas segmentation of brain magnetic resonance images. NeuroImage 49: 2352–2365.
36. Lotjonen J, Wolz R, Koikkalainen J, Julkunen V, Thurfjell L, et al. (2011) Fast and robust extraction of hippocampus from mr images for diagnostics of alzheimer's disease. NeuroImage 56: 185–196.
37. Van Leemput K, Maes F, Vandermeulen D, Suetens P (1999) Automated model-based tissue classification of MR images of the brain. IEEE Transactions on Medical Imaging 18: 897–908.
38. Lerch J, Evans A (2005) Cortical thickness analysis examined through power analysis and a population simulation. NeuroImage 24: 163–173.
39. Mazziotta J, Toga A, Evans A, Fox P, Lancaster J, et al. (2001) A probabilistic atlas and reference system for the human brain: International Consortium for Brain Mapping (ICBM). Philos Trans R Soc Lond B Biol Sci 356: 1293–1322.
40. Sled JG, Zijdenbos AP, Evans AC (1998) A nonparametric method for automatic correction of intensity nonuniformity in MRI data. IEEE Transactions on Medical Imaging 17: 87–97.
41. Smith SM (2002) Fast robust automated brain extraction. Hum Brain Mapp 17: 143–155.
42. Zijdenbos AP, Forghani R, Evans AC (1998) Automatic quantification of MS lesions in 3D MRI brain data sets: Validation of INSECT. In: III WMW, Colchester ACF, Delp SL, eds. MICCAI Springer, volume 1496 of Lecture Notes in Computer Science. pp 439–448.
43. Tohka J, Zijdenbos A, Evans A (2004) Fast and robust parameter estimation for statistical partial volume models in brain mri. NeuroImage 23: 84–97.
44. Kim JS, Singh V, Lee JK, Lerch J, Ad-Dab'bagh Y, et al. (2005) Automated 3-d extraction and evaluation of the inner and outer cortical surfaces using a laplacian map and partial volume effect classification. NeuroImage 27: 210–221.
45. Chung M, Taylor J (2004) Diffusion smoothing on brain surface via finite element method. In: ISBI IEEE. pp 432–435.

46. Brun CC, Lepor N, Pennec X, Lee AD, Barysheva M, et al. (2009) Mapping the regional inuence of genetics on brain structure variability – a tensor-based morphometry study. NeuroImage 48: 37–49.

47. Koikkalainen J, Lotjonen J, Thurfjell L, Rueckert D, Waldemar G, et al. (2011) Multi-template tensor-based morphometry: Application to analysis of alzheimer's disease. NeuroImage 56: 1134–1144.

48. Belkin M, Niyogi P (2003) Laplacian eigenmaps for dimensionality reduction and data representation. Neural Computation 15: 1373–1396.

49. Rueckert D, Sonoda LI, Hayes C, Hill DLG, Leach MO, et al. (1999) Nonrigid registration using free-form deformations: Application to breast MR images. IEEE Transactions on Medical Imaging 18: 712–721.

50. Wolz R, Heckemann RA, Aljabar P, Hajnal JV, Hammers A, et al. (2010) Measurement of hippocampal atrophy using 4D graph-cut segmentation: Application to ADNI. NeuroImage 52: 1009–1018.

51. Draper NR, Smith H (1998) Applied Regression Analysis (Wiley Series in Probability and Statistics). Wiley.

52. Krzanowski WJ (1988) Principles of Multivariate Analysis: A User's Perspective Oxford University Press.

53. Cortes C, Vapnik V (1995) Support-vector networks. Machine Learning 20: 273–297.

54. Vemuri P, Gunter JL, Senjem ML, Whitwell JL, Kantarci K, et al. (2008) Alzheimer's disease diagnosis in individual subjects using structural mr images: Validation studies. NeuroImage 39: 1186–1197.

55. Westman E, Simmons A, Zhang Y, Muehlboeck JS, Tunnard C, et al. (2011) Multivariate analysis of mri data for alzheimer's disease, mild cognitive impairment and healthy controls. NeuroImage 54: 1178–1187.

CSF and Brain Structural Imaging Markers of the Alzheimer's Pathological Cascade

Xianfeng Yang[1], Ming Zhen Tan[1], Anqi Qiu[1,2,3]*

1 Department of Bioengineering, National University of Singapore, Singapore, Singapore, **2** Singapore Institute for Clinical Sciences, the Agency for Science, Technology and Research, Singapore, Singapore, **3** Clinical Imaging Research Center, National University of Singapore, Singapore, Singapore

Abstract

Cerebral spinal fluid (CSF) and structural imaging markers are suggested as biomarkers amended to existing diagnostic criteria of mild cognitive impairment (MCI) and Alzheimer's disease (AD). But there is no clear instruction on which markers should be used at which stage of dementia. This study aimed to first investigate associations of the CSF markers as well as volumes and shapes of the hippocampus and lateral ventricles with MCI and AD at the baseline and secondly apply these baseline markers to predict MCI conversion in a two-year time using the Alzheimer's Disease Neuroimaging Initiative (ADNI) cohort. Our results suggested that the CSF markers, including Aβ42, t-tau, and p-tau, distinguished MCI or AD from NC, while the Aβ42 CSF marker contributed to the differentiation between MCI and AD. The hippocampal shapes performed better than the hippocampal volumes in classifying NC and MCI, NC and AD, as well as MCI and AD. Interestingly, the ventricular volumes were better than the ventricular shapes to distinguish MCI or AD from NC, while the ventricular shapes showed better accuracy than the ventricular volumes in classifying MCI and AD. As the CSF markers and the structural markers are complementary, the combination of them showed great improvements in the classification accuracies of MCI and AD. Moreover, the combination of these markers showed high sensitivity but low specificity for predicting conversion from MCI to AD in two years. Hence, it is feasible to employ a cross-sectional sample to investigate dynamic associations of the CSF and imaging markers with MCI and AD and to predict future MCI conversion. In particular, the volumetric information may be good for the early stage of AD, while morphological shapes should be considered as markers in the prediction of MCI conversion to AD together with the CSF markers.

Citation: Yang X, Tan MZ, Qiu A (2012) CSF and Brain Structural Imaging Markers of the Alzheimer's Pathological Cascade. PLoS ONE 7(12): e47406. doi:10.1371/journal.pone.0047406

Editor: Yong Fan, Institution of Automation, CAS, China

Received April 13, 2012; **Accepted** September 13, 2012; **Published** December 19, 2012

Funding: The work was supported by grants: a centre grant from the National Medical Research Council (NMRC/CG/NUHS/2010), the Young Investigator Award at the National University of Singapore (NUSYIA FY10 P07), and the National University of Singapore MOE AcRF Tier 1. The funders had no role in study design, data collection and analysis, decision to publish, or preparation of the manuscript.

Competing Interests: The authors have declared that no competing interests exist.

* E-mail: bieqa@nus.edu.sg

Introduction

Cerebral spinal fluid (CSF) and imaging markers have been suggested as biomarkers to augment existing diagnostic criteria of both mild cognitive impairment (MCI) and Alzheimer's disease (AD) [1,2,3,4,5,6]. Jack et al. [7] proposed a possible hypothetical model in which biomarkers were temporally arranged in order of abnormality along the pathological cascade of AD. In this model, abnormal CSF Aβ42 could occur two decades before the first dementia-related symptoms, reaching a plateau prior any manifestation of cognitive impairment. In comparison to trajectories of CSF tau, magnetic resonance imaging (MRI) markers surfaced much later and were well correlated with the severity of AD symptoms. However, this hypothetical model was directly derived from longitudinal studies, where statistical inferences were founded primarily on the rate of change of AD-related biomarkers over time. For instance, increased rates of ventricular expansion and brain atrophy in the medial temporal lobe were found to be significantly correlated with cognitive decline, with good predictions for MCI to AD conversion [8] [9] [10].

Beyond simple volumetric measures, morphological shape of the brain captures not only the degree of tissue loss but also its precise anatomical location. As such, brain shape measures have since

been suggested as improved predictors for MCI conversion to AD. For instance, changes of hippocampal shapes between baseline and a 2-year follow-up predicted MCI-AD conversion up to 80% accuracy [11,12]. Unfortunately, to date, no clear, authoritative instruction on which structural MRI measures are to be associated with MCI and AD is available. This could be, partly, a result of the extensive variety of image analysis techniques available. In addition, while recent studies [13,14] have tested the feasibility of baseline structural volumes and CSF in predicting conversion from MCI to AD, performance of baseline structural shapes with CSF markers for MCI-AD conversion remains relatively unknown.

In this paper, we first evaluated the hypothetical model suggested by Jack et al. [7] through a cross-sectional study on the Alzheimer's Disease Neuroimaging Initiative (ADNI) cohort. For this, we employed a supervised, multivariate classification method, support vector machine (SVM), to distinguish MCI and AD from normal aging. Features used include CSF biomarkers and the shapes and volumes of hippocampus and lateral ventricles. The hippocampi and lateral ventricles were chosen for their well-validated status as prominent hallmarks of AD [8,15,16,17,18,19,20]. Subsequently, we aim to predict MCI conversion to AD over a two-year follow-up period using baseline

CSF and MRI measures. In particular, both volumetric and shape analyses were applied to compare their sensitivity and specificity in the prediction of MCI conversion to AD.

Methods

The ADNI was launched in 2003 by the National Institute on Aging (NIA), the National Institute of Biomedical Imaging and Bioengineering (NIBIB), the Food and Drug Administration [21], private pharmaceutical companies and non-profit organizations, as a $60 million, 5-year public–private partnership. The primary goal of ADNI has been to test whether serial MRI, PET, other biological markers, and clinical and neuropsychological assessments can be combined to measure the progression of MCI and early AD. Determination of sensitive and specific markers of very early AD progression is intended to aid researchers and clinicians to develop new treatments and monitor their effectiveness, as well as lessen the time and cost of clinical trials.

ADNI is the result of efforts of many coinvestigators from a broad range of academic institutions and private corporations, and subjects have been recruited from over 50 sites across the U.S. and Canada. The initial goal of ADNI was to recruit 800 adults, ages 55 to 90, to participate in the research — approximately 200 cognitively normal older individuals to be followed for 3 years, 400 people with MCI to be followed for 3 years, and 200 people with early AD to be followed for 2 years (see www.adni-info.org for up-to-date information). The data were analyzed anonymously, using publicly available secondary data from the ADNI study, therefore no ethics statement is required for this work.

Subjects

The ADNI general eligibility criteria are described at www.adni-info.org. Briefly, subjects are between 55–90 years of age, having a study partner able to provide an independent evaluation of functioning. Specific psychoactive medications will be excluded. General inclusion/exclusion criteria are as follows: 1) healthy subjects: Mini-Mental State Examination (MMSE) scores between 24–30, a Clinical Dementia Rating (CDR) of 0, non-depressed, non-MCI, and nondemented; 2) MCI subjects: MMSE scores between 24–30, a memory complaint, having objective memory loss measured by education adjusted scores on Wechsler Memory Scale Logical Memory II, a CDR of 0.5, absence of significant levels of impairment in other cognitive domains, essentially preserved activities of daily living, and an absence of dementia; and 3) mild AD: MMSE scores between 20–26, CDR of 0.5 or 1.0, and meets the National Institute of Neurological and Communicative Disorders and Stroke and the Alzheimer's Disease and Related Disorders Association (NINCDS/ADRDA) criteria for probable AD.

In this study, 383 subjects were chosen from our previous study [22]. Within this group, 218 have both MRI and CSF baseline data (age: 74.4±7.2 years), with 72 normal controls (NC), 35 AD subjects, and 111 MCI patients. Amongst these 383 subjects, 25 subjects with MCI converted to AD within 24 months.

Structural MR scans were collected across a variety of scanners with protocols individualized for each scanner, as defined at www.loni.ucla.edu/ADNI/Research/Cores/index.shtml. The CSF Aβ42, t-tau and p-tau data were downloaded from the ADNI web site (www.loni.ucla.edu/ADNI).

MRI analysis

Figure 1 illustrates the MRI data processing that is detailed below.

Structural Delineation. We automatically delineated the hippocampus (HC) and lateral ventricles (LV) from the intensity inhomogeneity corrected T1-weighted MR images using Free-Surfer [23]. Due to the lack of constraints on structural shapes, this process introduced irregularities and topological errors (e.g. holes) at the hippocampal and ventricular boundary. This would increase shape variation and thus reduces statistical power to detect group differences. To avoid this pitfall, we generated the hippocampal or ventricular shape of each individual subject with the properties of smoothness and correct topology by injecting an atlas shape into them using the large deformation diffeomorphic metric image mapping algorithm [24]. The hippocampal and lateral ventricular atlas shapes were created from 41 manually labeled hippocampi and lateral ventricles via a large deformation diffeomorphic atlas generation algorithm [25]. Each hippocampal (or lateral ventricular) volume was approximated by the transformed atlas through the LDDMM transformation. The reader is referred to [26] for the mathematical derivation of this atlas injection procedure and its evaluation as well as the segmentation accuracy on the hippocampus and lateral ventricles. This delineation approach has been successfully applied to investigate the hippocampus and other subcortical shapes in AD [22].

We constructed the surface representation of the hippocampus and lateral ventricles by composing the LDDMM transformation on the corresponding atlas surfaces [27]. The left and right hippocampal surfaces were respectively constructed using 2364 triangles with 1184 vertices and 2458 triangles with 1231 vertices, while the left and right lateral ventricular surfaces were respectively composed of 6966 triangles with 3485 vertices and 7890 triangles with 3947 vertices. The average triangle area and edge length of the hippocampal surfaces were respectively 0.59 mm^2 and 1.2 mm, while those of the ventricular surfaces were respectively 0.64 mm^2 and 1.1 mm. Hence, the size of the triangles was comparable to the image resolution (1 mm^3).

ISOMAP Shape Embedding. Unlike the scalar volume measure, structural shapes lie on a high dimensional space, which makes it challenging for statistical inference. In this study, we employed ISOMAP [28] to embed the shapes of the hippocampus and lateral ventricles into a Euclidean space with a few dimensions such that this low-dimensional embedding is quasi-isometric to the shapes in the high dimensional space. For this, we first computed diffeomorphic metric distances between any two shapes using their first order approximation described in [29] and constructed a pairwise distance matrix. ISOMAP then found a Euclidean low-dimensional representation of the shapes that preserved the relationship of any two shapes described in the pair-wise distance matrix. These Euclidean coordinates were obtained by finding eigenvectors corresponding to the largest eigenvalues of the kernel matrix stemmed from the distance matrix reshaped by a centering matrix [28]. The dimension of the eigenvectors is the same as the number of subjects, and each eigenvector is one component or one dimension of the ISOMAP shape embedding. Using this approach with all 383 subjects, the bilateral hippocampal shapes can be characterized using the first 20 ISOMAP components whose Euclidean distance matrix is highly correlated with the pair-wise metric distance matrix generated using the first order approximation of the diffeomorphic metric (Pearson's Correlation: r = 0.91). The bilateral lateral ventricular shapes can be represented using the first 20 ISOMAP components whose Euclidean distance matrix is very much similar to the pair-wise metric distance matrix (Pearson's Correlation: r = 0.97).

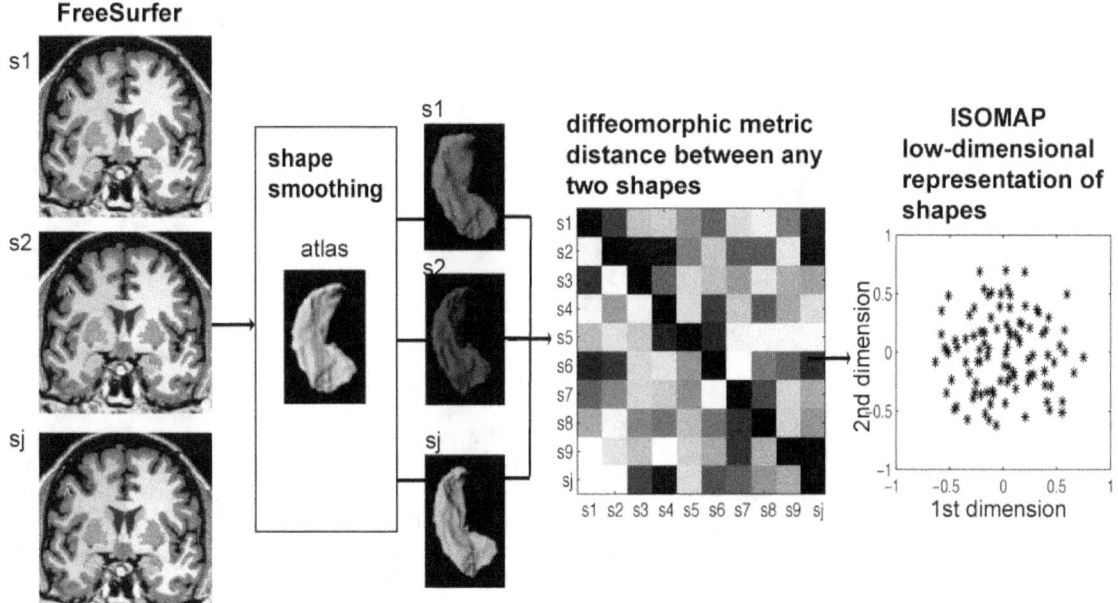

Figure 1. Schematic of MRI data processing.
doi:10.1371/journal.pone.0047406.g001

Statistical Analysis

A linear support vector machine (SVM) [30] was employed to identify diagnosis of subjects from any two groups (NC, MCI, and AD). The SVM classifier seeks the optimal decision boundary that has a maximal margin closest to the training samples such that generalization error bound can be minimized. Hence, the SVM classifier is robust to outliers. In our study, we independently and jointly considered volumes (or shapes) of the hippocampus, lateral ventricles and CSF markers as the SVM input features to identify subjects with MCI and AD from NC and MCI from AD. Shape features comprise only of ISOMAP components with significant group differences based on Student t-tests.

Our study had fewer AD subjects as compared to the NC or MCI groups. To resolve any influences of unequal sample sizes among the NC, MCI, and AD groups on the classification accuracy, we employed random sampling to reduce the number of NC and MCI subjects such that all three groups have equal sample sizes. This was repeated for 100 times. For each trial, leave-one-out cross-validation was adopted to estimate the classification accuracy. The confidence interval of the classification accuracy was computed.

Moreover, we also applied the SVM to test the sensitivity and specificity for predicting MCI conversion in a two-year time window when volumes (or shapes) of the hippocampus and lateral ventricles as well as CSF markers assessed at the baseline were independently or jointly considered as features in the SVM.

Results

Demographic Information

Demographic information for different diagnosis groups at baseline are shown in **Table 1**. No significant differences in age were found among the NC, MCI, and AD groups (ANOVA, $p = 0.454$). 25 out of 111 MCI subjects were diagnosed as AD at the two-year follow up and were denoted as the MCI-c group. Rest of the MCI subjects were placed in the MCI-s group. No significant MMSE difference was found between the two MCI groups at baseline ($p = 0.10$).

Markers at Stages of MCI an AD

Hippocampal volume and shape markers. Bilateral hippocampal volumes distinguished MCI and AD subjects from normal controls at an accuracy of 61.9% and 65.5% respectively, with relatively high specificity (MCI: 66.1%; AD: 73.3%) but low sensitivity (MCI: 57.7%; AD: 57.8%) (**Table 2**). However, the hippocampal volumes lost statistical power in the separation of subjects with MCI and AD (classification accuracy: 42.3%; sensitivity: 45.3%; specificity: 39.2%, **Table 2**).

In shape analysis, the first 20 ISOMAP components characterized bilateral hippocampal shapes among all 383 subjects. The 1st, 2nd, 3rd, 4th, 9th, 13th, 18th components contributed to hippocampal shape differences between NC and AD. Among these components, most of them (the 1st, 2nd, 3rd, 7th, 13th) also contributed to shape differences between NC and MCI (**Table 3**). Interestingly, only the 4th and 9th components showed shape differences between MCI and AD. Moreover, among these ISOMAP components, the 1st and 2nd components were highly correlated with the hippocampal volume (Pearson correlations: $r = 0.7$, $p < 0.01$ for the 1st component; $r = 0.5$, $p < 0.01$ for the 2nd component), which were dominant components for group differences in hippocampal shapes between NC and MCI. This is illustrated as relatively homogeneous shrinkage over the bilateral hippocampi in **Figure 2 (a,b)**. But the 4th and 9th components were not associated with the hippocampal volume ($p > 0.05$), suggesting that only local hippocampal shapes contributed to the difference between MCI and AD, as seen in **Figure 2 (c,d)**. This can be further supported by evidence of increased classification accuracy rates for the classifications between NC and AD (79.2%), NC and MCI (67.4%), and MCI and AD (57.2%) (**Table 2**) when the ISOMAP embedding of hippocampal shapes were used in the SVM classifiers.

Lateral ventricular volume and shape markers. The volumes of bilateral lateral ventricles distinguished subjects with MCI and AD from normal controls at the accuracy of 63.1% and 65.5% respectively, with relatively high specificity (MCI: 75.3%; AD: 72.3%) but low sensitivity (MCI: 50.9%; AD: 58.8%) (**Table 2**). However, volumes of the lateral ventricles lost statistical

Table 1. Demographic information for each of the diagnosis groups (normal controls (NC), mild cognitive impairment (MCI), and Alzheimer's disease (AD)) at the baseline.

Group	Subjects *n*	Age (mean±SD)	Gender (female/male)	MMSE (mean±SD)
NC	72	75.2±5.2	35/37	29±1
MCI-s	86	74±7.7	28/58	26.7±1.8
MCI-c	25	73.5±6.9	6/19	26.1±1.5
AD	35	74.6±9.3	15/20	22.9±1.8

Note: SD – standard deviation; MMSE – mini-mental state examination; MCI-s – subjects with MCI who remained as MCI at the two-year follow up; MCI-c – subjects with MCI who converted as AD at the two-year follow up.
doi:10.1371/journal.pone.0047406.t001

power in separating subjects with MCI and AD (classification accuracy: 30.4%; sensitivity: 21.2%; specificity: 39.7%, **Table 2**).

In shape analysis, the first 20 ISOMAP components characterized bilateral lateral ventricular shapes among all 383 subjects. The 1st, 7th, 8th, 9th, 17th, 19th components contributed to hippocampal shape differences between NC and AD. Among these components, several of them (the 1st, 8th) also contributed to shape differences between NC and MCI (**Table 3**). Interestingly, only the 9th, 13th, and 17th components showed the shape differences between MCI and AD. Moreover, among these ISOMAP components, the 1st component was highly correlated with the ventricular volume (Pearson correlations: r = 0.98, p<0.01), though it was not the only component contributing to shape differences between NC and MCI, as illustrated in **Figure 3 (a,b)**. However, the 9th, 13th, and 17th components were not associated with the lateral ventricular volume (p>0.05), suggesting that only local ventricular shapes contributed to the difference between MCI and AD. This can also be seen in **Figure 3 (c,d)**. Unlike the hippocampus, the lateral ventricular shapes did not lead to better classification accuracy rates between NC and AD

(61.5%), and between NC and MCI (59%) when compared with the lateral ventricular volumes (see **Table 2**). However, the ventricular shapes achieved markedly better accuracy in distinguishing MCI and AD (60.1%) (**Table 2**).

CSF Markers. Student's *t*-tests revealed that all three CSF markers, Aβ42, t-tau, and p-tau, showed statistically significant differences between NC and AD and between NC and MCI (**Table 3**). However, only Aβ42 showed group differences between MCI and AD (**Table 3**). The SVM classification revealed that the CSF markers can distinguish NC and AD at the classification accuracy of 81.4%, higher than those based on the hippocampal or ventricular imaging markers (**Table 2**). Additionally, the CSF markers achieved similar accuracy in distinguishing NC and MCI, and MCI and AD subjects in comparison with hippocampal and ventricular shapes. Interestingly, the CSF markers gave higher sensitivities than the imaging markers (**Table 2**).

The combination of the Imaging and CSF Markers. Combining the CSF markers and the volumes of the hippocampus and lateral ventricles as features in the SVM

Table 2. The classification accuracy, sensitivity, and specificity of the support vector machine (SVM) classifiers are given for distinguishing normal controls (NC) and subjects with Alzheimer's disease (AD), NC and subjects with mild cognitive impairment (MCI), and subjects with MCI and AD.

	NC.vs. AD	NC.vs. MCI	MCI.vs. AD
Hippocampal Volumes and Shapes			
Hp volumes	65.5% (CI: 64.4%~66.6%) Sensitivity = 57.8%, Specificity = 73.3%	61.9% (CI: 61%~62.8%) Sensitivity = 57.7%, Specificity = 66.1%	42.3% (CI:32.2%~52.3%) Sensitivity = 45.3%, Specificity = 39.2%
Hp shapes	79.2% (CI: 78.5%~80%) Sensitivity = 75.8%, Specificity = 82.8%	67.4% (CI: 66.2%~68.6%) Sensitivity = 64%, Specificity = 70.8%	57.2% (CI: 51.7%~62.8%) Sensitivity = 59.9%, Specificity = 54.5%
Lateral Ventricular Volumes and Shapes			
LV volumes	65.5% (CI: 64.9%~66.1%) Sensitivity = 58.8% Specificity = 72.3%	63.1% (CI: 62%~64.2%) Sensitivity = 50.9%, Specificity = 75.3%	30.4% (CI: 18.8%~42%) Sensitivity = 21.2% Specificity = 39.7%
LV shapes	61.5% (CI: 59.2%~63.9%) Sensitivity = 59.2%, Specificity = 63.9%	59% (CI: 56.1%~62%) Sensitivity = 53.6%, Specificity = 64.4%	60.1% (CI:57.1%~63.1%) Sensitivity = 62%, Specificity = 58.3%
CSF			
CSF markers	81.4% (CI: 80.3%~82.5%) Sensitivity = 87.4%, Specificity = 74.9%	68.4% (CI: 67.8%~69%) Sensitivity = 66.7%, Specificity = 70.1%	61.3% (CI: 59.4%~63.2%) Sensitivity = 84.3%, specificity = 38.3%
Combination			
CSF, Hp volumes, LV volumes	85.4% (CI: 84.3%~86.5%) Sensitivity = 88.8%, Specificity = 82%	72% (CI: 70.5%~73.5%) Sensitivity = 70.1%, Specificity = 73.9%	60.9% (CI: 59.1%~62.8%) Sensitivity = 80.4%, Specificity = 41.4%
CSF, Hp shapes, LV shapes	92.2% (CI: 91%~93.5%) Sensitivity = 94.7%, Specificity = 89.8%	70.3% (CI: 68.6%~72.9%) Sensitivity = 69.5%, specificity = 71.9%	69.6% (CI: 66.4%~72.8%) Sensitivity = 70.7%, Specificity = 68.6%

The volumes and shapes of the hippocampus (Hp) and lateral ventricles (LV) as well as cerebral spinal fluid (CSF) markers are respectively used as features in the SVM.
doi:10.1371/journal.pone.0047406.t002

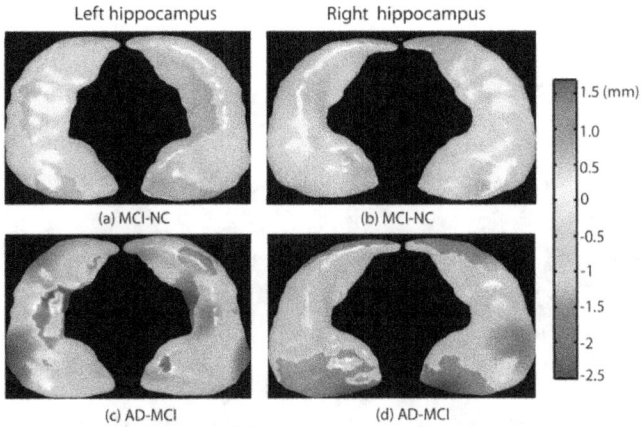

Figure 2. Hippocampal shape differences among normal controls (NC), mild cognitive impairment (MCI), and Alzheimer's Disease (AD). Panels (a,b) respectively show group differences in the left and right hippocampal surface deformations between MCI and NC. Panels (c,d) respectively show group differences in the left and right hippocampal surface deformations between AD and MCI. Warm color denotes regions where structures have surface outward-deformation in the former group when compared with the latter group, while cool color denotes regions where structures have surface inward-deformation in the former group when compared with the latter group.
doi:10.1371/journal.pone.0047406.g002

increased the classification accuracies between NC and AD (85.4%) and between NC and MCI (72%) when compared to those achieved using only one type of markers (see **Table 2**). Nevertheless, there was no improvement on the classification accuracy between MCI and AD when compared with that using the CSF markers alone.

Combining the CSF markers and the shapes of the hippocampus and lateral ventricles as features in the SVM increased the classification accuracies between NC and AD (92.2%), between NC and MCI (70.3%), and between MCI and AD (69.6%) when compared to those achieved using only one type of the markers (see Table 2).

Shapes of the two structures with the CSF markers performed better in separating NC and MCI ($p<0.001$) or NC and AD ($p<0.001$) when compared to features combining the volumes and CSF markers. However, shapes of the two structures with the CSF markers performed worse in separating NC and MCI when compared to features combining the volumes and CSF markers ($p = 0.013$).

Prediction of the MCI Conversion

To predict MCI conversion at a two-year follow-up, we trained an NC and AD classifier using the CSF and imaging markers before applying it to the 25 MCI converters and 86 MCI non-converters. Again, combination of the CSF markers with the hippocampus and lateral ventricles shapes at baseline showed the best prediction (66.7%) and sensitivity (82%) for identifying the MCI converters when compared to individual imaging or CSF markers (**Table 4**).

Discussion

Our study demonstrated the dynamic trajectories of the CSF, hippocampal and lateral ventricular markers in the Alzheimer's pathological cascade using a cross-sectional ADNI sample and also showed the feasibility of predicting future MCI-to-AD conversion using baseline CSF and imaging markers. The CSF markers, including Aβ42, t-tau, and p-tau, distinguished MCI or AD from NC, while only the Aβ42 CSF marker contributed to the differentiation between MCI and AD. The hippocampal shapes performed better than the hippocampal volumes in classifying NC and MCI, NC and AD, as well as MCI and AD. Interestingly, as compared to the ventricular shape, ventricular volume performed better in distinguishing MCI or AD from NC. The ventricular shape, however, showed better accuracy in the classification for MCI and AD. As the CSF and structural markers were complementary, their combination showed great improvement in the classification accuracies at all the stages of AD. Moreover, the combination of these baseline markers also showed high sensitivity but low specificity for predicting MCI conversion to AD during a two-year period.

Our findings supported the conclusion drawn in previous studies [31]; [32], where abnormality of both CSF Aβ42 and neurodegenerative biomarkers, including CSF tau and MRI markers, precedes clinical symptoms; all these markers showed significant differences between NC and MCI groups. However, our findings did not support the hypothesis where CSF Aβ42 reaches a plateau before the appearance of MRI atrophy and cognitive symptoms, and remain static thereafter [7]. In our study, CSF Aβ42 continued to show appreciable power discriminant between MCI and AD. In contrast, CSF tau lost its discriminating power in distinguishing MCI and AD patients, suggesting that CSF Aβ42 reaches its plateau after CSF tau in the Alzheimer's pathological cascade.

MCI and AD patients were not well-separated using hippocampal volume, implying that the overall tissue loss in the hippocampus may not be a good marker for monitoring AD progression. However, we may not conclude that the hippocampus

Table 3. ISOMAP components of the hippocampus and lateral ventricles as well as CSF markers contribute to the group differences between normal controls (NC) and subjects with Alzheimer's disease (AD), NC and subjects with mild cognitive impairment (MCI), and subjects with MCI and AD.

	NC.vs. AD	NC.vs. MCI	MCI vs AD
Imaging Markers			
	ISOMAP components	ISOMAP components	ISOMAP components
hippocampal shapes	1,2,3,4,9,13,18	1,2,3,7,13	4,9
lateral ventricular shapes	1,7,8,9,17,19	1,8,12,14	9, 13,17
CSF Markers			
CSF Aβ42, t-tau, p-tau	Aβ42, t-tau, p-tau	Aβ42, t-tau, p-tau	Aβ42

doi:10.1371/journal.pone.0047406.t003

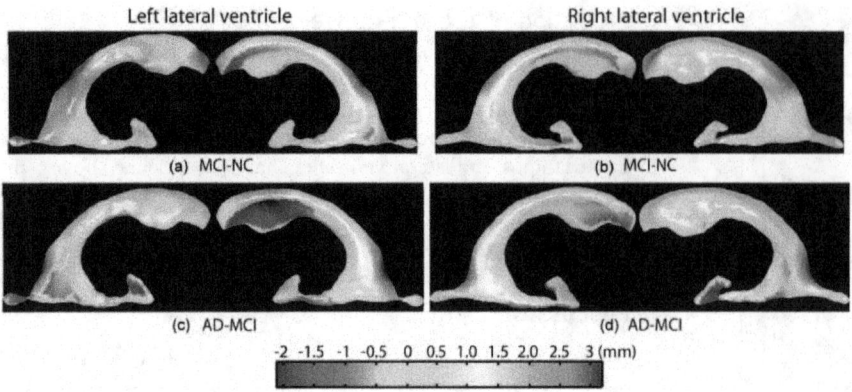

Left lateral ventricle   Right lateral ventricle

(a) MCI-NC   (b) MCI-NC

(c) AD-MCI   (d) AD-MCI

-2 -1.5 -1 -0.5 0 0.5 1.0 1.5 2.0 2.5 3 (mm)

Figure 3. Shape differences of the lateral ventricles among normal controls (NC), mild cognitive impairment (MCI), and Alzheimer's Disease (AD). Panels (a,b) respectively show group differences in the left and right lateral ventricular surface deformations between MCI and NC. Panels (c,d) respectively show group differences in the left and right lateral ventricular surface deformations between AD and MCI. Warm color denotes regions where structures have surface outward-deformation in the former group when compared with the latter group, while cool color denotes regions where structures have surface inward-deformation in the former group when compared with the latter group.
doi:10.1371/journal.pone.0047406.g003

reached its abnormality peak before the late stage of AD, as its local shape variations were significantly associated with progression from MCI to AD. Our results also showed that such local shape markers aided the hippocampal markers in achieving slightly better accuracy than the CSF markers in the prediction for MCI conversion to AD. This was also supported by previous studies, suggesting that MRI markers (e.g. cortical thickness of the medial temporal lobe) correlate well with severity of cognitive impairment and have greater predictive power than the CSF tau [33]. Based on these evidences, we may conclude that the hippocampal shape marker reaches its plateau after CSF tau. However, the order in which the CSF Aβ42 and MRI markers reach their abnormality peaks is still unclear based on our current study.

The volume of the lateral ventricles cannot distinguish MCI and AD patients. Interestingly, the overall expansion of the lateral ventricles showed better performance in identifying MCI or AD from NC when compared with their shapes. This result agrees with previous studies, suggesting that rates of ventricular expansion were significantly different between AD (or MCI) and NC groups [8]. This implies that complicated shape analysis might not always be necessary to provide better structural morphological

markers when compared to volumetric analysis. Even for the same structure, its markers can be different at different stages of AD. Again, we may not conclude that the lateral ventricles reached their abnormality peak before the late stage of AD, as their local shape variations were significantly associated with progression from MCI to AD. Likewise, ventricular shape markers slightly outperformed CSF markers in the prediction for MCI conversion to AD, as verified by previous studies [34], wherein clearer correlation was observed for ventricular volumes against worsening cognitive indices, as compared to CSF biomarkers.

Our study showed that the CSF and structural markers are complementary to each other in the AD pathological cascade. This suggests that the CSF markers, (Aβ42, t-tau, and p-tau) with the volumes of the hippocampus and lateral ventricles, is a good combination for distinguishing NC and MCI, while CSF Aβ42 marker with the shape of the hippocampus and lateral ventricles is a good combination for identifying MCI and AD.

As the shapes of the hippocampus and lateral ventricles contributed more to the difference between MCI and AD than their volumes, our study further showed that the combination of the CSF markers and the shapes of the two structures at baseline predicted MCI conversion to AD in the two-year follow up at an

Table 4. The accuracy, sensitivity, and specificity for predicting the MCI converters are listed when the volumes or shapes of the hippocampus (Hp) or the lateral ventricles (LV), or the CSF markers, or their combination were used as features in the classification.

Markers	Accuracy (95% CI)	Sensitivity	Specificity
Hippocampal volumes and Shapes			
Hp volumes	54%(53.1%~54.9%)	54.4%	53.6%
Hp shapes	63%(62.1%~64%)	74.9%	51.2%
Lateral Ventricular Volumes and Shapes			
LV volumes	55.6%(54.7%~56.5)	63.7%	47.5%
LV shapes	62.7%(61.5%~63.9%)	67.9%	57.5%
CSF			
CSF markers	62.2%(61.3%~63.1%)	80.4%	44%
Combination			
CSF, Hp volumes, LV volumes	59.2%(58.3%~60%)	81.1%(80.5%~81.6%)	37.2%(35.6%~38.9%)
CSF, Hp shapes, LV shapes	66.7%(65.7%~67.8%)	82%(81.5%~82.6%)	51.4% (49.4%~53.3%)

doi:10.1371/journal.pone.0047406.t004

improved accuracy of 66.7%. Previous studies [35] achieved similar prediction accuracy (68.5%) for the MCI conversion within a three-year follow up, with suggestions claiming that multiple predictors, including the CSF markers, hippocampal volume, entorhinal cortex thickness, etc. would not perform better than a single predictor. This differs from the conclusion derived from our findings, possibly because structural shape measures contain more complementing features than structural volume measures. The combination of the shapes and CSF markers achieved high classification accuracy (92.2%) between NC and AD, improving by more than 10% over the CSF markers. This result is comparable to those previously reported where CSF, MRI and PET imaging markers were combined [36].

In summary, we conclude that it is feasible to employ a cross-sectional sample to investigate dynamic associations of the CSF and imaging markers with MCI and AD and to predict future MCI conversion to AD. In particular, volumetric information may be good for the early stages of AD while morphological shapes should be considered as markers in the prediction of MCI conversion to AD together with the CSF markers.

Acknowledgments

Data used in preparation of this article were obtained from the Alzheimer's Disease Neuroimaging Initiative (ADNI) database (adni.loni.ucla.edu). As such, the investigators within the ADNI contributed to the design and implementation of ADNI and/or provided data but did not participate in analysis or writing of this report. A complete listing of ADNI investigators can be found at: http://adni.loni.ucla.edu/wp-content/uploads/how_to_apply/ADNI_Acknowledgement_List.pdf.

Author Contributions

Conceived and designed the experiments: XY MZT AQ. Performed the experiments: XY MZT AQ. Analyzed the data: XY MZT AQ. Contributed reagents/materials/analysis tools: XY MZT AQ. Wrote the paper: XY MZT AQ.

References

1. Jack CR, Jr., Albert MS, Knopman DS, McKhann GM, Sperling RA, et al. (2011) Introduction to the recommendations from the National Institute on Aging-Alzheimer's Association workgroups on diagnostic guidelines for Alzheimer's disease. Alzheimers Dement 7: 257–262.

2. McKhann GM, Knopman DS, Chertkow H, Hyman BT, Jack CR, Jr., et al. (2011) The diagnosis of dementia due to Alzheimer's disease: recommendations from the National Institute on Aging-Alzheimer's Association workgroups on diagnostic guidelines for Alzheimer's disease. Alzheimers Dement 7: 263–269.

3. Albert MS, DeKosky ST, Dickson D, Dubois B, Feldman HH, et al. (2011) The diagnosis of mild cognitive impairment due to Alzheimer's disease: recommendations from the National Institute on Aging-Alzheimer's Association workgroups on diagnostic guidelines for Alzheimer's disease. Alzheimers Dement 7: 270–279.

4. Sperling RA, Aisen PS, Beckett LA, Bennett DA, Craft S, et al. (2011) Toward defining the preclinical stages of Alzheimer's disease: recommendations from the National Institute on Aging-Alzheimer's Association workgroups on diagnostic guidelines for Alzheimer's disease. Alzheimers Dement 7: 280–292.

5. Ferrarini L, Palm WM, Olofsen H, van der Landen R, van Buchem MA, et al. (2008) Ventricular shape biomarkers for Alzheimer's disease in clinical MR images. Magnetic resonance in medicine : official journal of the Society of Magnetic Resonance in Medicine/Society of Magnetic Resonance in Medicine 59: 260–267.

6. Ferrarini L, Frisoni GB, Pievani M, Reiber JH, Ganzola R, et al. (2009) Morphological hippocampal markers for automated detection of Alzheimer's disease and mild cognitive impairment converters in magnetic resonance images. Journal of Alzheimer's disease : JAD 17: 643–659.

7. Jack CR, Jr., Knopman DS, Jagust WJ, Shaw LM, Aisen PS, et al. (2010) Hypothetical model of dynamic biomarkers of the Alzheimer's pathological cascade. Lancet Neurol 9: 119–128.

8. Jack CR, Jr., Lowe VJ, Weigand SD, Wiste HJ, Senjem ML, et al. (2009) Serial PIB and MRI in normal, mild cognitive impairment and Alzheimer's disease: implications for sequence of pathological events in Alzheimer's disease. Brain 132: 1355–1365.

9. Davatzikos C, Bhatt P, Shaw LM, Batmanghelich KN, Trojanowski JQ (2011) Prediction of MCI to AD conversion, via MRI, CSF biomarkers, and pattern classification. Neurobiol Aging 32: 2322 e2319–2327.

10. Kantarci K, Weigand SD, Przybelski SA, Shiung MM, Whitwell JL, et al. (2009) Risk of dementia in MCI: combined effect of cerebrovascular disease, volumetric MRI, and 1H MRS. Neurology 72: 1519–1525.

11. Qiu A, Younes L, Miller MI, Csernansky JG (2008) Parallel transport in diffeomorphisms distinguishes the time-dependent pattern of hippocampal surface deformation due to healthy aging and the dementia of the Alzheimer's type. Neuroimage 40: 68–76.

12. Costafreda SG, Dinov ID, Tu Z, Shi Y, Liu CY, et al. (2011) Automated hippocampal shape analysis predicts the onset of dementia in mild cognitive impairment. Neuroimage 56: 212–219.

13. Westman E, Muehlboeck JS, Simmons A (2012) Combining MRI and CSF measures for classification of Alzheimer's disease and prediction of mild cognitive impairment conversion. Neuroimage.

14. Cui Y, Liu B, Luo S, Zhen X, Fan M, et al. (2011) Identification of conversion from mild cognitive impairment to Alzheimer's disease using multivariate predictors. PLoS One 6: e21896.

15. Cardenas VA, Du AT, Hardin D, Ezekiel F, Weber P, et al. (2003) Comparison of methods for measuring longitudinal brain change in cognitive impairment and dementia. Neurobiol Aging 24: 537–544.

16. Ridha BH, Barnes J, Bartlett JW, Godbolt A, Pepple T, et al. (2006) Tracking atrophy progression in familial Alzheimer's disease: a serial MRI study. Lancet Neurol 5: 828–834.

17. Apostolova LG, Dutton RA, Dinov ID, Hayashi KM, Toga AW, et al. (2006) Conversion of mild cognitive impairment to Alzheimer disease predicted by hippocampal atrophy maps. Arch Neurol 63: 693–699.

18. Fox NC, Warrington EK, Freeborough PA, Hartikainen P, Kennedy AM, et al. (1996) Presymptomatic hippocampal atrophy in Alzheimer's disease. A longitudinal MRI study. Brain 119 (Pt 6): 2001–2007.

19. Wang L, Swank JS, Glick IE, Gado MH, Miller MI, et al. (2003) Changes in hippocampal volume and shape across time distinguish dementia of the Alzheimer type from healthy aging. Neuroimage 20: 667–682.

20. Apostolova LG, Dinov ID, Dutton RA, Hayashi KM, Toga AW, et al. (2006) 3D comparison of hippocampal atrophy in amnestic mild cognitive impairment and Alzheimer's disease. Brain 129: 2867–2873.

21. Alves Fda S, Figee M, Vamelsvoort T, Veltman D, de Haan L (2008) The revised dopamine hypothesis of schizophrenia: evidence from pharmacological MRI studies with atypical antipsychotic medication. Psychopharmacol Bull 41: 121–132.

22. Qiu A, Fennema-Notestine C, Dale AM, Miller MI, Initiative AsDN (2009) Regional shape abnormalities in mild cognitive impairment and Alzheimer's disease. Neuroimage 45: 656–661.

23. Fischl B, Salat DH, Busa E, Albert M, Dieterich M, et al. (2002) Whole Brain Segmentation: Automated Labeling of Neuroanatomical Structures in the Human Brain. Neuron 33: 341–355.

24. Miller MI, Qiu A (2009) The emerging discipline of Computational Functional Anatomy. Neuroimage 45: S16–39.

25. Qiu A, Brown T, Fischl B, Ma J, Miller MI (2010) Atlas Generation for Subcortical and Ventricular Structures with Its Applications in Shape Analysis. IEEE Transactions on Image Processing 19: 1539–1547.

26. Qiu A, Miller MI (2008) Multi-structure network shape analysis via normal surface momentum maps. Neuroimage 42: 1430–1438.

27. Qiu A, Brown T, Fischl B, Ma J, Miller MI (2010) Atlas generation for subcortical and ventricular structures with its applications in shape analysis. IEEE Trans Image Process 19: 1539–1547.

28. Tenenbaum JB, de Silva V, Langford JC (2000) A global geometric framework for nonlinear dimensionality reduction. Science 290: 2319–2323.

29. Yang X, Goh A, Qiu A (2011) Locally Linear Diffeomorphic Metric Embedding (LLDME) for surface-based anatomical shape modeling. Neuroimage 56: 149–161.

30. Vapnik VN (1995) The Nature of Statistical Learning Theory: Springer.

31. Chetelat G, Desgranges B, De La Sayette V, Viader F, Eustache F, et al. (2002) Mapping gray matter loss with voxel-based morphometry in mild cognitive impairment. Neuroreport 13: 1939–1943.

32. Shaw LM, Vanderstichele H, Knapik-Czajka M, Clark CM, Aisen PS, et al. (2009) Cerebrospinal fluid biomarker signature in Alzheimer's disease neuroimaging initiative subjects. Ann Neurol 65: 403–413.

33. Vemuri P, Wiste HJ, Weigand SD, Shaw LM, Trojanowski JQ, et al. (2009) MRI and CSF biomarkers in normal, MCI, and AD subjects: predicting future clinical change. Neurology 73: 294–301.

34. Vemuri P, Wiste HJ, Weigand SD, Knopman DS, Trojanowski JQ, et al. (2010) Serial MRI and CSF biomarkers in normal aging, MCI, and AD. Neurology 75: 143–151.

35. Ewers M, Walsh C, Trojanowski JQ, Shaw LM, Petersen RC, et al. (2010) Prediction of conversion from mild cognitive impairment to Alzheimer's disease dementia based upon biomarkers and neuropsychological test performance. Neurobiol Aging.

36. Zhang D, Wang Y, Zhou L, Yuan H, Shen D (2011) Multimodal classification of Alzheimer's disease and mild cognitive impairment. Neuroimage 55: 856–867.

Sensitivity and Specificity of Medial Temporal Lobe Visual Ratings and Multivariate Regional MRI Classification in Alzheimer's Disease

Eric Westman[1]*[9], Lena Cavallin[2,3][9], J-Sebastian Muehlboeck[2], Yi Zhang[2], Patrizia Mecocci[4], Bruno Vellas[5], Magda Tsolaki[6], Iwona Kłoszewska[7], Hilkka Soininen[8], Christian Spenger[2], Simon Lovestone[9,10], Andrew Simmons[9,10], Lars-Olof Wahlund[1], for the AddNeuroMed consortium

1 Department of Neurobiology, Care Sciences and Society, Karolinska Institutet, Stockholm, Sweden, 2 Department of Clinical Science, Intervention and Technology, Karolinska Institutet, Stockholm, Sweden, 3 Department of Radiology, Karolinska University Hospital, Stockholm, Sweden, 4 Institute of Gerontology and Geriatrics, University of Perugia, Perugia, Italy, 5 INSERM U 558, University of Toulouse, Toulouse, France, 6 Aristotle University of Thessaloniki, Thessaloniki, Greece, 7 Medical University of Lodz, Lodz, Poland, 8 University of Eastern Finland and University Hospital of Kuopio, Kuopio, Finland, 9 King's College London, Institute of Psychiatry, London, United Kingdom, 10 NIHR Biomedical Research Centre for Mental Health, London, United Kingdom

Abstract

Background: Visual assessment rating scales for medial temporal lobe (MTL) atrophy have been used by neuroradiologists in clinical practice to aid the diagnosis of Alzheimer's disease (AD). Recently multivariate classification methods for magnetic resonance imaging (MRI) data have been suggested as alternative tools. If computerized methods are to be implemented in clinical practice they need to be as good as, or better than experienced neuroradiologists and carefully validated. The aims of this study were: (1) To compare the ability of MTL atrophy visual assessment rating scales, a multivariate MRI classification method and manually measured hippocampal volumes to distinguish between subjects with AD and healthy elderly controls (CTL). (2) To assess how well the three techniques perform when predicting future conversion from mild cognitive impairment (MCI) to AD.

Methods: High resolution sagittal 3D T1w MP-RAGE datasets were acquired from 75 AD patients, 101 subjects with MCI and 81 CTL from the multi-centre AddNeuroMed study. An automated analysis method was used to generate regional volume and regional cortical thickness measures, providing 57 variables for multivariate analysis (orthogonal partial least squares to latent structures using seven-fold cross-validation). Manual hippocampal measurements were also determined for each subject. Visual rating assessment of MTL atrophy was performed by an experienced neuroradiologist according to the approach of Scheltens et al.

Results: We found prediction accuracies for distinguishing between AD and CTL of 83% for multivariate classification, 81% for the visual rating assessments and 89% for manual measurements of total hippocampal volume. The three different techniques showed similar accuracy in predicting conversion from MCI to AD at one year follow-up.

Conclusion: Visual rating assessment of the MTL gave similar prediction accuracy to multivariate classification and manual hippocampal volumes. This suggests a potential future role for computerized methods as a complement to clinical assessment of AD.

Citation: Westman E, Cavallin L, Muehlboeck J-S, Zhang Y, Mecocci P, et al. (2011) Sensitivity and Specificity of Medial Temporal Lobe Visual Ratings and Multivariate Regional MRI Classification in Alzheimer's Disease. PLoS ONE 6(7): e22506. doi:10.1371/journal.pone.0022506

Editor: Jerson Laks, Federal University of Rio de Janeiro, Brazil

Received April 14, 2011; **Accepted** June 22, 2011; **Published** July 21, 2011

Funding: This study was supported by InnoMed (Innovative Medicines in Europe) an Integrated Project funded by the European Union of the Sixth Framework program priority FP6-2004-LIFESCIHEALTH-5, Life Sciences, Genomics and Biotechnology for Health. AS and SL were supported by funds from the NIHR Biomedical Research Centre for Mental Health at the South London (www.nihr.ac.uk), Maudsley NHS Foundation Trust and Institute of Psychiatry, King's College, London. The funders had no role in study design, data collection and analysis, decision to publish, or preparation of the manuscript.

Competing Interests: The authors have the following competing interest: this study was supported by InnoMed (Innovative Medicines in Europe). There are no patents, products in development or marketed products to declare. This does not alter the authors' adherence to all the PLoS ONE policies on sharing data and materials, as detailed online in the guide for authors.

* E-mail: eric.westman@ki.se

⑨ These authors contributed equally to this work.

Introduction

Dementia is the third most common cause of death in society today, exceeded only by cancer and cardiovascular disorders and Alzheimer's disease (AD) is the most common form of dementia.

Biomarkers of AD based on non-invasive *in vivo* methods are highly desirable for diagnosis, monitoring disease progression and evaluating disease-modifying treatment strategies. An ideal biomarker would detect a fundamental feature of AD neuropathology, be diagnostically sensitive and specific, and produce accurate and reproducible results [1]. Magnetic Resonance Imaging (MRI), Positron Emission Tomography (PET), and cerebrospinal fluid (CSF) measures all allow different aspects of AD pathology to be studied. The new suggested research criterion for AD is centered on a clinical core of early and significant episodic memory impairment and at least one abnormal biomarker from MRI, PET and CSF [2] and the new suggested diagnostic criterion also utilize biomarkers [3].

Several groups including our own have proposed the use of multivariate techniques for analyzing multiple regional measures from MRI to aid diagnosis of AD and to predict future conversion from the prodromal stages of the disease often referred to as mild cognitive impairment (MCI) to AD. Previous studies have shown that computerized methods give high prediction accuracies when distinguishing between patient groups [4,5,6,7]. If computerized methods based on MRI are to be useful in clinical practice then they will need to be as good as or better than experienced neuroradiologists. Klöppel et al. previously compared the diagnostic accuracy of a computerized method (support vector machines (SVM)) with radiological expertise, concluding that SVM gives comparable results to a well-trained neuroradiologist [8]. The study had the strength of using neuropathologically confirmed images, however they did not use a validated and widely used clinical rating scale and they studied relatively small cohorts.

We recently used the multivariate method orthogonal partial least squares to latent structures (OPLS) with multiple regional volumes and cortical thickness measures as input to investigate patterns of atrophy and prediction accuracy in two large multicenter cohorts (AddNeuroMed and the Alzheimer's Disease Neuroimaging Initiative (ADNI)). The study included over a thousand patients and we found prediction accuracies between 83–87% when discriminating between AD and controls [9].

The aim of the current study is to compare the performance of the OPLS multivariate technique with that of an experienced neuroradiologist using data from the AddNeuroMed cohort (a part of InnoMed, (Innovative Medicines in Europe), an Integrated Project funded by the European Union Sixth Framework programme) [10,11]. The method used for visual rating assessment is the well established Scheltens method which uses a five point scale to grade atrophy in the medial temporal lobe [12]. To our knowledge this is the first comparison of the Scheltens visual rating scale for assessment of AD with a computerized method. Additionally our study uses a substantially larger cohort than the earlier study by Klöppel et al, and we also include subjects with mild cognitive impairment. For further evaluation we also aimed to compare the visual rating assessment with manual hippocampal measures. Manual measures have been used for AD diagnosis in research for many years and this region is one part of the visual rating assessment protocol described by Scheltens et al. However, manual hippocampal measurements are time consuming and not feasible in clinical practice. The different approaches were compared in two steps, firstly by distinguishing between AD and controls, and secondly by assessing how well the approaches predicted conversion of MCI subjects at baseline to AD at one year follow-up.

Materials and Methods

Ethics Statement

Written consent was obtained where the research participant had capacity, and in those cases where dementia compromised capacity then assent from the patient and written consent from a relative, according to local law and process, was obtained. This study was approved by ethical review boards in each participating country (local ethical review board at University of Perugia, University of Toulouse, Aristotle University of Thessaloniki, Medical University of Lodz, University of Eastern Finland and University Hospital of Kuopio and King's College London).

Study data and inclusion and diagnostic criteria

All patients originated from the AddNeuroMed project, part of InnoMed (Innovative Medicines in Europe), a European Union program designed to make drug discovery more efficient. The project is designed to develop and validate novel surrogate markers in Alzheimer's disease (AD) and includes a human neuroimaging strand [13,14] which combines MRI data with other biomarkers and clinical data. Data was collected from six different sites across Europe; University of Kuopio, Finland, University of Perugia, Italy, Aristotle University of Thessaloniki, Greece, King's College London, United Kingdom, University of Lodz, Poland and University of Toulouse, France. MRI images from a total of 252 subjects were included in this study; 75 AD patients, 101 MCI patients and 81 healthy controls. Demographics of the cohort are given in Table 1. All AD and MCI subjects were recruited from local memory clinics of the six participating sites while the control subjects were recruited from non-related members of the patient's families, caregiver's relatives or social centres for the elderly. The inclusion and exclusion criteria were as follows.

Alzheimer's disease. *Inclusion criteria*: 1) ADRDA/NINCDS and DSM- IV criteria for probable Alzheimer's disease. 2) Mini Mental State Examination score range between 12 and 28. 4) Age 65 years or above. *Exclusion criteria*: 1) Significant neurological or psychiatric illness other than Alzheimer's disease. This would exclude patients with vascular dementia or large infarcts. 2) Significant unstable systematic illness or organ failure. All AD subjects had a Clinical Dementia Rating (CDR) scale score of 0.5 or above.

Mild Cognitive Impairment and Controls. *Inclusion criteria*: 1) Mini Mental State Examination score range between 24 and 30. 2) Geriatric Depression Scale score less than or equal to 5. 3) Age 65 years or above. 4) Medication stable. 5) Good general health. *Exclusion criteria*: 1) Meet the DSM- IV criteria for Dementia. 2) Significant neurological or psychiatric illness other than Alzheimer's disease. 3) Significant unstable systematic illness or organ failure. The distinction between MCI and controls was based on two criteria: 1) subject scores 0 on Clinical Dementia

Table 1. Subject characteristics.

| | AddNeuroMed | | |
	CTL	MCI	AD
Number	81	101	75
Female/Male	45/36	52/49	50/25
Age	73.6±6.3	74.0±5.8	74.2±6.0
Education	11.0±4.8	8.7±4.3	8.3±4.2
MMSE	29.0±1.2	27.2±1.6	21.3±4.6
CDR	0	0.5	1.1±0.5
ADAS1	3.4±1.5	5.3±1.2	6.6±1.5

Data are represented as mean ± standard deviation. AD = Alzheimer's disease, MCI = Mild Cognitive Impairment, CTL = healthy control, Education in years, MMSE = Mini Mental State Examination, ADAS1 = Word list non-learning (mean), CDR = Clinical Dementia Rating.
doi:10.1371/journal.pone.0022506.t001

Rating Scale = control. 2) Subject scores 0.5 on Clinical Dementia Rating scale = MCI. For the MCI subjects it was preferable that the subject and informant reported occurrence of memory problems.

CDR, Mini-Mental State, and CERAD Cognitive Battery were assessed for each subject. The CERAD Cognitive Battery was replaced with the Alzheimer's Disease Assessment Scale (ADAS–Cog) for the AD subjects. This cognitive test battery is specially designed for AD trials [15]. Both the ADAS-cog and the CERAD battery use the same 10-word recall task. The only difference is that the scoring is inverted. The mean number of words not recalled in the CERAD word list immediate recall task was calculated. The variable obtained was named ADAS1, corresponding to the first subtest of ADAS-Cog. This was performed to obtain comparable measures between groups.

MRI

Data acquisition for the AddNeuroMed study was designed to be compatible with the Alzheimer Disease Neuroimaging Initiative (ADNI) [16]. The imaging protocol for both studies included a high resolution sagittal 3D T1-weighted MPRAGE volume (voxel size $1.1 \times 1.1 \times 1.2$ mm^3) and axial proton density/T2-weighted fast spin echo images. The MPRAGE volume was acquired using a custom pulse sequence specifically designed for the ADNI study to ensure compatibility across scanners [16]. Full brain and skull coverage was required for both of the latter datasets and detailed quality control carried out on all MR images from both studies according to the AddNeuroMed quality control procedure [13,14].

Regional volume segmentation and cortical thickness parcellation

We utilized a pipeline, developed by Fischl and Dale which produces regional cortical thickness and volumetric measures (Figure 1). Cortical reconstruction and volumetric segmentation includes removal of non-brain tissue using a hybrid watershed/ surface deformation procedure [17], automated Talairach transformation, segmentation of the subcortical white matter and deep grey matter volumetric structures (including hippocampus, amygdala, caudate, putamen, ventricles) [17,18,19] intensity normalization [20], tessellation of the grey matter white matter boundary, automated topology correction [21,22], and surface deformation following intensity gradients to optimally place the grey/white and grey/cerebrospinal fluid borders at the location where the greatest shift in intensity defines the transition to the other tissue class [23,24,25]. Once the cortical models are complete, registration to a spherical atlas takes place which utilizes individual cortical folding patterns to match cortical geometry across subjects [26]. This is followed by parcellation of the cerebral cortex into units based on gyral and sulcal structure [27,28]. Left and right sided volumes and thicknesses were averaged. The regional cortical thickness was measured from 34 areas and the regional volumes were measured from 23 areas. All volumetric measures from each subject were normalized by the subject's intracranial volume. This segmentation approach has been used for multivariate classification of Alzheimer's disease and healthy controls [7], neuropsychological-image analysis [29,30,31], imaging-genetic analysis [32,33] and biomarker discovery [34].

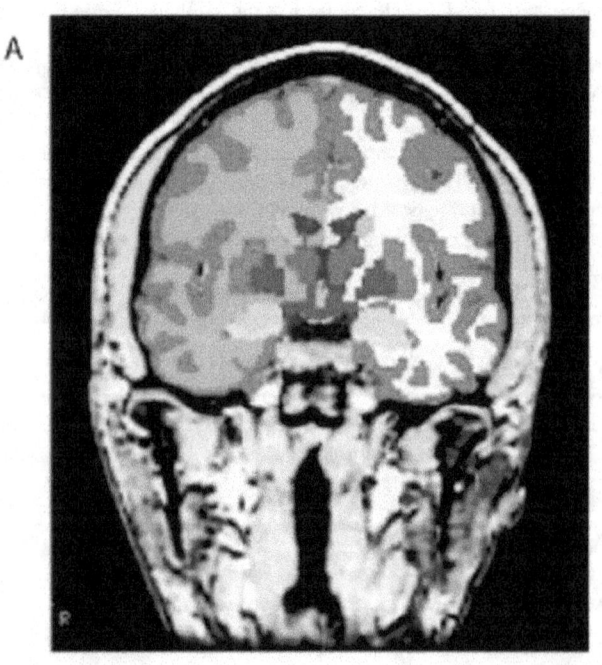
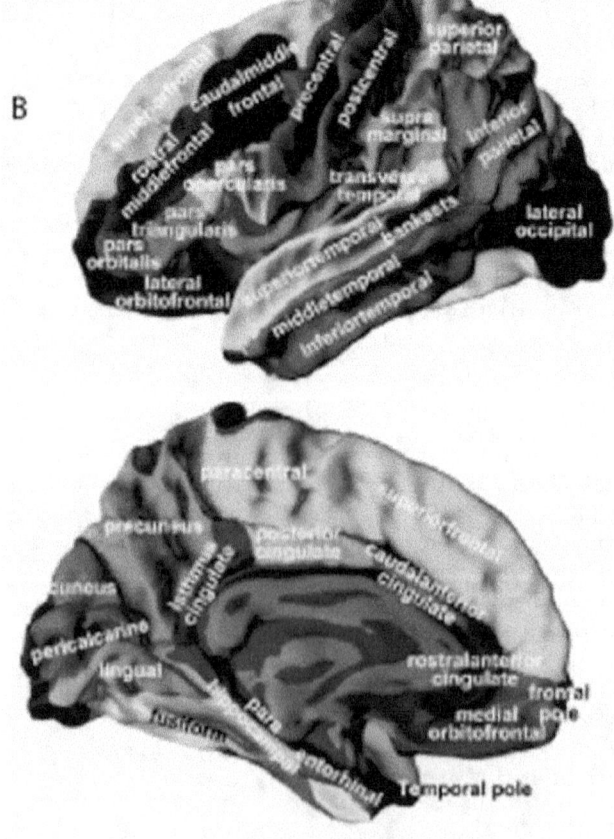

Figure 1. Representations of ROIs included as candidate input variables in the multivariate OPLS model. (A) Regional volumes. (B) Regional cortical thickness measures.
doi:10.1371/journal.pone.0022506.g001

Visual rating assessment for medial temporal lobe atrophy

The 3D T1-weighted MPRAGE images were reoriented to an oblique coronal orientation perpendicular to the AC-PC (anterior commisure - posterior commisure) line suitable for both volumetric and visual assessment. Visual assessment of the medial temporal lobe atrophy was performed on a single MR-slice posterior to the amygdala and the mamillary bodies positioned such that the hippocampus, the pons and the cerebral peduncles are all covered by the slice. The rating scheme used here was first proposed by Scheltens et al. [12] and is based on a visual estimation of volume of the medial temporal lobe. The visual assessment includes hippocampus proper, dentate gyrus, subiculum, parahippocampal gyrus, entorhinal cortex and surrounding CSF spaces such as the temporal horns and choroid fissure. The right and left sides are rated separately. Scores range from 0 (no atrophy) to 4 (end stage atrophy) as detailed in Table 2 and Figure 2. For subjects <75 years, a MTA score of 2 or more is considered abnormal, while for subjects >75 years, a MTA score of 3 or more is considered abnormal (http://www.radiologyassistant.nl/en/43dbf6d16f98d). The rater (LC) was blinded to diagnosis, gender and age. Intra-rater reliability of the visual assessment of the medial temporal lobe atrophy was tested in 100 randomly selected subjects by repeated assessment with an interval of one week. Intra-rater reliability was 0.81 on right side and on left side 0.78. Weighted kappa was 0.93 on both sides.

Manual segmentation of hippocampus

Manual measurements of hippocampal volume were performed on a HERMES workstation (Nuclear Diagnostics, Stockholm, Sweden). Each measurement was performed with constant parameters by a neuroradiologist (YZ) who was blinded to clinical information. A ROI tool was used within the HERMES Multimodality software package, to manually delineate the hippocampal formation using previously defined anatomical landmarks [35]. Intra-rater reliability of the measurements was tested in 15 randomly selected subjects by repeated measurements with an interval of one month. The intra class correlation coefficients (ICC) of the measurements were >0.93. The total hippocampal volume from each subject was normalized by the subjects' intracranial volume.

Multivariate data analysis

MRI measures were analyzed using orthogonal partial least squares to latent structures (OPLS) [6,7,36,37,38,39], a supervised multivariate data analysis method included in the software package SIMCA (Umetrics AB, Umea, Sweden). A very similar method, partial least square to latent structures (PLS) has

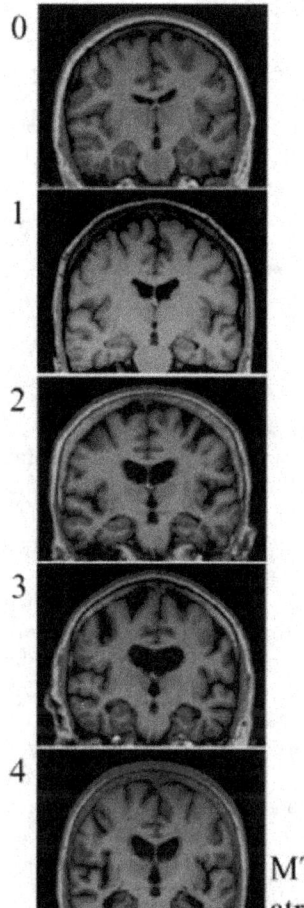

MTA 0-4 increasing atrophy

Figure 2. Visual assessment of the medial temporal lobe atrophy was performed on a single MR-slice posterior to the amygdala and the mamillary bodies. The was positioned so the hippocampus, the pons and the cerebral peduncles were all visible. The visual assessment included hippocampus proper, dentate gyrus, subiculum, parahippocampal gyrus, entorhinal cortex and surrounding CSF spaces such as temporal horn and choroid fissure. The right and left side were rated separately. Scores range from 0 (no atrophy) to 4 (end stage atrophy).
doi:10.1371/journal.pone.0022506.g002

previously been used in several studies to analyze MR-data [40,41,42,43,44]. OPLS and PLS give the same predictive accuracy, but the advantage of OPLS is that the model created to compare groups is rotated, which means that the information related to class separation is found in the first component of the model, the predictive component. The other orthogonal components in the model, if any, relate to variation in the data not connected to class separation. Focusing the information related to class separation on the first component makes data interpretation easier [39].

Pre-processing was performed using mean centring and unit variance scaling. Mean centring improves the interpretability of the data, by subtracting the variable average from the data. By doing so the data set is repositioned around the origin. Large variance variables are more likely to be expressed in modeling than low variance variables. Consequently, unit variance scaling was selected to scale the data appropriately. This scaling method calculates the standard deviation of each variable. The inverse standard deviation is used as a scaling weight for each MR-measure.

Table 2. Visual rating of the medial temporal lobe.

Scale	Width of Choroid fissure	Width of temporal horn	Hippocampal thickness
0	N	N	N
1	↑	N	N
2	↑ ↑	↑	↓
3	↑ ↑ ↑	↑ ↑	↓ ↓
4	↑ ↑ ↑	↑ ↑ ↑	↓ ↓ ↓

Scheltens et al., 1992.
doi:10.1371/journal.pone.0022506.t002

The results from the OPLS analysis are visualized in a scatter plot by plotting the predictive component, which contains the information related to class separation. Components are vectors, which are linear combinations of partial vectors and are dominated by the input variables (x). The first and second components are by definition orthogonal to each other and span the projection plane of the points. Each point in the scatter plot represents one individual subject. The predictive component receives a $Q^2(Y)$ value that describes its statistical significance for separating groups. $Q^2(Y)$ values >0.05 are regarded as statistically significant [45], where

$$Q^2(Y) = 1 - PRESS/SSY \qquad (1)$$

where PRESS (predictive residual sum of squares) = $\Sigma(y_{actual} - y_{predicted})^2$ and SSY is the total variation of the Y matrix after scaling and mean centring [45]. $Q^2(Y)$ is the fraction of the total variation of the Ys (expected class values) that can be predicted by a component according to cross validation (CV). Cross validation is a statistical method for validating a predictive model which involves building a number of parallel models. These models differ from each other by leaving out a part of the data set each time. The data omitted is then predicted by the respective model. In this study we used seven fold cross-validation, which means that 1/7th of the data is omitted for each cross-validation round. Data is omitted once and only once. Variables were plotted according to their importance for the separation of groups. The plot shows the MRI measures and their corresponding jack-knifed confidence intervals. Jack-knifing is used to estimate the bias and standard error. Measures with confidence intervals that include zero have low reliability [39]. Covariance is plotted on the y-axis, where

$$Cov(t, X_i) = t^T X_i / (N - 1) \qquad (2)$$

where t is the transpose of the score vector t in the OPLS model, i is the centered variable in the data matrix X and N is the number of variables [39]. A measure with high covariance is more likely to have an impact on group separation than a variable with low covariance. MRI measures below zero in the scatter plot have lower values in controls compared to AD subjects, while MRI measures above zero are higher in controls compared to AD subjects in the model.

Altogether 57 variables were used for OPLS analysis. No feature selection was performed, meaning all measured variables were included in the analysis. A model containing age was also created to test if there were any significant differences between the diagnostic groups in relation to the variable. We investigated whether age would increase the predictive power of the models using it as an x-variable.

Sensitivity and specificity were calculated from the cross-validated prediction values of the OPLS models and for the visual assessment. Finally, the positive and negative likelihood ratios (LR+ = sensitivity/(100−specificity) and LR− = (100−sensitivity)/specificity) were calculated. A positive likelihood ratio between 5–10 or a negative likelihood ratio between 0.1–0.2 increases the diagnostic value in a moderate way, while a value above 10 or below 0.1 significantly increases the diagnostic value of the test [46].

Finally the AD vs. CTL models were used as training sets to investigate how well they could predict conversion from MCI to AD after one year follow-up and how they compare to the visual assessment. To easily compare the performance of the three methods we also calculated the sensitivity (MCI-c predicted as AD) at a fixed specificity (MCI-s predicted as CTL). We set the specificity for all three methods for this comparison to that of the visual assessment since this can not be changed and recalculated the sensitivity and specificity for the other two methods.

Results

Subject cohort

252 subjects were included in this study: 75 AD patients, 101 MCI patients and 81 control subjects. Using age as an x-variable in the OPLS models did not have any effect on the predictive power of the models separating the groups when all image variables were included. Therefore, age was excluded from further analysis. All MRI volumetric measures were normalised by dividing by each subject's intracranial volume. As expected, performance on the MMSE, CDR and ADAS1 was poorest among AD patients and best among controls (Table 1). The MCI group had scores between the AD and the control groups (Table 1).

OPLS modelling and quality

Two models were created using (1) total hippocampal volume (2) automated regional volume and cortical thickness measures to compare AD vs. controls. The first model using the total manual hippocampal volume accounted for 100% of the variance of the original data $(R^2(X))$ and its' cross validated predictability, $Q^2(Y) = 0.61$. The second model using regional MRI measures resulted in one predictive component with $R^2(X) = 60\%$ and cross validated predictability $Q^2(Y) = 0.45$.

Classification accuracy of the different techniques

The separation between patients with AD and controls and the predictive power of the models $Q^2(Y)$ can be seen in Figure 3A using automated regional volume and cortical thickness measures as input. As can be observed there is a distinct separation between AD and controls. This model resulted in a prediction accuracy of 82.7% (accuracy, sensitivity, specificity, positive likelihood ratio and negative likelihood ratio given in Table 3). Figure 3B illustrates the variables of importance for the distinction between the two groups. The pattern of atrophy, including hippocampus, amygdala and entorhinal cortex among other temporal lobe regions, together with volume measures of CSF is as expected very similar to previous analyses of the AddNeuroMed cohort using regional MRI measures and an OPLS model [9]. Visual rating assessment using the Scheltens scale resulted in a prediction accuracy of 80.8%. Finally, total hippocampal volume yielded a prediction accuracy of 89.1%. The best predictive result was obtained from manual hippocampal measures closely followed by the automated image pipeline with OPLS and lastly the visual rating assessment.

Predicting conversion from MCI at baseline to AD at one year follow-up

Finally, we wanted to investigate how the three different approaches would predict conversion from MCI at baseline to AD at one year clinical follow-up. All MCI subjects were classified as either AD or control like using OPLS models (AD vs. CTL). The visual assessment for the MCI subjects were performed in the same way, using the same cut offs as described previously, resulting in an assessment of abnormal or normal brain changes with respect to age. The results are shown in Table 4 demonstrating that 68% of the MCI converters (MCI-c) were classified as more AD-like and 68% of the MCI stable (MCI-s) classified as more control-like at baseline using visual rating assessment. Using automated regional MRI measures as input to the OPLS model, 74% of the MCI-c

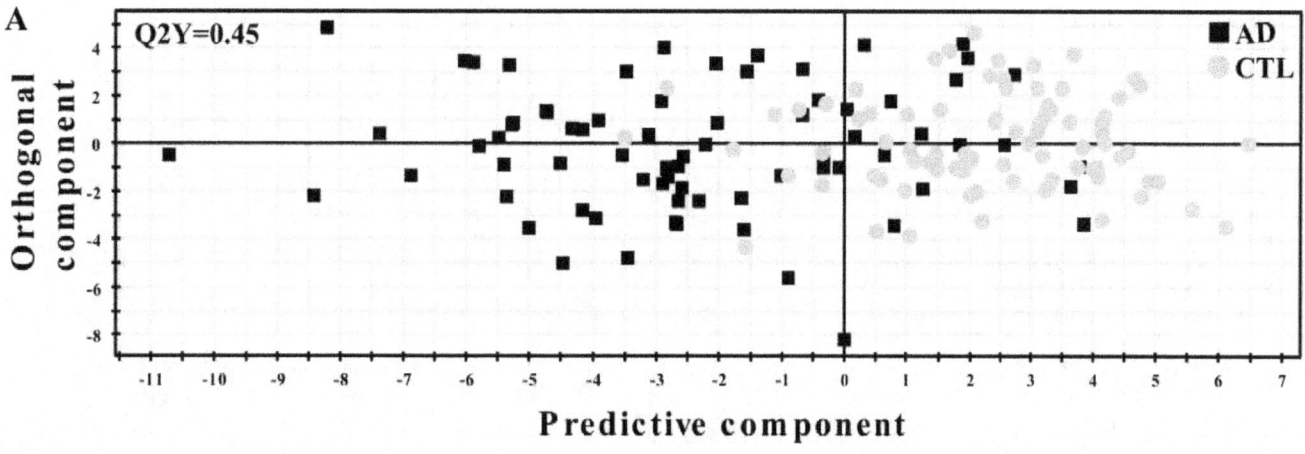

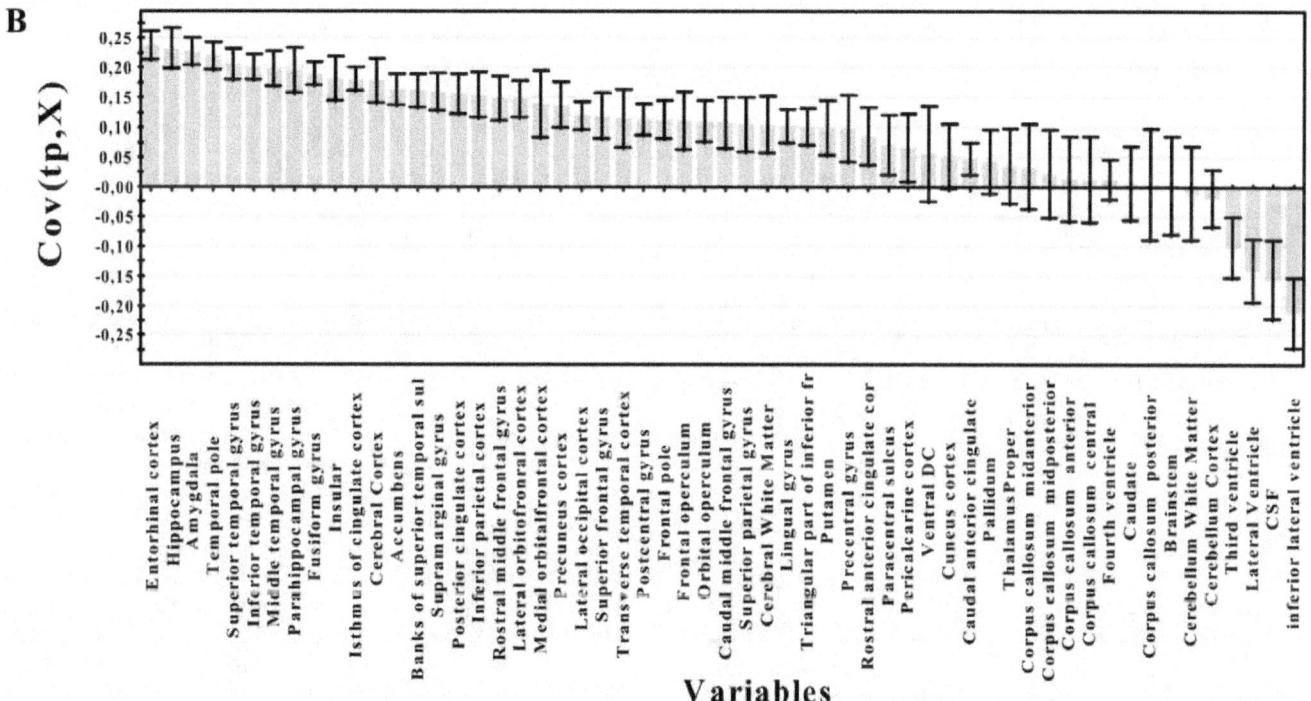

Figure 3. OPLS cross validated score plots and MRI measures of importance for the separation between AD and CTL. (A) The scatter plot visualises group separation and the predictability of the AD vs. CTL model. Each black square represents an AD subject and each gray circle a control subject. Control subjects to the left of zero and AD subjects to the right of zero are falsely predicted. Q²(Y)>0.05 (statistically significant model). (B) Measures above zero have a larger value in controls compared to AD and measures below zero have a lower value in controls compared to AD. A measure with a high covariance is more likely to have an impact on group separation than a measure with a low covariance. Measures with jack knifed confidence intervals that include zero have low reliability.
doi:10.1371/journal.pone.0022506.g003

subjects who converted to AD at one year follow-up were predicted as more AD-like and 70% of the MCI-s were predicted as more control-like at baseline. For the total hippocampal volume, 79% of the MCI-c subjects who converted to AD at one year follow-up were predicted as more AD-like and 54% of the MCI-s were predicted as more control-like. When we set the specificity (MCI-s predicted as CTL) to a fixed value (the specificity of the visual assessment) to make the comparison of the methods easier, the results were slightly altered (Table 4). The best results were obtained from the OPLS model with automated regional MRI measures as input, with 79% of MCI-c subjects who converted to AD at one year follow-up predicted as more AD-like,

compared to 68% for the manual hippocampal volumes and Scheltens visual assessment rating.

Discussion

Automated computerized MRI methods to aid in the diagnosis of AD will only be implemented in clinical practice if they are carefully investigated and validated. The aim of this study was to further validate the OPLS technique with fully automated MRI measures as input and compare it to the Scheltens scale for visual assessment of medial temporal lobe atrophy and to that of total hippocampal volume. To our knowledge this is the first time that

Table 3. Sensitivity/specificity and likelihood ratios for the different methods.

	Sensitivity	Specificity	Accuracy	LR+	LR−
Visual assessment	78.7 (68.1–86.4)	82.7 (73.1–89.4)	80.8 (73.9–86.2)	4.6 (2.8–7.4)	0.26 (0.16–0.40)
Fischl and Dale	77.3 (66.7–85.3)	87.7 (78.7–93.2)	82.7 (75.6–87.8)	6.3 (3.5–11.3)	0.26 (0.17–0.40)
Manual outlining	93.3 (85.3–97.1)	85.2 (75.9–91.3)	89.1 (83.2–93.1)	6.3 (3.7–10.7)	0.08 (0.03–0.18)

Confidence intervals within parentheses, LR+ = positive likelihood ratio and LR− = negative likelihood ratio.
doi:10.1371/journal.pone.0022506.t003

the Scheltens visual rating scale has been compared to a computerized method. We wanted to investigate which approach would distinguish between AD patients and controls with the highest accuracy and best predict conversion from MCI to AD. We have previously shown that combining a set of automated measures of the brain together with manual measures of hippocampus significantly improves the prediction accuracy using OPLS [6]. Manual measures of different brain regions are time consuming and operator dependent however and are hence not regularly used in a clinical settings. Therefore we further investigated the power of OPLS using only automated measures as input (using the same volumes and cortical thickness measures as used here) in two large cohorts (AddNeuroMed and Alzheimer's disease Neuroimaging Initiative (ADNI)). This was performed to investigate if similar patterns of atrophy and prediction accuracy could be obtained from two different large cohorts using the OPLS model [9] and we found good comparability between the two cohorts. We have also previously investigated the value of combining magnetic resonance spectroscopy (MRS) with automated regional MRI measures using OPLS [7] which showed a significant improvement compared with using either set of measures individually. The next natural step was to compare the OPLS technique with a well established visual rating assessment scale such as the Scheltens scale, performed by an experienced neuroradiologist, as we describe here.

Table 4. MCI prediction.

Method	Number	AD-like	CTL-like
Visual assessment converters	19	68% (13)	32% (6)
Fischl and Dale converters	19	74% (14)	26% (5)
Manual hippocampal volume converters	19	79% (15)	21% (4)
Visual assessment non-converters	82	32% (26)	68% (56)
Fischl and Dale non-converters	82	30% (24)	70% (58)
Manual hippocampal volume non-converters	82	46% (38)	54% (44)

Results for fixed specificity	Number	MCI-c as AD	MCI-s as CTL
Visual assessment	101	68%	68%
Fischl and Dale	101	79%	68%
Manual hippocampal volume	101	68%	68%

AD = Alzheimer's disease, MCI = Mild Cognitive Impairment, CTL = healthy control, MCI-c = MCI converters and MCI-s = MCI stable. To better compare the performance of the three methods we also calculated the sensitivity (MCI-c predicted as AD) at a fixed specificity (MCI-s predicted as CTL). We set the specificity to that of the visual rating assessment and recalculated the sensitivity and specificity of the other two methods used.
doi:10.1371/journal.pone.0022506.t004

Classification accuracy of the different techniques

The results suggest that the OPLS technique with fully automated regional MRI measures as input performs better than the visual rating assessments made by an experienced neuroradiologist. The sensitivity of the two methods is similar resulting in identical negative likelihood ratios (77.3%, 0.26 and 78.7%, 0.26 respectively), while the specificity was higher for the OPLS technique than the visual assessment (87.7% and 82.7%) yielding a higher positive likelihood ratio (6.3 and 4.6). The overall accuracy was higher for the OPLS technique compared to the visual rating scale (82.7% and 80.8%). When the specificity was fixed for all three methods at the value of the visual rating assessments, the sensitivity of the OPLS analysis (79%) was better than the other two methods (both 68%). Although the manually measured total hippocampal volume still yielded the best prediction accuracy, the time consuming nature of manual measures makes them impractical in a clinical settings. Manual measurements can also be operator dependent and it can be hard to compare such measures across sites and within sites if different operators are used. If only positive likelihood ratios are considered then the OPLS method with fully automated image measures performs as well as the manually measured total hippocampal volume. The results from the OPLS method using the fully automated MRI measures and the results from the hippocampal volumes are in line with our earlier results from the AddNeuroMed cohort and have been discussed and compared to that of other groups previously [6,9]. Comparing the results from the current study with previously published work we found only one similar study which compared a computerized technique (SVM) with neuroradiologist evaluations [8]. In this prior study, two small cohorts of AD patients and controls were evaluated (40 subjects in the first cohort and 28 subjects in the second cohort). The SVM and visual assessments gave prediction accuracies of 95% vs. 88.8% respectively, for the first cohort, and 92.9% vs. 82.5% for the second cohort. The SVM results were better than the OPLS results that we report here for both cohorts, with the result from the visual rating assessment results higher for their first cohort than our study, but similar to our study for their second cohort. The cohorts included in the study by Klöppel et al. were neuropathologically confirmed and much smaller than the cohort investigated in the present study, which is a likely explanation for the higher prediction accuracy. Klöppel et al. also published another paper [5] using pathologically confirmed data to distinguish between AD and CTL using SVM. High prediction accuracies were again obtained, up to 96% but the sample sizes were again smaller (maximum 20 in each group). They also had a slightly larger cohort (33 AD and 57 CTL) with probable mild AD subjects. Using no feature selection, they obtained a prediction accuracy of 81.1% (sensitivity 60.6% and specificity 93.0%). Prediction accuracies can sometimes be misleading, especially if one group is much smaller than the other. In this present study using the OPLS method with no feature selection on the automated measure, we found an accuracy of 82.7% (sensitivity 77.3% and specificity 87.7%). As can be observed the accuracy of the latter study by Kloppel et al is very similar to ours, but their sensitivity is much lower. It is important that computerized analysis techniques are validated in large cohorts, since it is easy for such methods to fix onto features that may be different between small cohorts, but are not generalizable to larger cohorts. Although neuropathologically confirmed data is preferred when evaluating these types of automated models, it is very difficult to obtain large neuropathologically confirmed datasets in practice. This is even more pronounced when studying the prodromal stages of the disease. MCI subjects are typically diagnosed approximately 10–15 years before death, which makes longitudinal follow-up very difficult and the acquisition of large neuropathologically confirmed datasets with recent MRI an exceedingly difficult endeavor. At the moment it is necessary to choose between small data sets which are neuropathologically confirmed, but potentially not representative of the heterogeneity and complexity of Alzheimer's disease, and larger datasets such as ours, which are more representative but not neuropathologically confirmed. A further advantage of our study, compared to that of Klöppel et al. is that the images acquired in our study are ADNI compatible, making our findings generalizable to other large ADNI compatible cohorts.

The new research and diagnostic criterion have a strong focus on the use of biomarkers including MRI, PET and CSF [2,3]. Although individual markers such as MRI can be powerful in AD, we believe that combining different markers is an attractive approach, particularly if considering differential diagnosis amongst different forms of dementia. Neurodegeneration in AD is estimated to start 20–30 years before the clinical diagnosis is given [47] and so if diagnosis is to be made at the prodromal stage of the disease then it may be necessary to combine several different markers of disease. Previously we have shown that combining regional MRI measures with magnetic resonance spectroscopy results improves classification results, doubling the positive likelihood ratio [7].

Predicting conversion from MCI at baseline to AD at one year follow-up

At one year follow-up 19 of the 101 subjects with mild cognitive impairment converted from MCI to AD while 82 remained stable. One of the aims of this study was to compare how the three methods performed in predicting conversion from MCI to AD. The accuracy of predicting conversion varied from 68–79%. Total manual hippocampal volume gave the best results, followed by the OPLS approach including automated MRI measures and finally the visual rating assessment. It is however difficult to confidently state that one method is better than the other due to the small numbers of subject converting. The three methods predict 15/19, 14/19 and 13/19 converters respectively as more AD like, which is a small absolute difference that has a larger impact on the percentage accuracy. The accuracy of the different models in correctly predicting stable MCI subjects varied between from 54–

70%. Although the OPLS method gave the best results, subjects diagnosed at baseline with MCI who are still classified as MCI at one year follow up may subsequently convert to AD at a later stage and thus assessing whether subjects will eventually convert to AD may require longer follow up times. Further large studies with longer follow up times are warranted to investigate this issue. To make the comparison of the performance of the three methods easier we calculated the sensitivity (MCI-c predicted as AD) at a fixed specificity (MCI-s predicted as CTL). This yielded the best sensitivity for the OPLS model with automated regional MRI measures as input. This model predicted 79% of the MCI-c subjects who converted to AD at one year follow-up as more AD-like, compared to 68% of the other two methods. Although the number of converters is relatively small, a likely explanation for these results is that combining multiple regions across the brain aids in the prediction of MCI conversion.

Conclusion

Visual rating assessment of the medial temporal lobe gave similar prediction accuracy to computerized multivariate classification and both accuracies are comparable to that of manual hippocampal volume measurements. While manual hippocampal volumes are a valuable research tool and have found utility in clinical trials, they are not however practical for use in routine clinical work. Our results demonstrate that computerized multivariate classification is as good as expert radiological review of MRI using a validated and widely used visual rating scale, which suggests a potential future role for computerized methods as a complement to clinical assessment. Improving classification models by adding other biomarkers will hopefully increase the predictive power of the models and improve our understanding of the etiology of the disease. Two limitations of the current study are however that the data is not neuropathologically confirmed and that the follow-up of the MCI subjects was for one year.

In conclusion we believe that this study and previous work [6,7,9] has shown that the OPLS model with automated MRI measures as input has the potential to serve as a complement to clinical assessment of AD, and to target appropriate populations for clinical trials.

Acknowledgments

The authors thank the Gamla Tjänarinnor Foundation, the Swedish Alzheimer's Association, Swedish Brain Power, Health Research Council of Academy of Finland and Stockholm Medical Image Laboratory and Education (SMILE).

Author Contributions

Conceived and designed the experiments: EW LC AS L-OW HS CS J-SM YZ PM BV MT IK SL. Performed the experiments: AS HS PM BV MT IK EW J-SM. Analyzed the data: EW LC YZ AS. Contributed reagents/materials/analysis tools: EW LC AS L-OW HS CS J-SM YZ PM BV MT IK SL. Wrote the paper: EW LC AS L-OW.

References

1. Kantarci K (2005) Magnetic resonance markers for early diagnosis and progression of Alzheimer's disease. Expert Rev Neurother 5: 663–670.
2. Dubois B, Feldman HH, Jacova C, DeKosky ST, Barberger-Gateau P, et al. (2007) Research criteria for the diagnosis of Alzheimer's disease: revising the NINCDS-ADRDA criteria. The Lancet Neurology 6: 734–746.
3. McKhann GM, Knopman DS, Chertkow H, Hyman BT, Jack CR, Jr., et al. (2011) The diagnosis of dementia due to Alzheimer's disease: Recommendations from the National Institute on Aging-Alzheimer's Association workgroups on diagnostic guidelines for Alzheimer's disease. Alzheimers Dement 7: 263–269.
4. Davatzikos C, Resnick SM, Wu X, Parmpi P, Clark CM (2008) Individual patient diagnosis of AD and FTD via high-dimensional pattern classification of MRI. Neuroimage 41: 1220–1227.
5. Kloppel S, Stonnington CM, Chu C, Draganski B, Scahill RI, et al. (2008) Automatic classification of MR scans in Alzheimer's disease. Brain 131: 681–689.
6. Westman E, Simmons A, Zhang Y, Muehlboeck JS, Tunnard C, et al. (2011) Multivariate analysis of MRI data for Alzheimer's disease, mild cognitive impairment and healthy controls. Neuroimage 54: 1178–1187.

7. Westman E, Wahlund L-O, Foy C, Poppe M, Cooper A, et al. (2010) Combining MRI and MRS to distinguish between Alzheimer's disease and healthy controls. J Alzheimers Dis 22: 171–181.

8. Kloppel S, Stonnington CM, Barnes J, Chen F, Chu C, et al. (2008) Accuracy of dementia diagnosis: a direct comparison between radiologists and a computerized method. Brain 131: 2969–2974.

9. Westman E, Simmons A, Muehlboeck S, Mecocci P, Vellas B, et al. (2011) AddNeuroMed and ADNI: Similar Patterns of Alzheimer's Atrophy and Automated MRI Classification Accuracy in Europe and North America. NeuroImage, In press.

10. Lovestone S, Francis P, Kloszewska I, Mecocci P, Simmons A, et al. (2009) AddNeuroMed;The European Collaboration for the Discovery of Novel Biomarkers for Alzheimer's Disease. Annals of the New York Academy of Sciences 1180: 36–46.

11. Lovestone S, Francis P, Strandgaard K (2007) Biomarkers for disease modification trials–the innovative medicines initiative and AddNeuroMed. J Nutr Health Aging 11: 359–361.

12. Scheltens P, Leys D, Barkhof F, Huglo D, Weinstein HC, et al. (1992) Atrophy of medial temporal lobes on MRI in "probable" Alzheimer's disease and normal ageing: diagnostic value and neuropsychological correlates. J Neurol Neurosurg Psychiatry 55: 967–972.

13. Simmons A, Westman E, Muehlboeck S, Mecocci P, Vellas B, et al. (2011) The AddNeuroMed framework for multi-centre MRI assessment of longitudinal changes in Alzheimer's disease: experience from the first 24 months. Int J Geriatr Psychiatry 26(1): 75–82.

14. Simmons A, Westman E, Muehlboeck S, Mecocci P, Vellas B, et al. (2009) MRI Measures of Alzheimer's Disease and the AddNeuroMed Study. Annals of the New York Academy of Sciences 1180: 47–55.

15. Rosen WG, Mohs RC, Davis KL (1984) A new rating scale for Alzheimer's disease. Am J Psychiatry 141: 1356–1364.

16. Jack CR, Jr., Bernstein MA, Fox NC, Thompson P, Alexander G, et al. (2008) The Alzheimer's Disease Neuroimaging Initiative (ADNI): MRI methods. J Magn Reson Imaging 27: 685–691.

17. Segonne F, Dale AM, Busa E, Glessner M, Salat D, et al. (2004) A hybrid approach to the skull stripping problem in MRI. Neuroimage 22: 1060–1075.

18. Fischl B, Salat DH, Busa E, Albert M, Dieterich M, et al. (2002) Whole brain segmentation: automated labeling of neuroanatomical structures in the human brain. Neuron 33: 341–355.

19. Fischl B, Salat DH, van der Kouwe AJ, Makris N, Segonne F, et al. (2004) Sequence-independent segmentation of magnetic resonance images. Neuroimage 23 Suppl 1: S69–84.

20. Sled JG, Zijdenbos AP, Evans AC (1998) A nonparametric method for automatic correction of intensity nonuniformity in MRI data. IEEE Trans Med Imaging 17: 87–97.

21. Fischl B, Liu A, Dale AM (2001) Automated manifold surgery: constructing geometrically accurate and topologically correct models of the human cerebral cortex. IEEE Trans Med Imaging 20: 70–80.

22. Segonne F, Pacheco J, Fischl B (2007) Geometrically accurate topology-correction of cortical surfaces using nonseparating loops. IEEE Trans Med Imaging 26: 518–529.

23. Dale AM, Fischl B, Sereno MI (1999) Cortical surface-based analysis. I. Segmentation and surface reconstruction. Neuroimage 9: 179–194.

24. Dale AM, Sereno MI (1993) Improved Localizadon of Cortical Activity by Combining EEG and MEG with MRI Cortical Surface Reconstruction: A Linear Approach. Journal of Cognitive Neuroscience 5: 162–176.

25. Fischl B, Dale AM (2000) Measuring the thickness of the human cerebral cortex from magnetic resonance images. Proc Natl Acad Sci U S A 97: 11050–11055.

26. Fischl B, Sereno MI, Tootell RB, Dale AM (1999) High-resolution intersubject averaging and a coordinate system for the cortical surface. Hum Brain Mapp 8: 272–284.

27. Desikan RS, Ségonne F, Fischl B, Quinn BT, Dickerson BC, et al. (2006) An automated labeling system for subdividing the human cerebral cortex on MRI scans into gyral based regions of interest. NeuroImage 31: 968–980.

28. Fischl B, van der Kouwe A, Destrieux C, Halgren E, Segonne F, et al. (2004) Automatically parcellating the human cerebral cortex. Cereb Cortex 14: 11–22.

29. Liu Y, Paajanen T, Zhang Y, Westman E, Wahlund L-O, et al. (2011) Combination analysis of neuropsychological tests and structural MRI measures in differentiating AD, MCI and control groups-The AddNeuroMed study. Neurobiol Aging 32: 1198–1206.

30. Liu Y, Paajanen T, Zhang Y, Westman E, Wahlund L-O, et al. (2010) Analysis of regional MRI volumes and thicknesses as predictors of conversion from mild cognitive impairment to Alzheimer's disease. Neurobiology of Aging 31: 1375–1385.

31. Tunnard C, Whitehead D, Hurt C, Wahlund L-O, Mecocci P, et al. (2011) Apathy and cortical atrophy in Alzheimer's disease. Int J Geriatr Psychiatry 26: 741–748.

32. Liu Y, Paajanen T, Westman E, Wahlund L-O, Simmons A, et al. (2010) Effect of APOE epsilon4 allele on cortical thicknesses and volumes: the AddNeuroMed study. J Alzheimers Dis 21: 947–966.

33. Liu Y, Paajanen T, Westman E, Zhang Y, Wahlund L-O, et al. (2010) APOE epsilon2 allele is associated with larger regional cortical thicknesses and volumes. Dement Geriatr Cogn Disord 30: 229–237.

34. Thambisetty M, Simmons A, Velayudhan L, Hye A, Campbell J, et al. (2010) Association of plasma clusterin concentration with severity, pathology, and progression in Alzheimer disease. Arch Gen Psychiatry 67: 739–748.

35. Pantel J, O'Leary DS, Cretsinger K, Bockholt HJ, Keefe H, et al. (2000) A new method for the in vivo volumetric measurement of the human hippocampus with high neuroanatomical accuracy. Hippocampus 10: 752–758.

36. Bylesjo M, Eriksson D, Kusano M, Moritz T, Trygg J (2007) Data integration in plant biology: the O2PLS method for combined modeling of transcript and metabolite data. Plant J 52: 1181–1191.

37. Johan Trygg SW (2002) Orthogonal projections to latent structures (O-PLS). Journal of Chemometrics 16: 119–128.

38. Rantalainen M, Cloarec O, Beckonert O, Wilson ID, Jackson D, et al. (2006) Statistically integrated metabonomic-proteomic studies on a human prostate cancer xenograft model in mice. J Proteome Res 5: 2642–2655.

39. Wiklund S, Johansson E, Sjostrom L, Mellerowicz EJ, Edlund U, et al. (2008) Visualization of GC/TOF-MS-based metabolomics data for identification of biochemically interesting compounds using OPLS class models. Anal Chem 80: 115–122.

40. Levine B, Kovacevic N, Nica EI, Cheung G, Gao F, et al. (2008) The Toronto traumatic brain injury study: Injury severity and quantified MRI. Neurology 70: 771–778.

41. McIntosh AR, Lobaugh NJ (2004) Partial least squares analysis of neuroimaging data: applications and advances. Neuroimage 23: S250–S263.

42. Oberg J, Spenger C, Wang FH, Andersson A, Westman E, et al. (2007) Age related changes in brain metabolites observed by (1)H MRS in APP/PS1 mice. Neurobiol Aging 29(9): 1423–33.

43. Westman E, Spenger C, Oberg J, Reyer H, Pahnke J, et al. (2009) In vivo 1H-magnetic resonance spectroscopy can detect metabolic changes in APP/PS1 mice after donepezil treatment. BMC Neurosci 10: 33.

44. Westman E, Spenger C, Wahlund L-O, Lavebratt C (2007) Carbamazepine treatment recovered low N-acetylaspartate+N-acetylaspartylglutamate (tNAA) levels in the megencephaly mouse BALB/cByJ-Kv1.1mceph/mceph. Neurobiology of Disease 26: 221–228.

45. Eriksson L, Johansson E, Kettaneh-Wold N, Trygg J, Wiksröm C, et al. (2006) Multi- and Megavariate Data Analysis (Part I -Basics and Principals and Applications). Umeå: Umetrics AB.

46. Qizilbash N, Schneider L, Chui H, Tariot P, Brodaty H, et al. (2002) Evidenced-based Dementia Pratice. Oxford, UK: Blackwell Publishing. pp 20–23.

47. Blennow K, de Leon MJ, Zetterberg H (2006) Alzheimer's disease. The Lancet 368: 387–403.

MRI Markers for Mild Cognitive Impairment: Comparisons between White Matter Integrity and Gray Matter Volume Measurements

Yu Zhang[1,2]*, Norbert Schuff[1,2], Monica Camacho[1,2], Linda L. Chao[1,2], Thomas P. Fletcher[3], Kristine Yaffe[4], Susan C. Woolley[5], Catherine Madison[5], Howard J. Rosen[6], Bruce L. Miller[6], Michael W. Weiner[1,2]

1 Center for Imaging of Neurodegenerative Diseases, San Francisco VA Medical Center, San Francisco, California, United States of America, 2 Department of Radiology and Biomedical Imaging, University of California San Francisco, San Francisco, California, United States of America, 3 The Scientific Computing and Imaging Institute at the University of Utah, Salt Lake City, Utah, United States of America, 4 Department of Psychiatry, Neurology and Epidemiology, San Francisco VA Medical Center and University of California San Francisco, San Francisco, California, United States of America, 5 Department of Neurology, California Pacific Medical Center, San Francisco, California, United States of America, 6 Department of Neurology, University of California San Francisco, San Francisco, California, United States of America

Abstract

The aim of the study was to evaluate the value of assessing white matter integrity using diffusion tensor imaging (DTI) for classification of mild cognitive impairment (MCI) and prediction of cognitive impairments in comparison to brain atrophy measurements using structural MRI. Fifty-one patients with MCI and 66 cognitive normal controls (CN) underwent DTI and T1-weighted structural MRI. DTI measures included fractional anisotropy (FA) and radial diffusivity (DR) from 20 predetermined regions-of-interest (ROIs) in the commissural, limbic and association tracts, which are thought to be involved in Alzheimer's disease; measures of regional gray matter (GM) volume included 21 ROIs in medial temporal lobe, parietal cortex, and subcortical regions. Significant group differences between MCI and CN were detected by each MRI modality: In particular, reduced FA was found in splenium, left isthmus cingulum and fornix; increased DR was found in splenium, left isthmus cingulum and bilateral uncinate fasciculi; reduced GM volume was found in bilateral hippocampi, left entorhinal cortex, right amygdala and bilateral thalamus; and thinner cortex was found in the left entorhinal cortex. Group classifications based on FA or DR was significant and better than classifications based on GM volume. Using either DR or FA together with GM volume improved classification accuracy. Furthermore, all three measures, FA, DR and GM volume were similarly accurate in predicting cognitive performance in MCI patients. Taken together, the results imply that DTI measures are as accurate as measures of GM volume in detecting brain alterations that are associated with cognitive impairment. Furthermore, a combination of DTI and structural MRI measurements improves classification accuracy.

Citation: Zhang Y, Schuff N, Camacho M, Chao LL, Fletcher TP, et al. (2013) MRI Markers for Mild Cognitive Impairment: Comparisons between White Matter Integrity and Gray Matter Volume Measurements. PLoS ONE 8(6): e66367. doi:10.1371/journal.pone.0066367

Editor: Yong Fan, Institution of Automation, CAS, China

Received October 10, 2012; **Accepted** May 7, 2013; **Published** June 6, 2013

Funding: This research was supported in part by National Institutes of Health/National Institute on Aging grants P01AG19724, P01AG12435 and grant from NIH/National Center for Research Resources P41RR023953, which were administered by the Northern California Institute for Research and Education, and with resources of the Veterans Affairs Medical Center, San Francisco, California. The funders had no role in study design, data collection and analysis, decision to publish, or preparation of the manuscript.

Competing Interests: The authors have declared that no competing interests exist.

* E-mail: Yu.Zhang@ucsf.edu

Introduction

Mild cognitive impairment (MCI) is a transitional stage between normal aging and early Alzheimer's disease (AD), though not all individuals with a diagnosis of MCI convert to AD [1]. Accurate identification of patients with MCI who are at increased risk of developing AD may facilitate timely initiation of treatments and possible prevention of dementia. While clinical assessments remain the standard diagnostic criteria for MCI, various imaging and biomarker measures have been proposed as complementary tests to improve diagnosis. Proposed measures include: MRI measured atrophy of the hippocampus and entorhinal cortex [2], 18F-fluorodeoxyglucose PET measured temporoparietal cortical hypometabolism, brain amyloid PET [3], and abnormal level of cerebrospinal fluid markers (amyloid-β42, total tau, and phosphorylated tau) [4,5]. Among these proposed markers, MRI has

attracted considerable interest, in part because of the low risk, non-invasive examinations and broad availability nowadays.

Aside from MRI measurements of brain atrophy [6–14], diffusion tensor imaging (DTI), a variant of MRI that is sensitive to microstructural tissue changes, has also shown promise in characterizing MCI [15–24]. DTI studies in MCI generally rely on diffusion summary measures, such as fractional anisotropy (FA), an index of the spatial directionality of tissue water diffusion and mean diffusivity (MD), a measure of the diffusion magnitude. These measures uniquely detect abnormalities in white matter (WM) regions. In particular, FA alterations in MCI – though often subtle [15,17,25–28] – have been found in limbic circuits (including posterior and parahippocampal tracts and fornix) [19,29–32] and posterior callosal areas [33,34]. To gain further insight into WM alterations in MCI, DTI studies have computed axial (DA) and radial (DR) diffusivity data in addition to FA. DR reflects the diffusion magnitude along the orthogonal directions of the diffusion tensor. In particular, an increase in DR has been associated with demyelination and axonal degeneration [35]. Some DTI studies using DR have demonstrated distinct zones of WM alterations in MCI where changes were barely seen with FA [22,36]. However, aside from a previous work [19] in our laboratory, few studies [25,37,38] have compared the accuracy of DTI measurements with structural imaging measurements in characterizing brain alterations in MCI. It is not clear whether the various indices of DTI are superior to, or provide complementary information to structural MRI measures of brain atrophy for accurately classifying MCI and predicting cognitive deficits.

The aims of the study were: 1) to determine to what extent GM atrophy measured by structural MRI and WM alterations measured by DTI in prominent brain regions affected in AD are also associated with MCI; 2) to test whether WM alterations based on DTI improve the classification of MCI, in comparison to classifications based on GM volume; 3) to compare the accuracies of using GM volume and DTI measures for prediction of cognitive performance in MCI.

Materials and Methods

Subjects and Clinical Assessments

One hundred and seventeen subjects participated in the study. Subjects were recruited between May 2005 and October 2010 either by memory clinics in the San Francisco Bay Area, including the Memory Disorders Clinic at the San Francisco Veterans Affairs Medical Center, the Memory and Aging Center at the University of California, San Francisco, and the Memory Clinic at the California Pacific Medical Center or by posting flyers and advertisements in local newspapers. All subjects gave written informed consent, approved by the institutional review boards of the University of California San Francisco and the San Francisco VA Medical Center.

All subjects received the same research MRI examinations, medical and neurological examinations and neuropsychological testing. Domains assessed during baseline neuropsychological testing included: general cognitive ability (i.e., Mini-Mental State Examination, (MMSE) [39]), global cognitive functioning (i.e., Clinical Dementia Rating, (CDR) [40]), phonemic verbal fluency (D words) and semantic fluency (Animal Naming) [41] California Verbal Learning Test - Short Form (CVLT II) [42] including Immediate Recall (sum of trials 1–4 correct scores with total 36 items), 9-item Long Delay Free Recall and Long Delay Cued Recall. To facilitate predictions of accuracies, the 3 CVLT II recall scores (immediate recall, long free and cued recalls) were further composited as one CVLT score because they are correlated with each other.

None of the subject met the clinical diagnostic criteria for dementia. Fifty-four subjects were diagnosed with MCI by clinicians based on clinical criteria established by Peterson et al., or by the Alzheimer's Disease Cooperative Study (ADCS), or if the subject met the MCI core diagnostic features, which include: subjective memory complaints and memory difficulties that are qualified by an informant; memory impairment which exceeds normal aging, as indexed by low cognitive performance on one or more neuropsychological tests which assess learning or recall (for example, delayed recall, word list); a MMSE score greater than or equal to 24/30; a CDR score of 0.5 (but not demented); intact activities of daily living; and no dementia. All MCI subjects, with the exception of three whose diagnostic details were missing, were further divided into two groups: amnestic MCI (aMCI, if the MCI

subjects had predominant memory impairments) and non-amnestic MCI (naMCI, if the MCI subjects had predominant non-memory impairments, such as executive, language, visual, behavioral, motor, or other deficits). Sixty-six cognitively normal subjects, whose neuropsychological scores were no worse than one standard deviation below the mean on standardized tests, but also not better than 2 standard deviations above the mean were included as controls. Exclusion criteria for all participants included any poorly controlled illness, use of medication or recreational drugs that could affect brain function, a history of brain trauma, brain surgery, ischemic events, or skull defects.

MRI Acquisitions

All scans were preformed on a 4 Tesla (Bruker/Siemens) MRI system with a single housing birdcage transmit and 8-channel receiver head coil. T1-weighted images were obtained using a 3D volumetric magnetization prepared rapid gradient echo (MPRAGE) sequence with TR/TE/TI $= 2300/3/950$ ms, 7-degree flip angle, $1.0 \times 1.0 \times 1.0$ mm^3 resolution, 157 continuous sagittal slices. In addition, FLAIR (fluid attenuated inversion recovery) images (TR/TE/TI $= 5000/355/1900$ ms) and T2-weighted images (TR/TE $= 4000/30$ ms) were acquired for clinical reading. DTI was acquired based on a dual-refocused spin-echo EPI sequence supplemented with twofold parallel imaging acceleration (GRAPPA) [43] to reduce susceptibility distortions. Other DTI parameters were TR/TE $= 6000/77$ ms, field of view 256×224 cm, 128×112 matrix size, yielding 2×2 mm^2 in-plane resolution, and 40 contiguous slices each 3 mm thick. One reference image ($b = 0$) and six diffusion-weighted images ($b = 800$ s/mm^2, along 6 noncollinear directions) were acquired.

GM Volume Data Processing

Automated cortical volume measures, cortical parcellation, and subcortical segmentation were performed with FreeSurfer software package, version 4.5 (surfer.nmr.mgh. harvard.edu/fswiki).

For a full description of the FreeSurfer processing steps, see Fischl et al [44,45]. In the first step, each T1-weighted volume was first corrected for head motion, then transformed into Talairach space using affine transformations (12 degrees of freedom), corrected for intensity non-uniformity, and separated from non-brain tissue. The remaining brain image volume was further normalized to match the intensity of a probabilistic atlas with 40 anatomical labeled regions of interest (ROI) per hemisphere before the atlas image was nonlinearly warped to the individual brain space to facilitate atlas-based tissue segmentation and anatomic labeling of subcortical structures, brain stem, cerebellum, and cerebral cortex. In the second step, FreeSurfer was used to generate topological cortical surface representations per hemisphere with theoretical surface bounded by the GM interface to white matter at the inner side and CSF at the outer side. Each hemisphere's cortical surface representation was mapped to the spherical coordinate system of the anatomical-labeled atlas, allowing an automated anatomical parcellation of cortex into gyral regions. The surface parcellation was then extended to GM volume, yielding parcellation of GM tissue sheet, volume and averaged thickness in each cortical and subcortical ROI. The anatomical accuracy of FreeSurfer processing was visually reviewed by trained readers with neuroanatomic knowledge but no corrections were performed by manual editing to avoid rater bias. Instead, data that did not pass the quality control of FreeSurfer processing were not included in the study.

Based on previous MRI reports of prominent brain alterations in AD and MCI [46–48], GM volumes were evaluated in 21 anatomical ROIs, including 3 callosal regions (anterior, middle and posterior corpus callosum), 8 medial temporal regions (bilateral hippocampus, entorhinal cortex, parahippocampal cortex and amygdala), 6 parietal regions (bilateral precuneus, posterior and isthmus cingulate gyrus) and 4 subcortical regions (bilateral thalamus and putamen) (Figure 1A). Although several other ROIs, such as inferior, middle and superior temporal cortex as well as inferior parietal cortex have been reported in the literature, we were unable to obtain reliable values from these regions across all subjects with the automated Freesurfer procedure due to limited image quality. Thus the study was limited in the above 21 ROIs in which FreeSurfer measurements were available for all participants. Regional values of the GM volume were normalized to total intracranial volume (ICV), to account for variations in head size.

DTI Data Processing

Preprocessing of the DTI data included skull-striping, motion and eddy-current correction with FSL package (http://www.fmrib.ox.ac.uk/fsl/), and geometric distortion correction based on a variational matching algorithm [49]. After FA and DR images were created for each participant, these images underwent an automated region of interest (ROI) extraction procedure: 1) All FA images were resliced to the SPM8 white matter (WM) template using a rigid-body transformation (dimensions: $121 \times 145 \times 121$ voxels, resolution: 1.5 mm^3). 2) The 'JHU ICBM-DTI-81' atlas package (cmrm.med.jhmi.edu/), which includes a probabilistic FA atlas and anatomical labels of 44 deep WM ROIs from the DTI data of 81 subjects, was imported into SPM8, and also resliced to the SPM8 WM template using a rigid-body transformation. 3) The resliced FA images were warped nonlinearly to an intensity-averaged FA template generated from all subjects using a diffeomorphic registration algorithm (DARTEL). Consequently,

all individual FA images and the 'JHU ICBM-DTI-81' FA and labeled atlas were spatially normalized onto a common space of the averaged FA template. 4) After that, a 'reversed warping' procedure was applied to assign the 'JHU ICBM-DTI-81' labeled atlas from the DARTEL common space to each individual FA space. 5) In subject's individual space, FA and DR were extracted from all labeled ROIs. To avoid inclusion of surrounding GM or CSF tissues, DTI values were obtained only in voxels with FA values greater than 0.20. Furthermore, data quality was reviewed and ROIs which contained visual mis-registration or WM hyperintensities were excluded. The decision to exclude ROIs with dominant WM hyperintensities was based on detection of a skewed FA distribution within the ROI toward very low FA values (<0.2) in combination with the visual inspection of the corresponding structural MRI for WM lesions.

Based on previous DTI reports [32,50], FA and DR of 20 anatomical ROIs were measured, including 3 regions of the commissural tracts (genu, body and splenium of the corpus callosum), 9 regions of the limbic tracts (fornix and bilateral Fornix (cres) with Stria terminalis, posterior and isthmus cingulum, and hippocampal cingulum) and 8 regions of the association tracts (bilateral inferior and superior longitudinal fasciculi, inferior fronto-occipital fasciculi and bilateral uncinate fasciculi) (Figure 1B).

Statistics

Differences between patients and controls were tested using a t-test for each ROI and MRI modality after effects of age and gender were linearly regressed out. For the rest of the analysis, FA, DR, and GM volume measures were centered and normalized to their respective standard deviations (i.e. transformed to z-scores) to eliminate scaling differences across the ROIs and MRI modalities. In addition, a non-parametric test using permutations of the

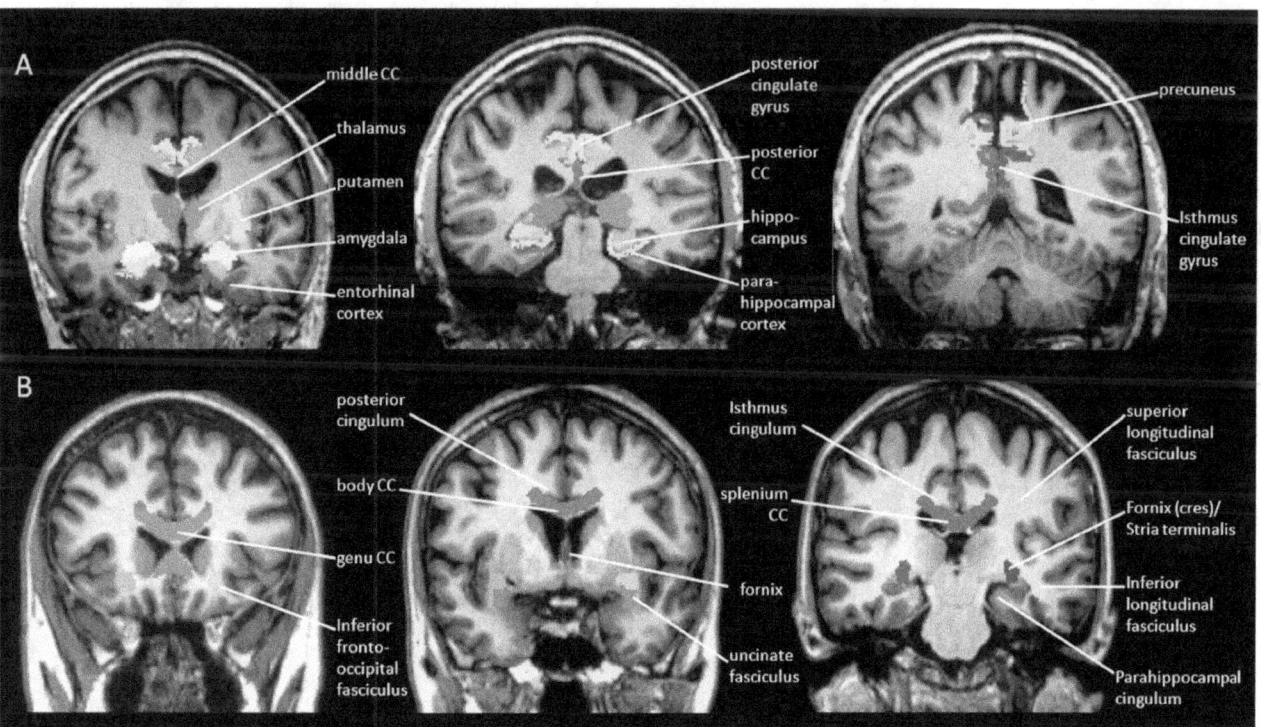

Figure 1. GM and WM parcellations. A. Automated parcellation of 21 cortical and subcortical ROIs for GM measurement, performed by Freesurfer software. B. Automated parcellation of 20 deep WM ROIs for DTI measurement, performed by SPM8.
doi:10.1371/journal.pone.0066367.g001

Table 1. Subjects and clinical characteristics.

| | Control | MCI | MCI subtypes | |
			naMCI	aMCI
Subject Number	66	51	17	31
Age (years)	67.2±10.0	72.8±8.7 [†]	71.9±10.9	73.1±7.5
Sex	**31 M : 35 F**	**30 M : 21 F**	**9 M : 8 F**	**20 M : 11 F**
Years of Education*	16.7±2.4	18.6±12.4	22.1±21.5	17.5±2.4
MMSE*	29.4±1.0	27.8±1.9 [‡]	28.5±1.7	27.5±1.9
Immediate Recall (Trials 1–4)	28.2±4.1	19.1±6.8 [‡]	21.6±6.0	17.1±6.8 [†]
Long Delay Free Recall	7.12±1.5	4.52±2.7 [‡]	5.76±1.9	3.93±2.8 [†]
Long Delay Cued Recall	7.45±1.3	4.65±2.4 [‡]	5.94±1.9	3.87±2.5 [†]
Verbal Fluency* (D-words)	14.6±5.6	13.4±6.0	14.3±5.9	12.9±6.1
Semantic Fluency* (Animal Naming)	21.6±6.1	15.7±6.2 [‡]	18.9±7.0	13.9±5.3 [†]
ICV (cm^3)	1076±125	1091±147	1046±111	1108±164
Total GM/ICV	0.40±0.04	0.37±0.04 [†]	0.38±0.03	0.36±0.04
Total WM/ICV	0.41±0.05	0.39±0.05	0.39±0.05	0.39±0.05

*6 subjects' years of education was missing. 4 subjects' MMSE was missing. 28 subjects' verbal fluency and semantic fluency were missing. Note, smaller scores of neurocognitive measures indicate greater impairment.
Significance of group differences between paired groups (MCI vs. Control, aMCI vs. naMCI):
[†]0.05<p≤0.001,
[‡]p<0.001.
doi:10.1371/journal.pone.0066367.t001

diagnostic labels was applied to determine whether the heterogeneity of MCI has to be taken into account for findings of differences between uniform MCI and CN. The concept of false discovery rate (FDR) was used to account for the multiple comparisons problem [51]. An adjusted level of p<0.05 was selected as threshold of significance. The classification accuracy of FA, DR, and GM volume was tested using regularized logistic regressions with all respective ROIs included simultaneously as factors. An L2-norm regularization term (Ridge regression) was used to control for overfitting [52]. The classification accuracy of FA, DR, and GM were then compared pairwise by testing differences in the area under the curve of an operator characteristics analysis (ROC) based on bootstraping (using the roc.test function in the pROC package of R, URL: http://www.r-project.org/index.html). Similarly, to test the accuracy of FA, DR, and GM volume in predicting neurocognitive performance, regularized linear regressions were used with cognitive scores as outcomes and with all respective ROIs included simultaneously as factors. Accuracy was expressed as the root mean square error (RMSE) between predicted and clinical values, where a smaller RMSE indicating a more accurate prediction. Differences in RMSE distributions of FA, DR, and GM volume where compared using t-tests. Lastly, classifications and predictions were performed with 5-fold cross-validation and bootstrapping to estimate reliability in terms of 95% confidence intervals (CI).

Results

Demographic and Clinical Characteristics

The clinical and demographic characteristics of the subjects as well as global brain volumes are summarized by diagnostic group in Table 1. Differences in gender and years of education between MCI patients and CN subjects were not significant. However, MCI patients were older than CN subjects and performed worse on most neuropsychological tests as expected, with the exception of verbal fluency (D-words). The MCI patients had, on average, less total GM volume (normalized to ICV) than CN, while differences in total WM volume (also normalized to ICV) were not significant.

Group differences based on GM volume and DTI measurements

Mean and standard error of group differences in MRI measurements for all ROIs are depicted in Figure 2A, separately for diffusion and volume. As for DTI, mean FA was significantly reduced in MCI as compared to controls in the splenium of the corpus callosum, the left isthmus cingulum and the fornix. Interestingly, FA of the left inferior longitudinal fasciculus was increased in MCI. DR was increased in MCI as compared to controls in the splenium of the corpus callosum, the left isthmus cingulum and bilaterally in the uncinate fasciculi, consistent with reduced FA in these regions. As for GM volume, the most prominent volume losses in MCI patients compared to controls involved bilateral hippocampi, the left entorhinal cortex, the right amygdala, and the thalamus bilaterally. The most prominent regions of cortical thinning in MCI included the left entorhinal cortex. The effect sizes of significant group differences based on FA and DR were similar (effect size = 0.42–0.61) to those based on GM volumes and thickness (effect size = 0.42–0.61). Differences between the left and the right side of the brain were not significant (p>0.65).

Differences between MCI subgroups in MRI measurements for all ROIs are depicted in Figure 2B, separately for diffusion and volume. As for DTI, significant differences between the MCI subgroups were found in bilateral posterior cingulum, right superior longitudinal fasciculus and left inferior longitudinal fasciculus. In these regions, DTI (FA/DR) values of the naMCI group were more abnormal than those of the aMCI group, while the values of the aMCI group was on average not different from those of controls. The difference between the two MCI subgroups was dominated by better than normal values in the aMCI group.

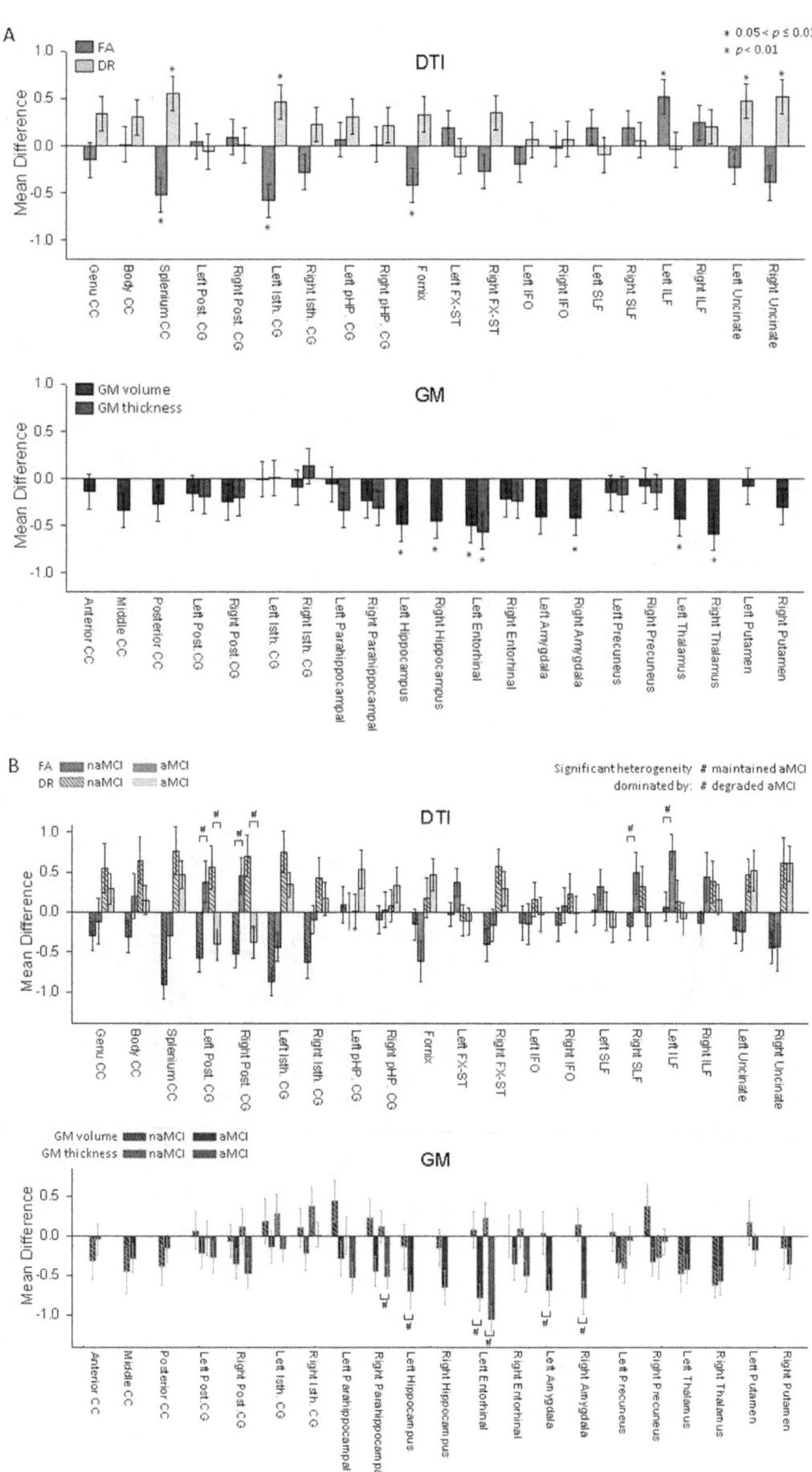

Figure 2. Mean differences of the DTI and GM measures between MCI and control. A. Mean differences and standard errors of regional DTI and GM measures, expressed as Z-scores, between MCI patients and controls for each ROI. Abbreviations:CC = corpus callosum; Post. CG = posterior cingulum; Isth. CG = isthmus cingulum; FX-ST = fornix (cres) and stria terminalis; IFO = inferior fronto-occipital fasciculus; SLF = superior longitudinal fasciculus; ILF = inferior longitudinal fasciculus. B. Mean differences and standard errors of regional DTI and MRI measures between aMCI, naMCI group and controls for each ROI. DTI and GM measures in ROIs with significant heterogeneities between aMCI and naMCI groups were labeled as "#".
doi:10.1371/journal.pone.0066367.g002

As for GM measures, significant differences between the MCI subgroups were found in the right hippocampus, left entorhinal cortex, bilateral amygdale, and the right parahippocampal cortex. In these regions, the difference between the two MCI subgroups was dominated by more GM loss and cortical thinning in the aMCI group. Hence, variations in the aMCI group dominated differences between MCI overall and controls.

Relations between DTI and GM volume in MCI

Relationships between regional DTI alterations in white matter and atrophy of GM in MCI were investigated using Pearson correlation coefficients. The significance of regional correlations are illustrate in Figure 3, separate for FA and DR measures in relation to GM volumes. Significant DTI-volume correlations were found between the limbic structures and the corpus callosum, whereas other regions showed no significant relationships.

Group classifications

Classification accuracy of MCI and control subjects based on either FA, DR, GM volume alone or in combinations is summarized in Table 2. The corresponding receiver operating characteristic curves of each classification are illustrated in Figure 4. The table indicates that classifications based on FA or DR alone were significant (lower bound of the confidence interval >50%) in contrast to classifications based on GM volumes that were not better than chance. However, using either DR or FA together with GM volume further improved accuracy.

Predictions of Cognitive Deficits

The accuracy of each FA, DR, or GM volume in predicting clinical scores of cognitive deficits is illustrated in Figure 5, showing the distribution of root mean square errors for each measure. The three imaging measures achieved similar levels of accuracy for predicting MMSE and CVLT.

Discussion

The main findings of this study are: 1) MCI is associated with significant alterations of FA and DR as well as GM volume loss in specific regions, in agreement with previous findings. 2) FA and DR achieve better classification accuracy than GM volume alone, and using DTI and GM volume together further improves classification. 3) FA, DR and GM volume are similarly accurate in predicting cognitive performance. Taken together, the results imply that DTI of WM alterations is as accurate as structural MRI of GM volume in detecting brain alterations that associated with cognitive impairment. Furthermore, a combination of DTI and structural MRI measures improves accuracy.

DTI has been used in more than a hundred MRI reports of MCI and AD studies. However, the findings have been inconsistent [53], unlike structural MRI reports of medial temporal lobe atrophy in MCI and AD. Different methodologies in selecting regions of interest are a potential source of inconsistency in DTI findings. We used an automated region selection method to eliminate rater dependent bias and also evaluated all selected regions simultaneously for analysis to gain statistical power. Our findings of reduced FA and increased DR in

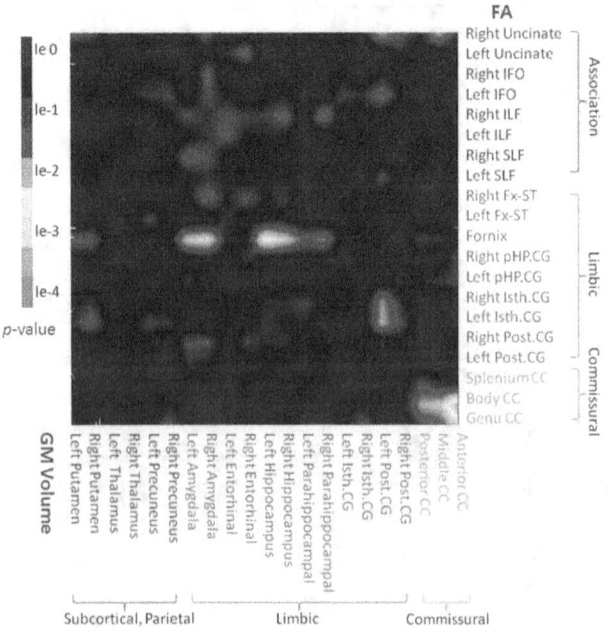
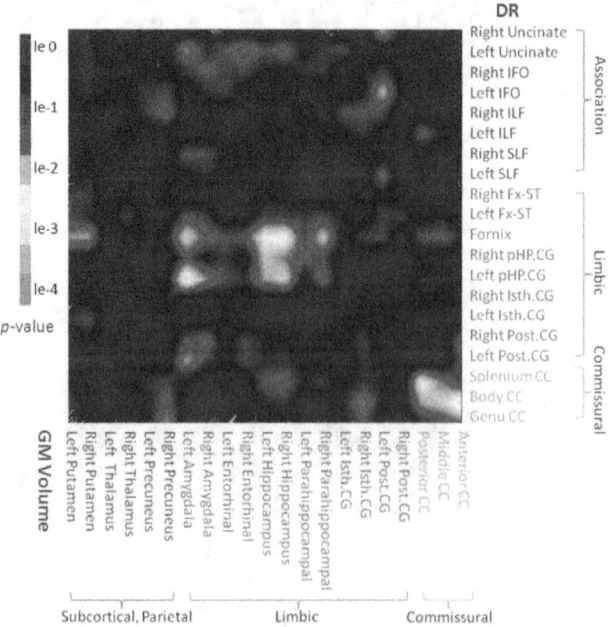

Figure 3. The correlations between DTI and GM volumes in MCI patients. The *p* value maps of the Pearson's correlation between DTI values and GM volumes. The green and warmer colors indicate significant correlations.
doi:10.1371/journal.pone.0066367.g003

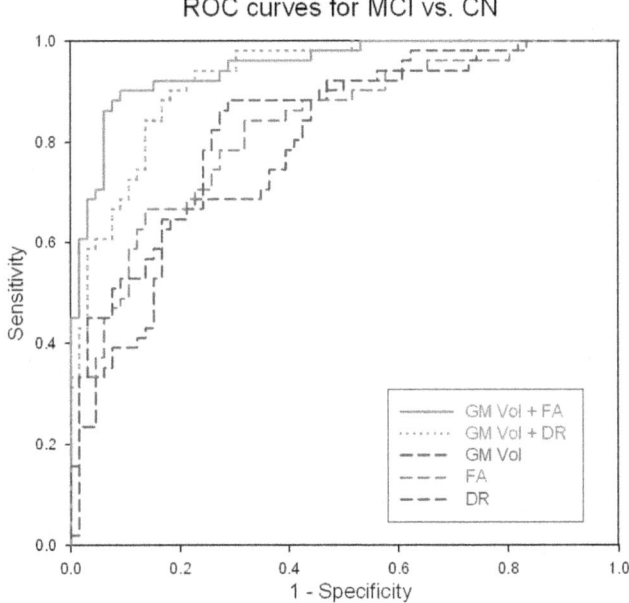

Figure 4. Classification accuracies based on DTI and GM volume measures. Receiver operator characteristic curves of classifications of MCI and control subjects based on DTI and GM volume measures used separately or together.
doi:10.1371/journal.pone.0066367.g004

the splenium, fornix isthmus cingulum, and uncinate fasciculi, are consistent with most other DTI studies with positive results [16,17,24,28,29,31,33,54,55]. However, our results conflict with some previous studies [15,18,25,56–58] that found no significant DTI alterations in some of these regions. The findings also do not fully replicate our previous results [19] that showed significant FA reduction in the parahippocampal cingulum of MCI subjects. The inconsistent DTI findings might results partially from methodological differences between the studies. In particular, simply artifacts of microscopic heterogeneity, such as crossing fibers, may explain some of the inconsistencies. Moreover, heterogeneous pathological underpinnings of study populations may also result different DTI findings. For example, increasing evidences indicate that cognitively normal elderly individuals show pathological features of AD (i.e., neuritic plaques and neurofibrillary tangles). If DTI is sensitive to capture already relevant pathologies in cognitively normal group, the group differentiation with DTI might be diminished. Nonetheless, our findings of abnormal DTI

in regions of the splenium, fornix, isthmus cingulum and uncinate fasciculus in MCI highlight a network of brain regions which are known to be vulnerable to AD pathology. The pattern of these regional DTI alterations suggests that regional degradation of WM matter integrity could be a sign of incipient AD pathology in MCI. An interesting finding is increased FA and decreased DR in the inferior longitudinal fasciculus in MCI. An increase in FA has been reported in other pathological conditions [59]. It has been proposed that reduced dendritic branching of the posterior parietal region may lead to an FA increase, though this hypothesis needs to be tested. However, increased FA could also be methodological artifacts induced by variations in the macroscopic architecture of the long association fibers [60]. The finding of increased FA of the inferior longitudinal fasciculus in MCI requires further investigations. In particular, DTI studies with more than six diffusion encoding directions need to be performed to achieve higher accuracy in measuring FA. In addition, the finding needs to be replicated in a separate population of MCI.

In contrast to DTI findings, our findings of GM atrophy in the medial temporal lobe and subcortical regions are generally in line with numerous other structural MRI studies of gray matter volume loss in MCI [6–12,14]. As for the relationship between regional alterations in DTI and GM atrophy, significant correlations were limited to limbic structures and the corpus callosum. Although this suggests that microstructural degeneration and macroscopic tissue loss are correlated, the neural processes underlying the relationship between cortical atrophy and decreased white matter integrity remain unclear. Both retrograde and anterograde neuronal degeneration [61] could be responsible for the finding. Longitudinal studies are needed to investigate the causal relationship between white matter degradations and cortical atrophy in MCI and AD.

The finding that DTI outperformed structural MRI GM volume in the classification of MCI is surprising, because brain atrophy is generally considered to be strongly associated with cognitive impairments. Some MRI studies in MCI, using regional brain volumes reported between 73% to 91% classification accuracy [62–69]. Thus, the 79.1% fitted accuracy under the ROC curve for classifying MCI and healthy controls reported in our study still appears to be consistent with the results in literature. However, these previous studies employed mostly a single or a small number of ROIs, such as the hippocampus or the entorhinal cortex, achieving reasonably high sensitivity but lacking specificity potentially because atrophy of the hippocampus and/or entorhinal cortex are not features unique to MCI. By utilizing multiple brain regions simultaneously for classifications, we may have captured the heterogeneity of the MCI population better than evaluating

Table 2. Group classifications based on either DTI or GM volume measures separately or used together.

Measure	Sensitivity (%)	Specificity (%)	Accuracy (%)	Fitted AUC (%)	Cross-validated AUC (%)		
					(95% CI Lower)	median	(95% CI Upper)
FA	70.6	77.2	74.4	82.8	51.5	70.8	90.0
DR	66.7	78.8	73.5	83.5	58.0	78.5	95.0
GM volume	64.7	83.3	75.2	79.1	49.5	67.3	86.2
FA + GM volume	88.2	90.9	89.7	94.9	63.9	82.3[a]	96.2
DR + GM volume	82.3	86.4	84.6	92.6	61.9	81.2[b]	96.2

AUC – area under a receiver operating characteristic curve. AUCs were tested using bootstrap (2000 boots):
[a]Differences between modalities (i.e. FA + GM volume vs. GM volume) were significant at 95% confidence interval.
[b]Differences between modalities (i.e. DR + GM volume vs. GM volume) were significant at 90% confidence interval.
doi:10.1371/journal.pone.0066367.t002

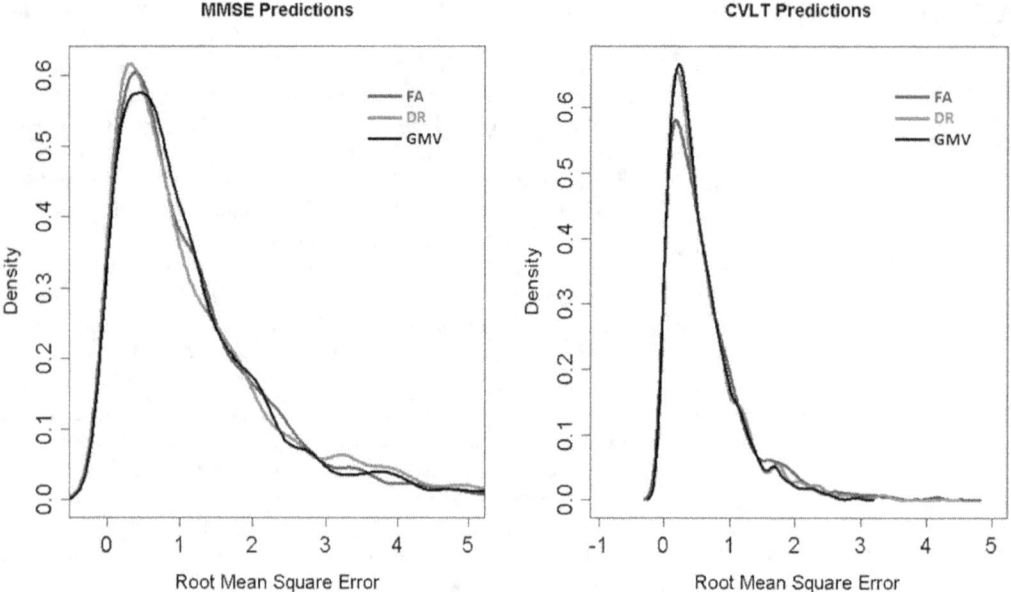

Figure 5. Accuracies of predicting cognitive scores based on DTI and GM volume measures. Distribution of root mean square errors in predicting MMSE and CVLT based on FA, DR or GM volume measures.
doi:10.1371/journal.pone.0066367.g005

each region separately. In contrast to studies that measured regional GM volumes, several DTI studies reported moderate classification accuracies (61–83%) of MCI [20,37,38,70] based on a pre-selected single ROI. However, a complication in interpreting previous DTI results is that the pre-selected single ROI were not in consistent anatomical locations and the regional variations in DTI across different brain locations were not considered. In this study we attempted to take regional variations into account by using all selected ROIs simultaneously for classifications. Thus the results are less dependent on pre-selection of regions and potentially more powerful. Our classification results, when considering multiple regions, have shown similar cross-validated accuracies as that reported in previous DTI studies. The findings that DTI outperformed GM volumes over the cross-validated accuracies imply that DTI measurement is as accurate as the GM volume measurement in classifying MCI from healthy elderly controls. Furthermore, another potential strength of the DTI measurement is that DTI improves the diagnostic accuracies when using together with GM volume measures, this finding reconfirms our previous report and other reports in literature [19,37,38].

Our finding that DTI and GM volume measures were similarly accurate in predicting cognitive performance in MCI has not been previously reported. Generally, cognitive performance has been associated with gray matter atrophy and less with white matter alterations [71–74]. In particular, measuring hippocampal volume loss has often been used as predictor of memory deficits in MCI, consistent with well-known role of the hippocampus for memory consolidation [75–77]. Mean diffusivity of the parahippocampi [15] or the posterior cinguli [26] was reported predictive for memory performance in previous DTI studies with small samples. The abnormalities reported by DTI may reflect WM insults such as myelin/axonal degeneration, oligodendrocytes death, reactive gliosis, and small infarctions that may occur secondarily to volume loss, which is known to be associated with memory deficits. Consequently, it is reasonable to consider DTI as a possible predictor to represent simultaneous though not identical neuro-pathological processes in addition to using GM volume. Although

we cannot determine in this cross-sectional study whether the predictions based on DTI reflect primary and secondary effects, our results imply that alterations in WM are similarly important for predictions of cognitive performance compared to GM volume loss. Moreover, by taking regional variations into account, we reduced bias toward localized alterations that may not be characteristic for MCI. We believe that our approach is more reliable and also provides more interpretable results than testing a few pre-determined regions separately. Our finding that DTI achieved similar power as GM volumes in predicting cognitive deficits highlights the potential value of DTI.

Our study has several limitations. It is possible that vascular factors contributed to FA, DR, and GM volume differences between MCI and controls [34,78], although we avoided brain areas with visual WM hyperintensities when selecting ROIs. On the other hand, some particular ROIs may include surrounding voxels that contain GM, CSF and crossing fibers that may have exaggerated group differences of DTI measures. Although in our study DTI measures were limited in ROIs that contain voxels of FA >0.2, there is no definition of a fiber boundary that enables fully exclusion of partial volume. The potential influence of vascular factors and partial volume effects on our results requires further investigation but is beyond the scope of this study. Second, the MCI group included not only subjects with memory complaints (amnestic MCI), but also those with executive, language or other deficits (non-amnestic MCI) as the dominant clinical symptoms. Correspondingly, the group may also be heterogeneous with respect to the pathological underpinnings of the clinical features. Furthermore, the number of subjects in this cohort, who converted to AD after 2-years clinical follow-up was too small to determine whether the DTI and GM volume alterations were linked to a conversion to AD with a reasonable level of confidence. Studies with longer follow-ups are needed to compare the predictive value of structural MRI and DTI for the development of AD. A methodological limitation was that we did not capture complete distributions of DTI and GM volume variations across the whole brain. This may have biased our results as well as reduced sensitivity as potential variations outside the regions of interest were ignored. Although recently advances have been made in processing all imaging voxels simultaneously, using machine learning algorithms [79], the methodological complexity of machine learning for MRI is not yet fully understood, especially when multiple imaging variables are used together. As machine learning methodologies in MRI become more robust, the comparisons between DTI and structural MRI should be repeated. Another methodological limitation is that DTI was performed with only 6 diffusion gradient directions, while more directions are known to stabilize tensor estimations. However, at the time this study was started, a DTI protocol with more diffusion directions was not available. It is therefore possible that our DTI results are confounded by larger error margins than recent DTI studies using more directions.

In conclusion, this study shows that DTI measures are as accurate as measures of GM volumes in characterizing brain alterations associated with cognitive impairment, and a combina-tion of DTI and structural MRI measurements improves classification accuracy.

Acknowledgments

The authors thank all the participants in this study. We also thank Mr. Matthew Nordstrom, Mr. Frank Ezekiel for the assistance with image processing, Mr. Derek Flenniken for clinical data organizing, and Mr. Philip Insel for the help with statistics.

Author Contributions

Conceived and designed the experiments: YZ NS MWW. Performed the experiments: YZ NS MC LLC. Analyzed the data: YZ NS MC LLC. Contributed reagents/materials/analysis tools: NS LLC TPF KY SCW CM HJR BLM MWW. Wrote the paper: YZ NS. Designed the software used in analysis: TPF. Results interpretation and manuscript editing: YZ NS LLC KY SCW CM HJR BLM MWW.

References

1. Albert MS, DeKosky ST, Dickson D, Dubois B, Feldman HH, et al. (2011) The diagnosis of mild cognitive impairment due to Alzheimer's disease: recommendations from the National Institute on Aging-Alzheimer's Association workgroups on diagnostic guidelines for Alzheimer's disease. Alzheimers Dement 7: 270–279.
2. Ramani A, Jensen JH, Helpern JA (2006) Quantitative MR imaging in Alzheimer disease. Radiology 241: 26–44.
3. Frisoni GB, Padovani A, Wahlund LO (2003) The diagnosis of Alzheimer disease before it is Alzheimer dementia. Arch Neurol 60: 1023; author reply 1023–1024.
4. Vemuri P, Wiste HJ, Weigand SD, Shaw LM, Trojanowski JQ, et al. (2009) MRI and CSF biomarkers in normal, MCI, and AD subjects: diagnostic discrimination and cognitive correlations. Neurology 73: 287–293.
5. Sluimer JD, Bouwman FH, Vrenken H, Blankenstein MA, Barkhof F, et al. (2010) Whole-brain atrophy rate and CSF biomarker levels in MCI and AD: a longitudinal study. Neurobiol Aging 31: 758–764.
6. Jack CR, Jr., Petersen RC, Xu YC, O'Brien PC, Smith GE, et al. (1999) Prediction of AD with MRI-based hippocampal volume in mild cognitive impairment. Neurology 52: 1397–1403.
7. Du AT, Schuff N, Amend D, Laakso MP, Hsu YY, et al. (2001) Magnetic resonance imaging of the entorhinal cortex and hippocampus in mild cognitive impairment and Alzheimer's disease. J Neurol Neurosurg Psychiatry 71: 441–447.
8. Kantarci K, Xu Y, Shiung MM, O'Brien PC, Cha RH, et al. (2002) Comparative diagnostic utility of different MR modalities in mild cognitive impairment and Alzheimer's disease. Dement Geriatr Cogn Disord 14: 198–207.
9. Grundman M, Jack CR, Jr., Petersen RC, Kim HT, Taylor C, et al. (2003) Hippocampal volume is associated with memory but not monmemory cognitive performance in patients with mild cognitive impairment. J Mol Neurosci 20: 241–248.
10. Pennanen C, Kivipelto M, Tuomainen S, Hartikainen P, Hanninen T, et al. (2004) Hippocampus and entorhinal cortex in mild cognitive impairment and early AD. Neurobiol Aging 25: 303–310.
11. Whitwell JL, Petersen RC, Negash S, Weigand SD, Kantarci K, et al. (2007) Patterns of atrophy differ among specific subtypes of mild cognitive impairment. Arch Neurol 64: 1130–1138.
12. Morra JH, Tu Z, Apostolova LG, Green AE, Avedissian C, et al. (2009) Automated 3D mapping of hippocampal atrophy and its clinical correlates in 400 subjects with Alzheimer's disease, mild cognitive impairment, and elderly controls. Hum Brain Mapp 30: 2766–2788.
13. Petersen RC (2009) Early diagnosis of Alzheimer's disease: is MCI too late? Curr Alzheimer Res 6: 324–330.
14. Frisoni GB, Fox NC, Jack CR, Jr., Scheltens P, Thompson PM (2010) The clinical use of structural MRI in Alzheimer disease. Nat Rev Neurol 6: 67–77.
15. Rogalski EJ, Murphy CM, deToledo-Morrell L, Shah RC, Moseley ME, et al. (2009) Changes in parahippocampal white matter integrity in amnestic mild cognitive impairment: a diffusion tensor imaging study. Behav Neurol 21: 51–61.
16. Kiuchi K, Morikawa M, Taoka T, Nagashima T, Yamauchi T, et al. (2009) Abnormalities of the uncinate fasciculus and posterior cingulate fasciculus in mild cognitive impairment and early Alzheimer's disease: a diffusion tensor tractography study. Brain Res 1287: 184–191.
17. Mielke MM, Kozauer NA, Chan KC, George M, Toroney J, et al. (2009) Regionally-specific diffusion tensor imaging in mild cognitive impairment and Alzheimer's disease. Neuroimage 46: 47–55.
18. Stahl R, Dietrich O, Teipel SJ, Hampel H, Reiser MF, et al. (2007) White matter damage in Alzheimer disease and mild cognitive impairment: assessment with diffusion-tensor MR imaging and parallel imaging techniques. Radiology 243: 483–492.
19. Zhang Y, Schuff N, Jahng GH, Bayne W, Mori S, et al. (2007) Diffusion tensor imaging of cingulum fibers in mild cognitive impairment and Alzheimer disease. Neurology 68: 13–19.
20. Fellgiebel A, Wille P, Muller MJ, Winterer G, Scheurich A, et al. (2004) Ultrastructural hippocampal and white matter alterations in mild cognitive impairment: a diffusion tensor imaging study. Dement Geriatr Cogn Disord 18: 101–108.
21. Bozoki AC, Korolev IO, Davis NC, Hoisington LA, Berger KL (2011) Disruption of limbic white matter pathways in mild cognitive impairment and Alzheimer's disease: A DTI/FDG-PET Study. Hum Brain Mapp 33: 1792–1802.
22. Oishi K, Akhter K, Mielke M, Ceritoglu C, Zhang J, et al. (2011) Multi-modal MRI analysis with disease-specific spatial filtering: initial testing to predict mild cognitive impairment patients who convert to Alzheimer's disease. Front Neurol 2: 54.
23. Teipel SJ, Meindl T, Grinberg L, Grothe M, Cantero JL, et al. (2010) The cholinergic system in mild cognitive impairment and Alzheimer's disease: an in vivo MRI and DTI study. Hum Brain Mapp 32: 1349–1362.
24. Zhuang L, Wen W, Zhu W, Trollor J, Kochan N, et al. (2010) White matter integrity in mild cognitive impairment: a tract-based spatial statistics study. Neuroimage 53: 16–25.
25. Walhovd KB, Fjell AM, Amlien I, Grambaite R, Stenset V, et al. (2009) Multimodal imaging in mild cognitive impairment: Metabolism, morphometry and diffusion of the temporal-parietal memory network. Neuroimage 45: 215–223.
26. Bozzali M, Giulietti G, Basile B, Serra L, Spano B, et al. (2011) Damage to the cingulum contributes to Alzheimer's disease pathophysiology by deafferentation mechanism. Hum Brain Mapp 33: 1295–1308.
27. Grambaite R, Selnes P, Reinvang I, Aarsland D, Hessen E, et al. (2011) Executive dysfunction in mild cognitive impairment is associated with changes in frontal and cingulate white matter tracts. J Alzheimers Dis 27: 453–462.
28. Pievani M, Agosta F, Pagani E, Canu E, Sala S, et al. (2010) Assessment of white matter tract damage in mild cognitive impairment and Alzheimer's disease. Hum Brain Mapp 31: 1862–1875.
29. Chua TC, Wen W, Chen X, Kochan N, Slavin MJ, et al. (2009) Diffusion tensor imaging of the posterior cingulate is a useful biomarker of mild cognitive impairment. Am J Geriatr Psychiatry 17: 602–613.
30. Fellgiebel A, Muller MJ, Wille P, Dellani PR, Scheurich A, et al. (2005) Color-coded diffusion-tensor-imaging of posterior cingulate fiber tracts in mild cognitive impairment. Neurobiol Aging 26: 1193–1198.
31. Choo IH, Lee DY, Oh JS, Lee JS, Lee DS, et al. (2010) Posterior cingulate cortex atrophy and regional cingulum disruption in mild cognitive impairment and Alzheimer's disease. Neurobiol Aging 31: 772–779.
32. Sexton CE, Kalu UG, Filippini N, Mackay CE, Ebmeier KP (2010) A meta-analysis of diffusion tensor imaging in mild cognitive impairment and Alzheimer's disease. Neurobiol Aging 32: 2322 e2325–2318.
33. Ukmar M, Makuc E, Onor ML, Garbin G, Trevisiol M, et al. (2008) Evaluation of white matter damage in patients with Alzheimer's disease and in patients with mild cognitive impairment by using diffusion tensor imaging. Radiol Med 113: 915–922.
34. Delano-Wood L, Bondi MW, Jak AJ, Horne NR, Schweinsburg BC, et al. (2010) Stroke risk modifies regional white matter differences in mild cognitive impairment. Neurobiol Aging 31: 1721–1731.

35. Song SK, Yoshino J, Le TQ, Lin SJ, Sun SW, et al. (2005) Demyelination increases radial diffusivity in corpus callosum of mouse brain. Neuroimage 26: 132–140.

36. Acosta-Cabronero J, Williams GB, Pengas G, Nestor PJ (2010) Absolute diffusivities define the landscape of white matter degeneration in Alzheimer's disease. Brain 133: 529–539.

37. Wang L, Goldstein FC, Veledar E, Levey AI, Lah JJ, et al. (2009) Alterations in cortical thickness and white matter integrity in mild cognitive impairment measured by whole-brain cortical thickness mapping and diffusion tensor imaging. AJNR Am J Neuroradiol 30: 893–899.

38. Cui Y, Wen W, Lipnicki DM, Beg MF, Jin JS, et al. (2011) Automated detection of amnestic mild cognitive impairment in community-dwelling elderly adults: a combined spatial atrophy and white matter alteration approach. Neuroimage 59: 1209–1217.

39. Folstein MF, Folstein SE, McHugh PR (1975) "Mini-mental state". A practical method for grading the cognitive state of patients for the clinician. J Psychiatr Res 12: 189–198.

40. Morris JC (1993) The Clinical Dementia Rating (CDR): current version and scoring rules. Neurology 43: 2412–2414.

41. Delis DC, Kaplan E, Kramer JH (2001) Delis-Kaplan Executive Function System. San Antonio: The Psychological Corporation.

42. Delis DC, Kramer JH, Kaplan E, Ober BA (2000) California Verbal Learning Test, 2nd Edition. San Antonio, TX: The Psychological Corporation.

43. Griswold MA, Jakob PM, Heidemann RM, Nittka M, Jellus V, et al. (2002) Generalized autocalibrating partially parallel acquisitions (GRAPPA). Magn Reson Med 47: 1202–1210.

44. Fischl B, Salat DH, Busa E, Albert M, Dieterich M, et al. (2002) Whole brain segmentation: automated labeling of neuroanatomical structures in the human brain. Neuron 33: 341–355.

45. Fischl B, van der Kouwe A, Destrieux C, Halgren E, Segonne F, et al. (2004) Automatically parcellating the human cerebral cortex. Cereb Cortex 14: 11–22.

46. Callen DJ, Black SE, Gao F, Caldwell CB, Szalai JP (2001) Beyond the hippocampus: MRI volumetry confirms widespread limbic atrophy in AD. Neurology 57: 1669–1674.

47. Jones BF, Barnes J, Uylings HB, Fox NC, Frost C, et al. (2006) Differential regional atrophy of the cingulate gyrus in Alzheimer disease: a volumetric MRI study. Cereb Cortex 16: 1701–1708.

48. Jacobs HI, Van Boxtel MP, Jolles J, Verhey FR, Uylings HB (2011) Parietal cortex matters in Alzheimer's disease: an overview of structural, functional and metabolic findings. Neurosci Biobehav Rev 36: 297–309.

49. Tao R, Fletcher PT, Gerber S, Whitaker RT (2009) A variational image-based approach to the correction of susceptibility artifacts in the alignment of diffusion weighted and structural MRI. Inf Process Med Imaging 21: 664–675.

50. Chua TC, Wen W, Slavin MJ, Sachdev PS (2008) Diffusion tensor imaging in mild cognitive impairment and Alzheimer's disease: a review. Curr Opin Neurol 21: 83–92.

51. Benjamini Y, Drai D, Elmer G, Kafkafi N, Golani I (2001) Controlling the false discovery rate in behavior genetics research. Behavioural Brain Research 125: 279–284.

52. Hastie T, Tibshirani RJ, Friedman J (2009) The Elements of Statistical Learning: Data Mining, Inference, and Prediction.: Springer.

53. Clerx L, Visser PJ, Verhey F, Aalten P (2012) New MRI markers for Alzheimer's disease: a meta-analysis of diffusion tensor imaging and a comparison with medial temporal lobe measurements. J Alzheimers Dis 29: 405–429.

54. Cho H, Yang DW, Shon YM, Kim BS, Kim YI, et al. (2008) Abnormal integrity of corticocortical tracts in mild cognitive impairment: a diffusion tensor imaging study. J Korean Med Sci 23: 477–483.

55. Ringman JM, O'Neill J, Geschwind D, Medina L, Apostolova LG, et al. (2007) Diffusion tensor imaging in preclinical and presymptomatic carriers of familial Alzheimer's disease mutations. Brain 130: 1767–1776.

56. Chen TF, Lin CC, Chen YF, Liu HM, Hua MS, et al. (2009) Diffusion tensor changes in patients with amnesic mild cognitive impairment and various dementias. Psychiatry Res 173: 15–21.

57. Bai F, Zhang Z, Watson DR, Yu H, Shi Y, et al. (2009) Abnormal integrity of association fiber tracts in amnestic mild cognitive impairment. J Neurol Sci 278: 102–106.

58. Rose SE, McMahon KL, Janke AL, O'Dowd B, de Zubicaray G, et al. (2006) Diffusion indices on magnetic resonance imaging and neuropsychological performance in amnestic mild cognitive impairment. J Neurol Neurosurg Psychiatry 77: 1122–1128.

59. Hoeft F, Barnea-Goraly N, Haas BW, Golarai G, Ng D, et al. (2007) More is not always better: increased fractional anisotropy of superior longitudinal fasciculus associated with poor visuospatial abilities in Williams syndrome. J Neurosci 27: 11960–11965.

60. Douaud G, Jbabdi S, Behrens TE, Menke RA, Gass A, et al. (2011) DTI measures in crossing-fibre areas: increased diffusion anisotropy reveals early white matter alteration in MCI and mild Alzheimer's disease. Neuroimage 55: 880–890.

61. Pearson RC, Powell TP (1987) Anterograde vs. retrograde degeneration of the nucleus basalis medialis in Alzheimer's disease. Journal of Neural Transmission Supplementum 24: 139–146.

62. Xu Y, Jack CR Jr., O'Brien PC, Kokmen E, Smith GE, et al. (2000) Usefulness of MRI measures of entorhinal cortex versus hippocampus in AD. Neurology 54: 1760–1767.

63. De Santi S, de Leon MJ, Rusinek H, Convit A, Tarshish CY, et al. (2001) Hippocampal formation glucose metabolism and volume losses in MCI and AD. Neurobiol Aging 22: 529–539.

64. Wolf H, Grunwald M, Kruggel F, Riedel-Heller SG, Angerhofer S, et al. (2001) Hippocampal volume discriminates between normal cognition; questionable and mild dementia in the elderly. Neurobiol Aging 22: 177–186.

65. Bottino CM, Castro CC, Gomes RL, Buchpiguel CA, Marchetti RL, et al. (2002) Volumetric MRI measurements can differentiate Alzheimer's disease, mild cognitive impairment, and normal aging. Int Psychogeriatr 14: 59–72.

66. Slavin MJ, Sandstrom CK, Tran TT, Doraiswamy PM, Petrella JR (2007) Hippocampal volume and the Mini-Mental State Examination in the diagnosis of amnestic mild cognitive impairment. AJR Am J Roentgenol 188: 1404–1410.

67. Colliot O, Chetelat G, Chupin M, Desgranges B, Magnin B, et al. (2008) Discrimination between Alzheimer disease, mild cognitive impairment, and normal aging by using automated segmentation of the hippocampus. Radiology 248: 194–201.

68. Jauhiainen AM, Pihlajamaki M, Tervo S, Niskanen E, Tanila H, et al. (2009) Discriminating accuracy of medial temporal lobe volumetry and fMRI in mild cognitive impairment. Hippocampus 19: 166–175.

69. Desikan RS, Cabral HJ, Hess CP, Dillon WP, Glastonbury CM, et al. (2009) Automated MRI measures identify individuals with mild cognitive impairment and Alzheimer's disease. Brain 132: 2048–2057.

70. Muller MJ, Greverus D, Weibrich C, Dellani PR, Scheurich A, et al. (2007) Diagnostic utility of hippocampal size and mean diffusivity in amnestic MCI. Neurobiol Aging 28: 398–403.

71. Grundman M, Sencakova D, Jack CR Jr., Petersen RC, Kim HT, et al. (2002) Brain MRI hippocampal volume and prediction of clinical status in a mild cognitive impairment trial. J Mol Neurosci 19: 23–27.

72. Loewenstein DA, Acevedo A, Potter E, Schinka JA, Raj A, et al. (2009) Severity of medial temporal atrophy and amnestic mild cognitive impairment: selecting type and number of memory tests. Am J Geriatr Psychiatry 17: 1050–1058.

73. Ystad MA, Lundervold AJ, Wehling E, Espeseth T, Rootwelt H, et al. (2009) Hippocampal volumes are important predictors for memory function in elderly women. BMC Med Imaging 9: 17.

74. Walhovd KB, Fjell AM, Dale AM, McEvoy LK, Brewer J, et al. (2010) Multimodal imaging predicts memory performance in normal aging and cognitive decline. Neurobiol Aging 31: 1107–1121.

75. Edison P, Archer HA, Hinz R, Hammers A, Pavese N, et al. (2007) Amyloid, hypometabolism, and cognition in Alzheimer disease: an [11C]PIB and [18F]FDG PET study. Neurology 68: 501–508.

76. Mosconi L, Brys M, Glodzik-Sobanska L, De Santi S, Rusinek H, et al. (2007) Early detection of Alzheimer's disease using neuroimaging. Exp Gerontol 42: 129–138.

77. Petersen RC, Jack CR Jr., Xu YC, Waring SC, O'Brien PC, et al. (2000) Memory and MRI-based hippocampal volumes in aging and AD. Neurology 54: 581–587.

78. Lee DY, Fletcher E, Martinez O, Ortega M, Zozulya N, et al. (2009) Regional pattern of white matter microstructural changes in normal aging, MCI, and AD. Neurology 73: 1722–1728.

79. Davatzikos C, Ruparel K, Fan Y, Shen DG, Acharyya M, et al. (2005) Classifying spatial patterns of brain activity with machine learning methods: application to lie detection. Neuroimage 28: 663–668.

Neuroimaging biomarkers: PET

65

Diagnosed Mild Cognitive Impairment Due to Alzheimer's Disease with PET Biomarkers of Beta Amyloid and Neuronal Dysfunction

Shizuo Hatashita*, Hidetomo Yamasaki

Neurology, Shonan-Atsugi Hospital, Atsugi, Japan

Abstract

The aim of this study is to identify mild cognitive impairment (MCI) due to Alzheimer's disease (AD) using amyloid imaging of beta amyloid (Aβ) deposition and FDG imaging of reflecting neuronal dysfunction as PET biomarkers. Sixty-eight MCI patients underwent cognitive testing, [11C]-PIB PET and [18F]-FDG PET at baseline and follow-up. Regions of interest were defined on co-registered MRI. PIB distribution volume ratio (DVR) was calculated using Logan graphical analysis, and the standardized uptake value ratio (SUVR) on the same regions was used as quantitative analysis for [18F]-FDG. Thirty (44.1%) of all 68 MCI patients converted to AD over 19.2±7.1 months. The annual rate of MCI conversion was 23.4%. A positive Aβ PET biomarker significantly identified MCI due to AD in individual MCI subjects with a sensitivity (SS) of 96.6% and specificity (SP) of 42.1%. The positive predictive value (PPV) was 56.8%. A positive Aβ biomarker in APOE ϵ4/4 carriers distinguished with a SS of 100%. In individual MCI subjects who had a prominent impairment in episodic memory and aged older than 75 years, an Aβ biomarker identified MCI due to AD with a greater SS of 100%, SP of 66.6% and PPV of 80%, compared to FDG biomarker alone or both PET biomarkers combined. In contrast, when assessed in precuneus, both Aβ and FDG biomarkers had the greatest level of certainty for MCI due to AD with a PPV of 87.8%. The Aβ PET biomarker primarily defines MCI due to AD in individual MCI subjects. Furthermore, combined FDG biomarker in a cortical region of precuneus provides an added diagnostic value in predicting AD over a short period.

Citation: Hatashita S, Yamasaki H (2013) Diagnosed Mild Cognitive Impairment Due to Alzheimer's Disease with PET Biomarkers of Beta Amyloid and Neuronal Dysfunction. PLoS ONE 8(6): e66877. doi:10.1371/journal.pone.0066877

Editor: Stephen D Ginsberg, Nathan Kline Institute and New York University School of Medicine, United States of America

Received February 8, 2013; **Accepted** May 10, 2013; **Published** June 14, 2013

Funding: The authors have no support or funding to report.

Competing Interests: GE Healthcare Ltd. (Little Chalfont, Buckinghamshire, HP7 9NA, United Kingdom) entered into the sublicense agreement with the Shonan-Atsugi Hospital to allow the use of the [11C]-PIB PET imaging. There are no further patents, products in development or marketed products to declare. This does not alter the authors' adherence to all the PLOS ONE policies on sharing data and materials, as detailed online in the guide for authors.

* E-mail: hatashita@shonan-atsugi.jp

Introduction

Mild cognitive impairment (MCI) has a multitude of causes, including predementia of Alzheimer's disease (AD) and non-AD as well as depression and various physical disorders. A recent study has shown that subjects with MCI are at increased risk of developing AD and that their overall rate of progression to AD is typically 10%−15% per year [1]. Identifying subjects with MCI who are most likely to decline in cognition over time is a major focus in AD research. Revised research criteria for the diagnosis of AD have been proposed, and a framework has been developed to capture the earliest stage of AD [2]. Recently, the National Institute on Aging (NIA) - Alzheimer's Association working group has proposed the diagnostic criteria for the symptomatic pre-dementia phase of AD, referred to a MCI due to AD [3]. The MCI due to AD could be used to identify individuals with AD pathophysiological processes as the primary cause of their progressive cognitive dysfunction.

The clinical research diagnosis of MCI due to AD is based on the Core Clinical Criteria used in all clinical settings without the need of highly specialized tests and the Clinical Research Criteria with the use of biomarkers. Some biomarker measurements directly reflect the pathology of AD, including positron emission tomography (PET) amyloid imaging and cerebrospinal fluid (CSF)

beta-amyloid (Aβ) 42, while other biomarkers reflect downstream neuronal injury associated with AD, including CSF tau (both total tau and phosphorylated tau), fluorodeoxyglucose (FDG)-PET imaging and MRI. The evidence of both Aβ deposition and neuronal injury together provide the greatest probability that the AD pathophysiological processes are present. A number of studies have compared the predictive value of two or more biomarkers at a time but findings have been inconsistent [4–6]. Some aspects of the clinical research criteria may be revised, as these criteria are put into practice and new findings become available.

The PET amyloid imaging with a tracer of [11C]-labeled Pittsburgh Compound-B ([11C]-PIB:N-methyl-[11C]2-[4′-methyl-laminophenyl]-6-hydroxybenzothiazole), which has a high affinity for fibrillar Aβ, is a reliable biomarker of underlying AD pathology [7,8]. On the other hand, a FDG-PET imaging for cerebral glucose metabolism, reflecting downstream neuronal injury, provides evidence about cognitive function and progression that can not be provided by amyloid PET imaging. We have recently demonstrated that a diagnostic framework with an Aβ deposition by [11C]-PIB PET, in different clinical stages of AD, allows for an earlier and more specific AD diagnosis [9]. In addition, our preliminary study with FDG-PET imaging showed that cerebral glucose metabolism starts to decrease in prodromal AD, and greater decrease correlates with greater cognitive impairment along the continuum from prodromal to AD dementia.

The present study was conducted to define the MCI due to AD using PET amyloid imaging of Aβ deposition and FGD-PET imaging of neuronal dysfunction as a biomarker. We sought to determine whether episodic memory impairment, age and apolipoprotein-E (APOE) genotype have an effect on progression to AD dementia.

Materials and Methods

Subjects

Sixty-eight Japanese participants were recruited from our memory clinic. All were between 50 and 90 years of age. They underwent neurological and neuropsychological assessment, and neuroimaging at baseline and once more after 12–24 months. Global cognitive status was assessed with the Mini-Mental-State Examination (MMSE) [10] and severity of dementia was rated on the Clinical Dementia Rating (CDR) scale [11]. The CDR sum of boxes (CDR SB) score was a simple sum of the score obtained in each of the 6 rated domains. A memory measure of immediate and delayed recall of a paragraph from the Wechsler Memory Scale-Revised (WMS-R) Logical Memory II was carried out as a simple episodic memory test [12]. The apolipoprotein E (APOE) genotype was determined from venous blood samples.

All 68 MCI patients met the Core Clinical Criteria for MCI, proposed by the NIA-Alzheimer's Association workgroup [3], including concern about a change in cognition, impairment in one or more cognitive domains, preservation of independence in functional abilities, and no dementia. Other systemic or brain diseases that could account for the decline in cognition, including degenerative, vascular, depressive, traumatic, medical comorbidities, or mixed disease were excluded. The MMSE score was greater than or equal to 24, and global CDR score was at least 0.5 in the memory domain. For the episodic memory measure, delayed recall of a paragraph from the WMS-R Logical Memory II (maximum score 25) was used with the following cutoff scores based on education: these scores were less than 8 for subject with ≥16 years of education, 4 for subjects with 8–15 years of education, and 2 for subjects with 0–7 years of education [12]. AD diagnosis was based on the criteria of the National Institute of Neurological and Communicative Disorders and Stroke-Alzheimer's Disease and Related Disorders Association (NINCDS-ADRDA) [13].

Each subject or their caregiver provided written informed consent for participation. The study protocol was approved by the Institutional Review Board of the Mirai Iryo Research Center Inc (Tokyo, Japan).

PET imaging

All PET scans were performed on the same day as the cognitive testing, using a Siemens ECAT ACCEL scanner in 3-dimensional scanning mode, providing 63 contiguous 2.46-mm slices with a 5.6-mm transaxial and a 5.4-mm axial resolution. All imaging data were reconstructed into a 128×128 matrix. The amyloid PET imaging was accomplished with the radiotracer [11C]-PIB, as previously described in detail [9]. Briefly, [11C]-PIB was produced in our PET center using the one-step [11C] methyl triflate approach. [11C]-PIB was injected intravenously as a bolus with a mean dose of 561.5±11.2 MBq (n = 68). Dynamic PET scanning was performed for 60 minutes according to a predetermined protocol. Sixty minutes following the completion of [11C]-PIB image, the subjects were injected intravenously with 249.9±28.8 MBq (n = 68) of [18F]-FDG and remained in a dark, quiet room.

Fifteen-minute static FDG-PET scans were acquired with the same camera after a 45-minute uptake period, and the image was reconstructed using the same image reconstruction techniques.

Image analysis

All subjects underwent T1-weighed MRI (1.5 T) for co-registration with the PET images. MRI-based correction of PET data for partial volume effects was carried out using the PMOD software (PMOD Technologies Ltd., Adliswil, Switzerland). Regions of interest were manually drawn on the co-registered MR image, including the following cortical regions: lateral temporal cortex, medial temporal cortex, frontal cortex, occipital cortex, parietal cortex, sensory motor cortex, anterior cingulate gyrus, posterior cingulate gyrus, precuneus cortex and cerebellar cortex.

Data management

Levels of PIB retention were determined by the distribution volume ratio (DVR) with Logan graphical analysis for 35 to 60 minutes with cerebellar gray matter as reference [14]. Regional DVR values of each cortical region and the cortical DVR value of the whole cortical regions were calculated. DVR PET images were created for visual inspection with a rainbow color scale. Scans of all subjects were visually assessed with 2 readers as amyloid-positive or amyloid-negative for cortical PIB retention. Amyloid-positive images showed greatly increased PIB retention in the cortex compared to white matter and a typical PIB pattern of cortical amyloid deposition, whereas amyloid-negative images showed no PIB retention in any of the cortical regions.

The same co-registration method was applied for quantification of [18F]-FDG. A standardized uptake value (SUV) of the same region was obtained and subsequently normalized to the cerebellar cortex as reference. Glucose metabolism was referred to as the SUV ratio (SUVR).

Statistical analysis

Group differences were evaluated with analysis of variance (ANOVA), followed by Bonferroni post hoc tests to assess the significance. Analysis correlation between DVR values, FDG SUV values, age, MMSE scores, CDR SB scores and WMS-R recall scores yielded Pearson's product moment correlation coefficient (r). Categorical variables were examined with Fisher's exact test. Paired t-tests were used to study changes between baseline and follow-up data. Results were considered significant at $p < 0.05$. Data are presented as means ± standard deviations (SD). Statistical analyses were performed with Statcel 3 software (OMS Inc. Japan).

Results

Clinical data and cognitive function

Thirty (44.1%) of the 68 patients with MCI converted to AD during the follow-up of 19.2±7.1 months (converters), while the remaining 38 (55.9%) did not progress to AD (stable patients). Twelve (50%) of 24 MCI patients aged 75–89 years converted to AD, compared to 18 (40.9%) of 44 MCI patients aged 50–74 years. Fourteen (50%) of 28 APOE ε4 carriers with MCI and 16 (40%) of 40 APOE ε4 non-carriers converted to AD. In particular, 5 (83.3%) of 6 APOE ε4/4 carriers with MCI converted to AD. Overall rate of MCI progression to AD was 23.4% per year.

The demographic characteristics of MCI converters and stable patients at baseline and follow-up are summarized in Table 1. The MMSE and CDR SB scores in MCI converters at baseline did not differ from those in stable patients. The mean MMSE score of

MCI converters decreased to 22.8±2.5 at follow-up and their CDR SB score increased to 2.5±1.0. The mean MMSE score of MCI converters decreased approximately 4 points whereas that of stable patients remained unchanged. There were no significant differences in age or sex between MCI converters and stable patients. None of the patients with MCI reverted to a normal status or converted to a non-AD dementia.

For the memory measure of WMS-R Logical Memory II Immediate and Delayed Recall, the mean delayed paragraph recall score at baseline was 1.7±2.0 for converters, which were significantly lower than the mean score for stable patients despite their having approximately the same level of education (Table 1). However, there was no significant difference in the mean immediate paragraph recall scores between MCI converters and stable patients.

Aβ deposition

Fifty-one (75%) of the 68 MCI patients had marked PIB retention in the frontal, parietal and lateral temporal cortical regions as well as the cingulate gyrus and precuneus, showing the typical AD pattern at baseline (Figure 1). Of 51 MCI patients who had Aβ deposition, 29 (56.8%) patients converted to AD during the follow-up period while the remaining 22 patients did not convert despite similar Aβ deposition. In contrast, 16 of 17 MCI patients who had no PIB retention in any cortical region were stable and only 1 MCI patient converted to AD.

Cortical PIB DVR values for MCI converters and stable patients are presented in Figure 2. At baseline, the mean value of cortical DVR in amyloid-positive converters (2.02±0.30, n = 29, p<0.01) was significantly higher than that in amyloid-negative stable patients (1.26±0.16, n = 16). In the amyloid-positive stable patients, in addition, the mean cortical DVR value (2.05±0.37, n = 22) was similar to amyloid-positive converters. Also, there were no significant differences in the regional DVR values of any cortical region between amyloid-positive converters and stable patients. The mean value of cortical DVR in amyloid-positive converters at follow-up (2.11±0.37, n = 29) was not significantly different from baseline (Figure 2). There were no significant changes in cortical DVR values between baseline and follow-up in amyloid-positive or amyloid–negative stable patients.

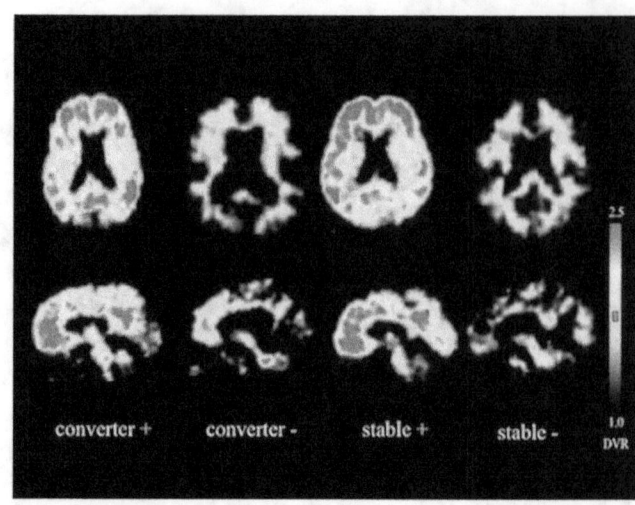

Figure 1. PIB-PET DVR images from 4 representative MCI converters and stable patients with (+) and without amyloid deposition (−) at baseline.
doi:10.1371/journal.pone.0066877.g001

Glucose metabolism

Fifty-seven (83.8%) of 68 MCI patients had reduced glucose metabolism (FDG SUVR ≤0.99) in whole cortical regions at baseline, 28 patients (49.1%) of whom progressed to AD during the follow-up period. A mean FDG SUVR value for the whole cortical regions in converters was 0.93±0.06 (n = 30, p<0.01) at baseline, significantly different from stable patients (0.98±0.06, n = 38). In cortical regions of the lateral temporal cortex, parietal cortex and precuneus, in particular, MCI converters had significantly lower regional FDG SUVR values at baseline compared to stable patients (Figure 3). At follow-up, MCI converters did not have significant decreases in mean values of FDG SUVR in whole cortical regions or each cortical region.

Table 1. Demographic Characteristics of Patients With MCI.

	Baseline		Follow up	
Characteristic	Converter	Stable	Converter	Stable
study popu	30	38	30	38
Education (yr)	12.2±2.4	12.0±2.0	12.2±2.4	12.0±2.0
MMSE	26.5±1.5	27.3±1.6	22.8±2.5*	27.3±1.6
global CDR	0.5	0.5	0.6±0.2	0.5
CDR SB	0.8±0.2	0.8±0.3	2.5±1.0*	0.7±0.4
Immediate Rec.	4.9±2.7	6.9±3.1	4.0±2.8	7.2±3.9
Delayed Rec.	1.7±2.0*	4.6±3.4	1.5±2.3	4.9±4.3
APOE ε4/4, ε4/3	14 (46.6%)	14 (36.8%)	14 (46.6%)	14 (36.8%)

MCI: mild cognitive impairment, MMSE: Mini-Mental State Examination, CDR: Clinical Dementia Rating, CDR SB: Clinical Dementia Rating sum of boxes score, study popu: number of patients in the study population, yr: years. Rec: WMS-R recall scores, APOE: apolipoprotein E, Data are presented as means ± SD, * Statistically significant difference from stable patients by multiple comparisons post hoc tests (p<0.05).
doi:10.1371/journal.pone.0066877.t001

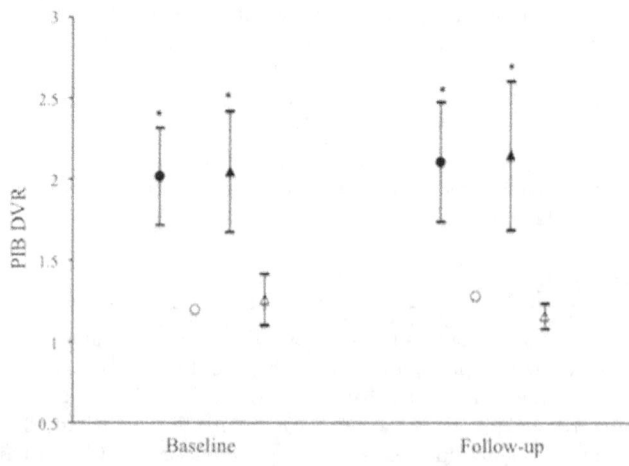

Figure 2. The cortical PIB DVR values in PIB-positive MCI converters (closed circles, n = 29), PIB-negative MCI converter (open circles, n = 1), PIB-positive stable MCI patients (closed triangles, n = 22), and PIB-negative stable MCI patients (open triangles, n = 16) at baseline and follow-up. Data are presented as mean ± SD. *Statistically significant difference from the PIB-negative stable MCI patients by multiple comparisons post hoc tests (p<0.01).
doi:10.1371/journal.pone.0066877.g002

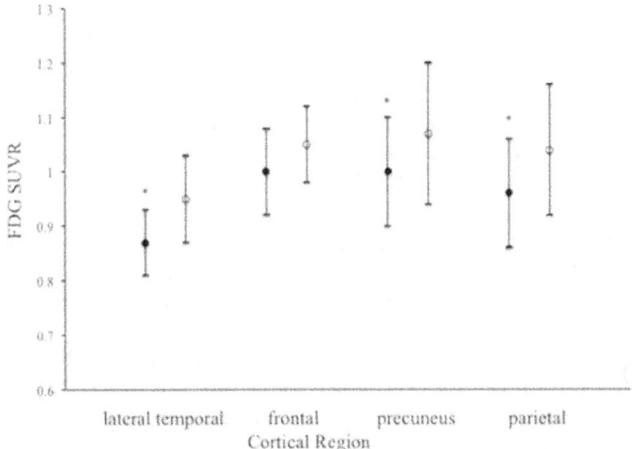

Figure 3. Regional FDG SUVR values in the lateral temporal cortex, frontal cortex, precuneus and parietal cortex of MCI converters (closed circles, n = 30) and stable patients (open circles, n = 38) at baseline. Data are presented as means ± SD. *Statistically significant difference from the stable patients by multiple comparisons post hoc tests (p<0.05).
doi:10.1371/journal.pone.0066877.g003

Comparison between Aβ deposition and glucose metabolism

Individual cortical FDG SUVR values were not correlated significantly with PIB DVR values in all MCI patients at baseline (r = −0.22, p = 0.06, n = 68). Also, there was also no significant correlation between regional FDG and DVR values in the lateral temporal cortex, frontal cortex, parietal cortex or precuneus.

Diagnostic value of PET biomarkers

The relationships between individual cortical PIB DVR and FDG SUVR values for all 68 MCI patients are shown in Figure 4. Individual PIB DVR values for 29 (96.6%) of 30 converters and 22 (57.8%) of 38 stable patients exceeded the lowest value of amyloid-positive subjects (DVR ≥1.49), which is used as a positive Aβ PET biomarker of Aβ deposition. On the other hand, individual FDG SUVR values were below the lower value (FDG SUVR ≤0.99), which is used as positive FDG PET biomarker, for 28 (93.3%) of 30 converters and 29 (76.3%) of 38 stable patients. Positive or negative value fell within the reliable range, as previously demonstrated [9], and standardization of biomarkers for both PET amyloid imaging and FDG-PET imaging was possible in our clinical setting.

We used a dichotomous test using chi-square analysis to assess the sensitivity (SS) and specificity (SP) of positive Aβ PET and FDG PET biomarkers for MCI due to AD (Table 2). A positive Aβ PET biomarker significantly identified MCI due to AD in individual MCI subjects with a sensitivity of 96.6% and a specificity of 42.1%, compared to negative Aβ PET biomarker (p<0.01). The positive predictive value (PPV) was 56.8%. A positive FDG PET biomarker had a sensitivity of 93.3% and a specificity of 23.6%. Combined positive Aβ and FDG biomarkers did not significantly discriminate MCI due to AD in individual MCI subjects.

In individual MCI subjects with APOE ε4, a positive Aβ PET biomarker significantly discriminated MCI due to AD (SS = 100%, SP = 28.5%) in addition to individual APOE ε4 non-carriers (SS = 93.7%, SP = 50%), compared to negative biomarker. In particular, a positive Aβ PET biomarker in the individual MCI subjects with APOE ε4/4 distinguished with a

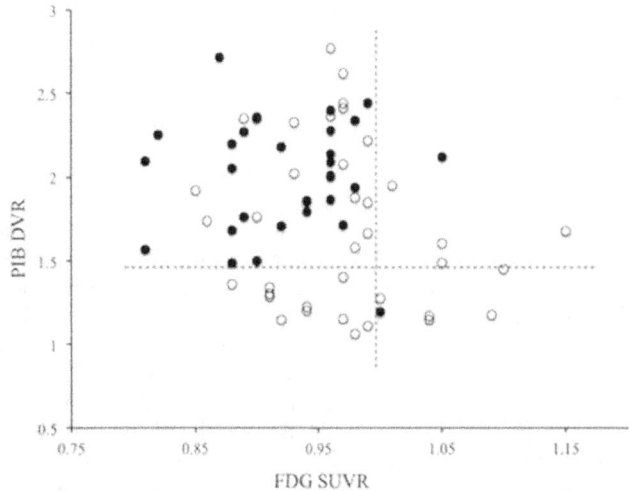

Figure 4. Scatter plot of the relationship between cortical PIB DVR and FDG SUVR values in individual MCI converters (closed circles, n = 30) and stable patients (open circles, n = 38). The horizontal dotted line indicates the greatest value of PIB DVR (≥1.49). The vertical dotted line indicates the lower value of FDG SUVR (≤0.99).
doi:10.1371/journal.pone.0066877.g004

sensitivity of 100% and a specificity of 0%. Combining Aβ and FDG PET biomarkers did not improve their sensitivity and specificity in individual APOE ε4 carriers and non-carriers.

When individual MCI patients, aged 75−89 years, had lower WMS-R Logical Memory (delayed recall score ≤4), a positive Aβ PET biomarker had greater sensitivity 100% and specificity 66.6% at identifying MCI due to AD (p<0.01), and the positive predictive value was 80%. However, combining positive Aβ and FDG PET biomarkers did not improve the discrimination of MCI due to AD compared to positive Aβ PET biomarker alone. In contrast, when assessed in a cortical region of precuneus, a combination of positive Aβ and FDG PET biomarkers discriminated MCI due to AD from individual MCI subjects with the

Table 2. Sensitivity and specificity of positive Aβ and/or FDG PET biomarkers for MCI due to AD in individual MCI patients.

Biomarker	SS	SP	PPV	NPV
aged 50–89				
Aβ PET	96.6	42.1	56.8	94.1
FDG PET	93.3	23.6	49.1	81.8
Aβ+ FDG PET	96.5	21.7	60.8	83.3
aged ≥75 years, lower delayed recall				
Aβ PET	100	66.6	80.0	100
FDG PET	91.6	44.4	68.7	80.0
Aβ+ FDG PET	100	60.0	84.6	100
APOE ε4 carriers				
Aβ PET	100	28.5	58.3	100
FDG PET	100	21.4	56.0	100
Aβ+ FDG PET	100	18.1	60.8	100

SS: sensitivity, SP: specificity, PPV: positive predictive value, NPV: negative predictive value, Aβ: β-amyloid, MCI: mild cognitive impairment, APOE: apolipoprotein E, Data are presented as percentages.
doi:10.1371/journal.pone.0066877.t002

greatest sensitivity of 96.6% and specificity of 73.3% (P<0.01). The combination had a higher positive predictive value of 87.8%.

Discussion

We demonstrated that 44.1% of 68 MCI patients converted to AD during a follow-up of 19.2 ± 7.1 months and the rate of MCI conversion was 23.4% per year. A recent study has reported that 48% of 31 subjects with MCI converted to AD during a follow-up period of 2.9 years [15]. The Alzheimer's Disease Neuroimaging Initiative has reported that 32.9% of 85 single-domain or multiple-domain amnestic MCI patients converted to AD during a follow-up period of 1.9 ± 0.4 years (an annual rate of 17.2%) [1]. Thus, conversion rates vary greatly depending on the criteria applied, the nature of the subject population and the period of observation.

In the present study, 50% of APOE ε4 carriers with MCI converted to AD while 40% of APOE ε4 non-carriers with MCI converted. This supports that the progressive value of genetic assessment alone is comparatively low although a high percentage of progressive MCI patients carry the APOE ε4 allele [18]. In contrast, this study showed that 83.3% of APOE ε4/4 carriers with MCI converted to AD. These findings indicate that the presence of the APOE ε4/4 in MCI patients is strongly associated with conversion to AD. The homozygous carriers of the APOE ε4 allele could have an increased risk of MCI progression to AD.

The present study demonstrated, using [11C]-PIB PET imaging, that 56.8% of 51 MCI patients with Aβ deposition converted to AD over 2 years, compared to 5.8% of 17 MCI patients without Aβ deposition. In addition, when MCI patients with Aβ deposition, aged 75−89 years, had an impaired episodic memory, the rate of MCI conversion was 80%. It has previously been reported that 82% of PIB-positive amnestic subjects with MCI converted to AD over a 3-year follow-up period [15], and 67% of MCI subjects with high PIB retention converted over 2 years [16]. These findings indicate that a high proportion of MCI patients with Aβ deposition convert to AD within a short period. In vivo detection of Aβ deposition with PET imaging is a useful prognostic tool for identifying MCI progression to AD.

We found that MCI converters had the regional hypometabolism in cortical regions of lateral temporal cortex, parietal cortex and precuneus at baseline compared to stable patients. Our results are consistent with the previous study that regional metabolic reduction, in temporoparietal or posterior cingulate cortices, was detected at baseline in MCI patients who converted to AD within 1 year, compared with non-converters [17]. The AD pathophysiological process has been demonstrated to be temporoparietal and/or precuneus hypometabolism, which is a topographic pattern characteristic of AD. Therefore, if a regional hypometabolism in the temporal, parietal and/or precuneus cortices is detected on FDG PET imaging, the progression to AD may occur within a few years.

An evaluation in predictive accuracy by combining different biomarkers and neuropsychological variables for the prediction of AD in MCI has been reported [19]. Inconsistencies in recent findings are likely due to a variability in neuroimaging processing techniques, CSF protein immunoassay techniques, setting cutoff

values for subject categorization, study design, and statistical analysis. To determine MCI due to AD, the biomarker in diagnosis reflecting Aβ and downstream neuronal injury has been proposed to be most important [3].

In the present study, we applied PET biomarkers to diagnose MCI due to AD in individual MCI subjects. An Aβ PET biomarker identified MCI due to AD with a sensitivity of 96.6% and a specificity of 42.1%. In individual APOE ε4/4 carriers with MCI, in particular, the Aβ PET biomarker distinguished MCI due to AD with greater certainty. Furthermore, when MCI subjects had a prominent impairment in episodic memory and aged older than 75 years, an Aβ PET biomarker provided a further increased level of certainty with a sensitivity of 100% and a specificity of 66.6%, compared to FDG PET biomarker alone or both PET biomarkers combined. A recent meta-analysis has shown that sensitivity and specificity of PIB-PET for predicting clinical progression to AD range from 83.3–100% and 41.7–76.8%, respectively [20]. These findings indicate that the sensitivity of an Aβ PET biomarker is high in the prediction of conversion to AD while the specificity is low. The Aβ PET biomarker is primarily required for diagnosing MCI due to AD in individual MCI subjects.

Furthermore, in this study, a positive FDG PET alone or combined positive Aβ and FDG biomarkers did not significantly discriminate MCI due to AD in individual MCI subjects. Although a FDG PET biomarker has been associated with the neuropathology of AD, it is not specific for AD. In contrast, when assessed in the precuneus with regional hypometabolism, both Aβ and FDG PET biomarkers had a greater level of certainty for MCI due to AD with the greatest sensitivity of 96.6% and specificity of 73.3%. The combination had the highest positive predictive value of 87.8%. We suggests that most individuals with a diagnosis of MCI due to AD, using Aβ and FDG PET biomarkers in a cortical region of precuneus, progress to AD even within a short period.

The MCI due to AD could be more certainly diagnosed in individual MCI subjects, based on core clinical criteria, with the conjugation of biomarkers of PET amyloid imaging and FDG-PET imaging. The clinical research diagnosis of MCI due to AD would have the greatest potential benefit for assessing risk level in single patients before the onset of the disease, providing a basis for earlier therapeutic and pharmacologic intervention, patient counseling, and the design of clinical trials.

Acknowledgments

GE Healthcare Ltd. (Little Chalfont, Buckinghamshire, HP7 9NA, United Kingdom) entered into the sublicense agreement with the Shonan-Atsugi Hospital to allow the use of the [11C]-PIB PET imaging. The authors thank all the patients and their relatives who have participated in this study, and the staff at Shonan-Atsugi Hospital.

Author Contributions

Conceived and designed the experiments: SH HY. Performed the experiments: SH HY. Analyzed the data: SH HY. Contributed reagents/materials/analysis tools: SH HY. Wrote the paper: SH HY.

References

1. Petersen RC, Aise PS, Beckett LA, Donohue MC, Gamst AC, et al. (2010) Alzheimer's Disease Neuroimaging Initiative (ADNI). Neurology 74: 201–209.
2. Dubois B, Feldman HH, Jacova C, Dekosky ST, Barberger-Gateauet P, et al. (2007) Research criteria for the diagnosis of Alzheimer's disease: revising the NINCDS-ADRDA criteria. Lancet Neurol 6: 734–746.
3. Albert MS, DeKosky ST, Diskson D, Dubois B, Feldman HH, et al. (2011) The diagnosis of mild cognitive impairment due to Alzheimer's disease: Recommendation from the National Institute on Aging-Alzheimer's Association workgroups on diagnostic guidelines for Alzheimer's disease. Alzheimers Dement 7: 270–279.
4. Forsberg A, Engler H, Almkvist O, Blomquist G, Hagman G, et al. (2008) PET imaging of amyloid deposition in patients with mild cognitive impairment. Neurobiol Aging 29: 1456–1465.

5. Jack CR, Lowe VJ, Weigand SD, Wiste HJ, Senjem ML, et al. (2009) Serial PIB and MCI in normal, mild cognitive impairment and Alzheimer's disease: implications for sequence of pathologic events in Alzheimer's disease. Brain 132: 1355–1365.

6. Landau SM, Harvey D, Madison CM, Reiman EM, Foster NL, et al. (2010) Comparing predictors of conversion and decline in mild cognitive impairment. Neurology 75: 230–238.

7. Mathis CA, Wang Y, Holt DP, Huang GF, Debnath ML, et al. (2003) Synthesis and evaluation of [11C]-labeled 6-substituted 2-arylbenzothiazoles as amyloid imaging agents. J Med Chem 46: 2740–2754.

8. Klunk WE, Engler H, Nordberg A, Wang Y, Blomqvist G, et al. (2004) Imaging brain amyloid in Alzheimer' disease with Pittsburgh Compound-B. Ann Neurol 55: 306–319.

9. Hatashita S, Yamasaki H (2010) Clinically different stages of Alzheimer's disease associated by amyloid deposition with [11C]-PIB PET imaging. J Alzheimers Dis 21: 995–1003.

10. Folstein MF, Folstein SE, McHugh PR (1975) 'Mini-mental state' A practical method for grading the cognitive state of patients for the clinician. J Psychiatr Res 12: 189–198.

11. Morris JC (1993) The clinical dementia rating (CDR): current version and scoring rules. Neurology 43: 2412–2414.

12. Wechsler DA (1987) Wechsler Memory Scale-Revised. New York: Psychological Corporation. New York.

13. Mckhann G, Drachman DA, Folstein M, KatzmanR, Price D, et al. (1984) Clinical diagnosis of Alzheimer's disease-report of the NINCDS-ADRDA work group under the auspices of Department of Health and Human Services Task Force on Alzheimer's disease. Neurology 34: 939–944.

14. Lopresti BJ, Klunk WE, Mathis CA, Hoge JA, Ziolko SK, et al. (2005) Simplified quantification of Pittsburgh Compound B amyloid imaging PET studies: a comparative analysis. J Nucl Med 46: 1959–1972.

15. Okello A, Koivumen J, Edison P, Acher HA, Turkheimer FE, et al. (2009) Conversion of amyloid positive and negative MCI to AD over 3 years: An [11C]-PIB PET study. Neurology 73: 754–760.

16. Villemagne VL, Pike KE, Chetelat G, Ellis KA, Mulligan RS, et al. (2011) Longitudinal Assessment of AB and cognition in Aging and Alzheimer Disease. Ann Neurol 69: 181–192.

17. Drzezga A, Lautenschlager N, Siebner H, Riemenschneider M, Willoch F, et al. (2003) Cerebral metabolic change accompanying conversion of mild cognitive impairment into Alzheimer's disease: a PET follow-up study. Eur J Nucl Med Mol Imaging 30: 1104–1113.

18. Drzezga A, Grimer T, Riemenschneider M, Lautenschlager N, Siebner H, et al. (2005) Prediction of individual clinical outcome in MCI by means of genetic assessment and [18F]-FDG PET. J Nucl Med 46: 1625–1632.

19. Ewers M, Walsh C, Trojanowski JQ, Shaw LM, Peterson RC, et al. (2012) Prediction of conversion from mil cognitive impairment to Alzheimer's disease dementia based upon biomarkers and neuropsychological test performance. Neurobiol Aging 33: 1203–1214.

20. Zhang S, Han D, Tan X, Feng J, Guo Y, et al. (2012) Diagostic accuracy of [18F]-FDG and [11C]-PIB-PET for prediction of short-term conversion to Alzheimer's disease in subjects with mild cognitive impairment. Int J Clin Pract 66: 185–198.

Regional Amyloid Deposition in Amnestic Mild Cognitive Impairment and Alzheimer's Disease Evaluated by [18F]AV-45 Positron Emission Tomography in Chinese Population

Kuo-Lun Huang[1,9], Kun-Ju Lin[2,3,9], Ing-Tsung Hsiao[2,3], Hung-Chou Kuo[1], Wen-Chuin Hsu[1], Wen-Li Chuang[1], Mei-Ping Kung[2,4], Shiaw-Pyng Wey[2,3], Chia-Ju Hsieh[2,3], Yau-Yau Wai[5], Tzu-Chen Yen[2]*, Chin-Chang Huang[1]*

1 Department of Neurology and Dementia Center, Chang Gung Memorial Hospital and Chang Gung University, Taoyuan, Taiwan, 2 Molecular Imaging Center and Department of Nuclear Medicine, Chang Gung University and Chang Gung Memorial Hospital, Taoyuan, Taiwan, 3 Healthy Aging Research Center and Department of Medical Imaging and Radiological Sciences, College of Medicine, Chang Gung University, Taoyuan, Taiwan, 4 Department of Radiology, University of Pennsylvania, Pennsylvania, United States of America, 5 Department of Radiology, Chang Gung Memorial Hospital, Taoyuan, Taiwan

Abstract

Background: To compare the neocortical amyloid loads among cognitively normal (CN), amnestic mild cognitive impairment (aMCI), and Alzheimer's disease (AD) subjects with [18F]AV-45 positron emission tomography (PET).

Materials and Methods: [18F]AV-45 PET was performed in 11 CN, 13 aMCI, and 12 AD subjects to compare the cerebral cortex-to-whole cerebellum standard uptake value ratios (SUVRs) of global and individual volumes of interest (VOIs) cerebral cortex. The correlation between global cortical [18F]AV-45 SUVRs and Mini-Mental State Examination (MMSE) scores was analyzed.

Results: The global cortical [18F]AV-45 SUVRs were significantly different among the CN (1.08 ± 0.08), aMCI (1.27 ± 0.06), and AD groups (1.34 ± 0.13) ($p=0.0003$) with amyloidosis positivity rates of 9%, 62%, and 92% in the three groups respectively. Compared to CN subjects, AD subjects had higher SUVRs in the global cortical, precuneus, frontal, parietal, occipital, temporal, and posterior cingulate areas; while aMCI subjects had higher values in the global cortical, precuneus, frontal, occipital and posterior cingulate areas. There were negative correlations of MMSE scores with SUVRs in the global cortical, precuneus, frontal, parietal, occipital, temporal, posterior cingulate and anterior cingulate areas on a combined subject pool of the three groups after age and education attainment adjustment.

Conclusions: Amyloid deposition occurs relatively early in precuneus, frontal and posterior cingulate in aMCI subjects. Higher [18F]AV-45 accumulation is present in parietal, occipital and temporal gyri in AD subjects compared to the aMCI group. Significant correlation between MMSE scores and [18F]AV-45 SUVRs can be observed among CN, aMCI and AD subjects.

Citation: Huang K-L, Lin K-J, Hsiao I-T, Kuo H-C, Hsu W-C, et al. (2013) Regional Amyloid Deposition in Amnestic Mild Cognitive Impairment and Alzheimer's Disease Evaluated by [18F]AV-45 Positron Emission Tomography in Chinese Population. PLoS ONE 8(3): e58974. doi:10.1371/journal.pone.0058974

Editor: Karl Herholz, University of Manchester, United Kingdom

Received November 28, 2012; **Accepted** February 8, 2013; **Published** March 14, 2013

Funding: This study was carried out with financial support from the National Science Council, Taiwan (Grant NSC-97-2314-B-182A-050, NSC-98-2314-B-182A-056, NSC-100-2314-B-182-003, NSC-100-2314-B-182A-091-MY3, and NSC-101-2314-B-182A-061-MY2), and Chang Gung Memorial Hospital (Grant CMRPG300071, CMRPG390793, and CMRPD1A0312). The funders had no role in study design, data collection and analysis, decision to publish, or preparation of the manuscript.

Competing Interests: The authors have declared that no competing interests exist.

* E-mail: cch0537@adm.cgmh.org.tw (CCH); yentc1110@gmail.com (TCY)

9 These authors contributed equally to this work.

Introduction

Alzheimer's disease (AD) is the most common cause of dementia and leads to progressive dysfunctions in memory and other cognitive domains. The diagnosis of AD is hampered by a lack of noninvasive biomarkers. Moreover, 67% of dementia patients with mild clinical symptoms may not be diagnosed by physicians [1]. The most widely accepted pathogeneses of AD include increased production or impaired clearance of amyloid-beta oligomers, resulting in excessive fibrillary amyloid plaque accumulation in the brain. Furthermore, the accumulation of amyloid plaques may precede the diagnosis of AD by 10 years [2]. Therefore, a reliable biomarker for determination of amyloid plaque aggregates could facilitate an early diagnosis and treatment of AD.

Molecular neuroimaging modalities such as positron emission tomography (PET) have a potential to provide functional information on the pathological process of AD. Several PET ligands have been investigated to determine their ability for detecting amyloid plaques, including [^{11}C]PIB [3], [^{11}C]SBI-13 [4], [^{11}C]BF-227 [5], [^{11}C]MeS-IMPY [6], [^{18}F]FDDNP [7], [^{18}F]AV-45 (florbetapir) [8], [^{18}F]AV-1 (florbetaben, BAY94-9172) [9], and [^{18}F]GE067 (flutemetamol) [10]. At present, the most widely researched imaging technique utilizes [^{11}C]PIB to detect amyloid plaques, but the short half-life of the carbon-11 (approximately 20.4 min) of [^{11}C]PIB limits its clinical application. On the other hand, PET tracers utilizing fluorine-18 have been designed to overcome this limitation since this isotope has a longer half-life of about 109.4 min, which makes off-site preparation and regional distribution easier. Among these tracers, [^{18}F]AV-45 has gained great attention as a PET imaging agent targeting amyloid plaques and been selected as the standard plaque imaging agent for the Alzheimer's Disease Neuroimaging Initiative (ADNI) [11]. [^{18}F]AV-45 shows good amyloid-binding affinity with a desirable pharmacokinetics. It remains at steady levels in the brain 30–90 min after injection, and a short imaging time (5–10 min) is sufficient [8]. A recent phase III study with 35 terminally ill participants was reported to compare [^{18}F]AV-45 imaging and postmortem amyloid immunohistochemistry. The results showed that [^{18}F]AV-45 imaging is well correlated with postmortem amyloid immunohistochemistry [12].

In this preliminary study, we aimed to compare the amyloid plaque distribution on [^{18}F]AV-45 PET scan in cognitively normal (CN), amnestic mild cognitive impairment (aMCI) and AD subjects, and correlate the cerebral cortical amyloid load with cognitive functioning among CN, aMCI and AD subjects. In addition, we aimed to determine a cutoff value to differentiate CN subjects from AD subjects in a Chinese population.

Methods

Participants

Thirty-six subjects were studied at the Center for Dementia of the Linkou Chang Gung Memorial Hospital (CGMH), Taiwan, including 11 CN, 13 aMCI, and 12 AD subjects. All subjects underwent a neurological examination, neurocognitive evaluation, and routine blood analysis. Study subjects were categorized on the basis of the consensus of panels composed of neurologists, neuropsychologists, neuroradiologists and experts in nuclear medicine. The CN subjects were volunteers with normal cognitive performance; the methods for CN subject recruitment have been described previously [8]. The diagnostic criteria for aMCI were based on those proposed by Petersen *et al* [13]: (1) subjective memory complaints by the patient or an informant, (2) relatively normal performance in other cognitive domains and (3) normal activities of daily living, (4) objective memory impairment on at least one neurocognitive test of memory performance, and (5) no dementia according to DSM-IV criteria [14]. No rigid cutoff score was applied to determine objective memory impairment, but aMCI was generally determined when memory measures fell 1.0–1.5 standard deviations below the means for age-matched norms in Taiwan. The diagnosis of AD was made when subjects fulfilled the National Institute of Neurological and Communicative Disorders and Stroke–Alzheimer's Disease and Related Disorders Association (NINCDS-ADRDA) criteria for probable AD [15]. A comprehensive battery of neurocognitive tests was administered to obtain objective evidence of cognitive impairment, including the Mini-Mental State Examination (MMSE) [16], Clinical Dementia Rating (CDR), logical memory in the Wechsler memory scale-revised (LM), visual-association memory test (VAMT), category verbal fluency test (CVFT), trail-making A test (TMAT), and clock-drawing test (CDT) [17]. Prior to enrollment, the study objectives and protocol were well informed to all subjects and also

their next of kin, caregivers or guardians if subjects were clinically suspected of AD. The written informed consent was obtained from all subjects before their participation in the study. In addition, the next of kin or guardians of 6 AD patients also gave their written informed consents since these patients' capacity to comprehend the study protocol was compromised or they could not sign their names clearly. The study protocol and the procedure of obtaining informed consents were approved by the institutional review board of Chang Gung Memorial Hospital and the Governmental Department of Health.

Magnetic Resonance Imaging (MRI) Acquisition

The MRI images were acquired on a 3T MR scanner (Magnetom Trio, a TIM system; Siemens, Erlangen, Germany). The scanning protocol included an axial fluid attenuation inversion recovery (FLAIR) sequence (TR = 9000 ms, TE = 87 ms, TI = 2500 ms, voxel size = $0.9 \times 0.7 \times 4$ mm^3) and a whole brain axial three-dimensional T1-weighted magnetization prepared rapid acquisition gradient echo (MP-RAGE) sequence (TR = 2000 ms, TE = 2.63 ms, TI = 900 ms, flip angle = 9°, voxel size = $1 \times 1 \times 1$ mm^3), which was subsequently reformatted as planes perpendicular to the long axis of the hippocampus in 2 mm slice thickness. An additional coronal T2-weighted turbo spin echo sequence (TR = 7400 ms, TE = 95 ms, voxel size = $0.4 \times 0.4 \times 2$ mm^3) was acquired with the identical geometric orientation with the reformatted coronal T1-weighted images [8].

[^{18}F]AV-45 PET Imaging

[^{18}F]AV-45 was synthesized at the cyclotron facility of Chang Gung Memorial Hospital following the method described previously [18]. In brief, [^{18}F]fluoride was obtained by bombardment of ^{18}O-enriched water with 12-MeV protons accelerated in a SHI-12S cyclotron (Sumitomo Heavy Industries, Tokyo, Japan). The [^{18}F]fluoride was then trapped on an Accel Plus QMA cartridge (Waters (Milford, MA) and eluted to a reaction vessel using a mixture of K_2CO_3, Kryptofix2.2.2 and acetonitrile. Following azeotropic distillation, the dehydrated [^{18}F]fluoride was reacted with AV-105, the precursor for synthesis of [^{18}F]AV-45 provided by Avid Radiopharmaceiticals (Philadelphia, PA), to form a fluorinated intermediate, N-Boc-[^{18}F]AV- 45, which was in turn to be hydrolyzed using HCl to remove the protection group. Product [^{18}F]AV- 45 was obtained after purification with semi-preparative HPLC. The radiochemical purity of [^{18}F]AV-45 was greater than 95%, and the specific activity was greater than 4000 TBq/mmol at the end of synthesis (EOS). The mean administered activity was 365 MBq (range, 325–394 MBq). The PET acquisition protocol and optimal scanning time were adapted from previous reports [8,19]. In brief, helical computed tomography images were obtained for attenuation correction at 40 min. Each PET acquisition consisted of two 5-min dynamic frames obtained 50–60 min post-injection in 3D mode [19] from the Biograph mCT PET/CT System (Siemens Medical Solutions, Malvern, PA, USA). PET projection data were iteratively reconstructed using 3-D OSEM algorithm of 4 iterations, 24 subsets, postsmoothed by a Gaussian filter of 2 mm FWHM and zoom = 3, and with CT-based attenuation correction. Scatter and random correction were also performed using the correction methods provided by the manufacture. The reconstructed images were with pixel size of 0.679 mm, and slice thickness of 2.027 mm. Individual frames of the [^{18}F]AV-45 PET dynamic series were realigned if motion was detected. Summed images were subsequently created for analysis [20].

[^{18}F]AV-45 Imaging Processing and Atlas-based Quantitative Volume of Interest (VOI) Analysis

Both PET and MRI images from each subject were co-registered first, and then MRI images were spatially normalized into the MNI T1 template as in Statistical Parametric Mapping 5 (SPM5) (Wellcome Department of Cognitive Neurology, University College London, London, UK). The transformation parameters of MR normalization were then applied to corresponding PET images. All the image data were processed in the PMOD software (version 3.2; PMOD Technologies Ltd., Zurich, Switzerland). For all subjects, a binary gray matter mask was first created by taking the non-zero pixels from an averaged gray matter probability map generated from the segmentation of the spatially normalized MR images from normal subjects. The final VOI template for VOI analysis was then obtained by taking the intersection of both the binary gray matter mask and the automated anatomic labeling (AAL) atlas (VOI template) for all subjects [21,22]; this step was performed to minimize the inclusion of both cerebrospinal fluid and white matter (and thus non-specific white matter [^{18}F]AV-45 retention) in the statistical measures of all VOIs [23]. The original AAL atlas which contains 116 regions was combined into the following 8 labeled VOIs for further analysis: the precuneus, frontal, parietal, occipital, temporal, posterior cingulate and anterior cingulate areas, and the whole cerebellum. The standard uptake value ratio (SUVR) was calculated by determining the ratios of the integrated activities between the target VOI (cortical regions) and whole cerebellum reference VOI.

Voxel-based statistical analysis was conducted with SPM5 [24]. The spatial normalization of individual [^{18}F]AV-45 images to MNI MRI T1-template space was performed in the same way as that for the VOI analysis described above. All voxels in the normalized [^{18}F]AV-45 images were divided by the mean [^{18}F]AV-45 uptake of the whole cerebellum VOI in each subject to form SUVR images. Moreover, all PET images in SPM analysis were smoothed by 8 mm FWHM Gaussian filtering. Voxel-wise [^{18}F]AV-45 uptake differences among the CN, aMCI, and AD subjects were assessed in SPM5. Statistical maps displaying group differences were shown at a significance value of p<0.01 and extent voxels of 100. Due to a relatively small sample size of our study, and to increase the sensitivity in the SPM analysis, the lower threshold of two-tailed p<0.01 under uncorrected statistics was applied here [25].

Determination of the Threshold for Cerebral Cortical Amyloidosis in [^{18}F]AV-45 Images

To quantitatively measure the threshold for global cerebral cortical amyloid burden, the [^{18}F]AV-45 images of the AD and CN groups were compared to derive the cutoff point with receiver operating characteristic (ROC) analysis. Subjects with a cortical SUVR level exceeding the threshold were categorized as positive for cerebral amyloidosis. In our cases, the threshold derived from the AD and CN groups was 1.178 with the area under the curve of 0.96 (p<0.001); the sensitivity and specificity were 92% and 91%, respectively.

Statistical Analyses

Data were expressed as means±SD or absolute numbers with proportions for descriptive statistics. Continuous variables were analyzed by non-parametric statistics with the Mann–Whitney U-test. Categorical data were analyzed using Fisher's exact test. Differences of [^{18}F]AV-45 cortical SUVRs between groups were assessed by non-parametric one-way analysis of variance (AN-OVA) using the Kruskal–Wallis test followed by Dunn's post hoc multiple comparison test. Correlations between cognitive test scores and cortical SUVRs were analyzed with both Pearson correlations and partial regression with adjustment for age and years of education. Statistical analyses were performed with SAS version 9.2 (SAS Institute Inc., New York, USA), and p<0.05 was considered significant.

Results

The study recruited 11, 13, and 12 subjects in the CN, aMCI, and AD groups, respectively. The demographic data were shown in Table 1. None of the subjects had adverse events directly related to [^{18}F]AV-45 administration.

VOI Analysis

The VOI analysis of [^{18}F]AV-45 images revealed significant differences in the global cortical SUVR among subjects with CN, aMCI and AD (Figure 1). Regarding to the differences in regional SUVRs, the precuneus, frontal, parietal, occipital, temporal, and posterior and anterior cingulate cortical SUVRs were also different among the three groups. In the post hoc analyses, all of these areas except the anterior cingulate had a higher SUVR of [^{18}F]AV-45 in AD subjects than CN subjects. Furthermore, the SUVRs of the global cortical, precuneus, frontal, occipital and posterior cingulate areas were higher in aMCI subjects than CN subjects. There was no difference in [^{18}F]AV-45 SUVRs of these predefined areas between aMCI and AD subjects. With the SUVR cutoff point of 1.178, the positive rate of cerebral cortical amyloidosis was 8%, 62%, and 92% for CN, aMCI and AD groups, respectively. Interestingly, there were varying degrees of [^{18}F]AV-45 retention in CN, aMCI negative for cerebral amyloidosis (aMCI (−)), aMCI positive for cerebral amyloidosis (aMCI (+)), and AD subjects, whose patterns closely followed the amyloid deposition distribution observed in post mortem brain tissue (Figure 2) [26].

SPM Analysis

The SPM analysis showed that aMCI subjects had significantly higher [^{18}F]AV-45 uptake than CN subjects in the frontal, temporal, parietal, occipital areas, as well as in the precuneus, which showed the most prominent differences (Figure 3A). These results were supported by the automated VOI analysis in which aMCI patients showed 15% increased [^{18}F]AV-45 uptake in the

Table 1. Demographic characteristics of the CN, aMCI, and AD groups.

	CN (n=11)	aMCI (n=13)	AD (n=12)	p
Gender (M/F)	6/5	5/8	3/9	0.35
Age, years	69.3 (6.6)	70.0 (11.2)	75.8 (5.7)	0.15
CDR	0.0 (0.0)	0.5 (0.0)*	1.1 (0.3)*	<0.0001
MMSE	27.9 (1.6)	19.7 (2.4)*	12.9 (3.7)*	<0.0001
Memory deficit duration, years	-	3.0 (1.2)	5.9 (2.2)	<0.001
Education level, years	9.4 (4.1)	6.2 (4.1)	7.2 (4.3)	0.19

*p<0.05 compared to the CN group.
Values were mean (SD) or numbers of patients.
CN, cognitively normal; aMCI, amnestic mild cognitive impairment; AD, Alzheimer's disease; CDR, clinical dementia rating; MMSE, mini-mental state examination.
doi:10.1371/journal.pone.0058974.t001

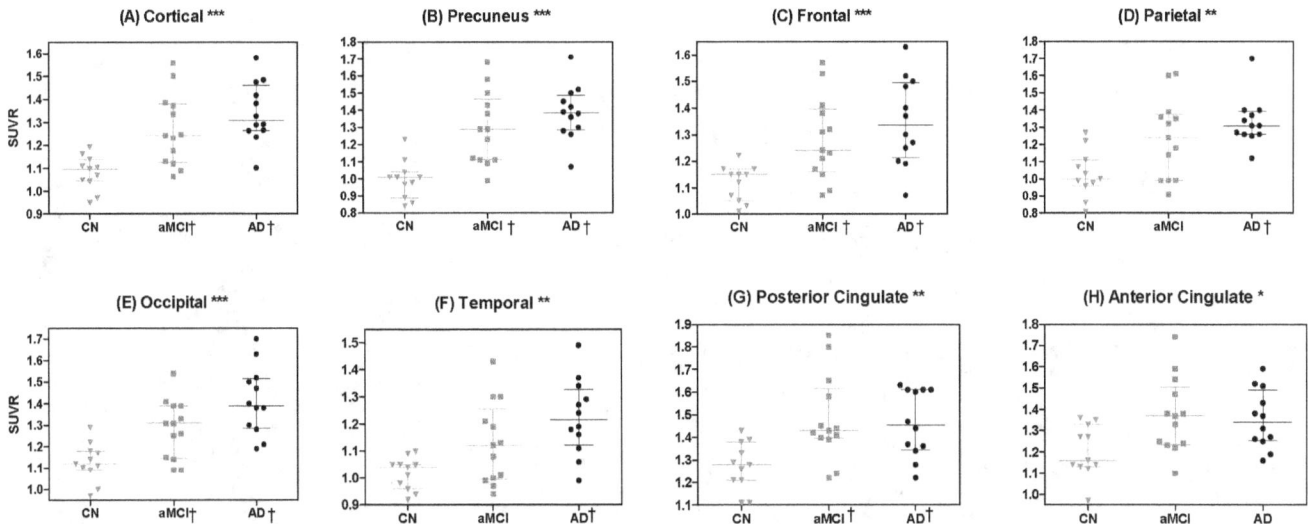

Figure 1. Scatter plots showing general and individual region-to-cerebellum ratios between different groups. Comparisons of [^{18}F]AV-45 SUVR in the predefined VOIs of the global cortical (A), precuneus (B), frontal (C), parietal (D), occipital (E), temporal (F), posterior cingulate (G) and anterior cingulate (H) areas among the cognitively normal (CN), amnestic mild cognitive impairment (aMCI), and Alzheimer's disease (AD) subjects. (* $p<0.05$, ** $p<0.005$, *** $p<0.0005$, when comparing SUVR among CN, aMCI and AD subjects with the Kruskal–Wallis ANOVA test. † $p<0.05$ versus CN subjects with Dunn's post hoc analysis).
doi:10.1371/journal.pone.0058974.g001

frontal cortex ($p<0.05$) and 30% in the precuneus ($p<0.005$) than the CN group. Individually, in the precuneus, 8 of 13 aMCI subjects had [^{18}F]AV-45 uptake values above 2 SD from the CN group mean. Comparing the SUVRs between AD and aMCI subjects, AD subjects had a slightly increased [^{18}F]AV-45 uptake over the frontal, temporal and parietal regions (Figures 3B and 3C). Correspondingly, the VOI analysis showed significant increase of [^{18}F]AV-45 in AD as compared to CN subjects in the additional brain regions including parietal (30% increase from the CN group mean, $p<0.01$), occipital (26% increase from the CN group mean, $p<0.01$), and temporal regions (20% increase from the CN group mean, $p<0.01$). Tables S1, S2 and S3 listed the peaks of the most significant increase in [^{18}F]AV-45 uptake obtained in this analysis with Talairach and Tournoux coordinates, x, y, and z in millimeters of these peaks, as well as the corresponding z scores.

Correlations between [^{18}F]AV-45 SUVRs and Cognitive Function

There was no association of the global cortical [^{18}F]AV-45 SUVR with age and education attainment. There was a negative correlation of the global cortical [^{18}F]AV-45 SUVR with the scores of MMSE (adjusted $R^2 = 0.44$), LM (adjusted $R^2 = 0.44$), CVFT (adjusted $R^2 = 0.37$), TMAT (adjusted $R^2 = 0.48$), CDT (adjusted $R^2 = 0.56$) and VAMT (adjusted $R^2 = 0.57$) with all p values <0.001 after adjustment for age and education. Furthermore, there was a negative correlation of MMSE scores with all the predefined VOI areas after adjustment for age and education (Figure 4).

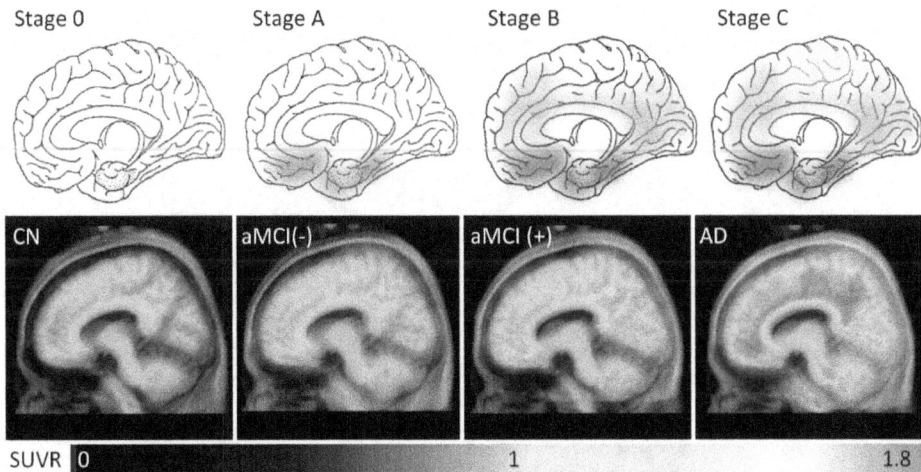

Figure 2. Representative sagittal [^{18}F]AV-45 PET images. Varying degrees of [^{18}F]AV-45 PET uptake in CN, aMCI negative for cerebral amyloidosis (aMCI (-)), aMCI positive for cerebral amyloidosis (aMCI (+)), and AD subjects (bottom row) were closely corresponding to the pathological amyloid deposition distribution adapted from Braak and Braak (top row) [26].
doi:10.1371/journal.pone.0058974.g002

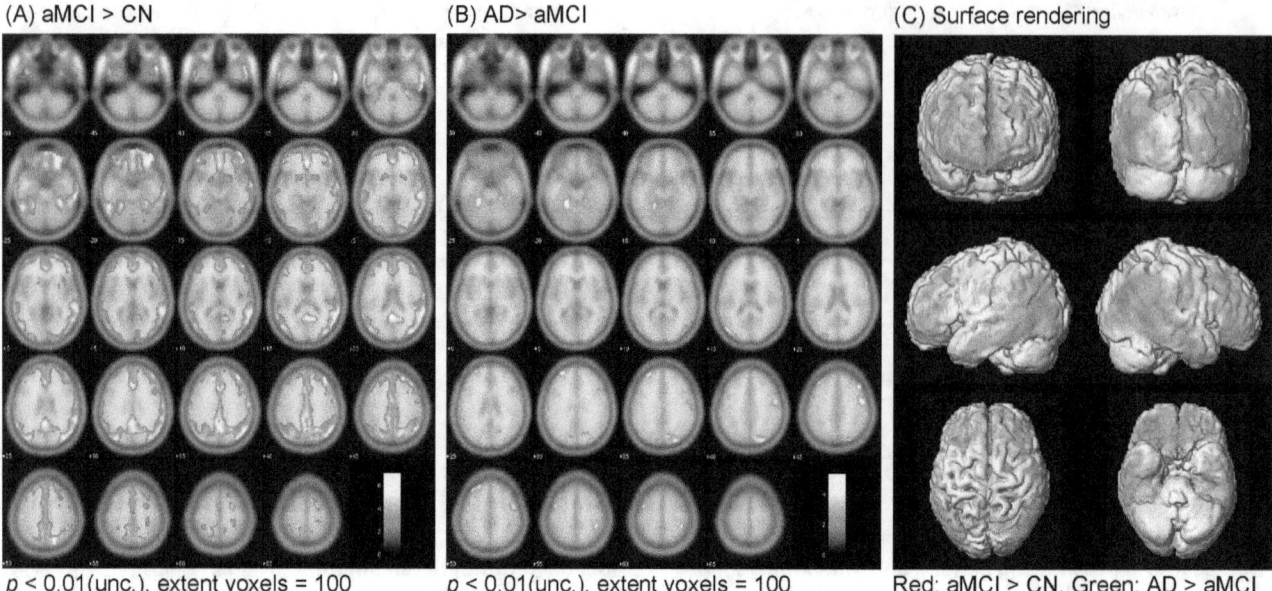

Figure 3. Statistical parametric mapping analysis: Localization of increased [^{18}F]AV-45 retention between CN, aMCI and AD subjects. Comparisons of [^{18}F]AV-45 SUVRs between cognitively normal (CN) and amnestic mild cognitively impairment (aMCI) subjects (A), and between aMCI and Alzheimer's disease (AD) subjects (B) (Uncorrected for multiple comparisons and the color bar values indicate the value of the T-statistic in each display). Surface rendering was used to illustrate the cortical areas where [^{18}F]AV-45 SUVRs were increased in aMCI than CN subjects (red) and increased in AD than aMCI subjects (green) (C).
doi:10.1371/journal.pone.0058974.g003

Discussion

Although the cause of AD is still unknown, the presence of amyloid plaques plays a pivotal role in the pathogenesis of the disease. Studies show that the presence of amyloid plaques in patients with mild cognitive impairment may increase the potential of conversion to AD [27]. Therefore, the development of imaging techniques to detect amyloid plaques in vivo would be helpful for early diagnosis and monitoring disease progress [28]. Several

fluorine-18-labeled radiotracers, including [^{18}F]AV-45 (florbetapir), [^{18}F]AV-1 (florbetaben) and [^{18}F]GE067 (flutemetamol), have been extensively employed for amyloid plaque detection both in vivo and ex vivo [29]. Although [^{11}C] PIB PET has been applied to compare the amyloid plaque distribution among CN, MCI and AD subjects in the Asian population [30], there are limited reports about fluorine-18-labeled amyloid PET studies in non-Caucasians [20,31,32]. In a recent report by Barthel *et al*, the Caucasian elderly normal subjects had higher SUVRs in different neocortical

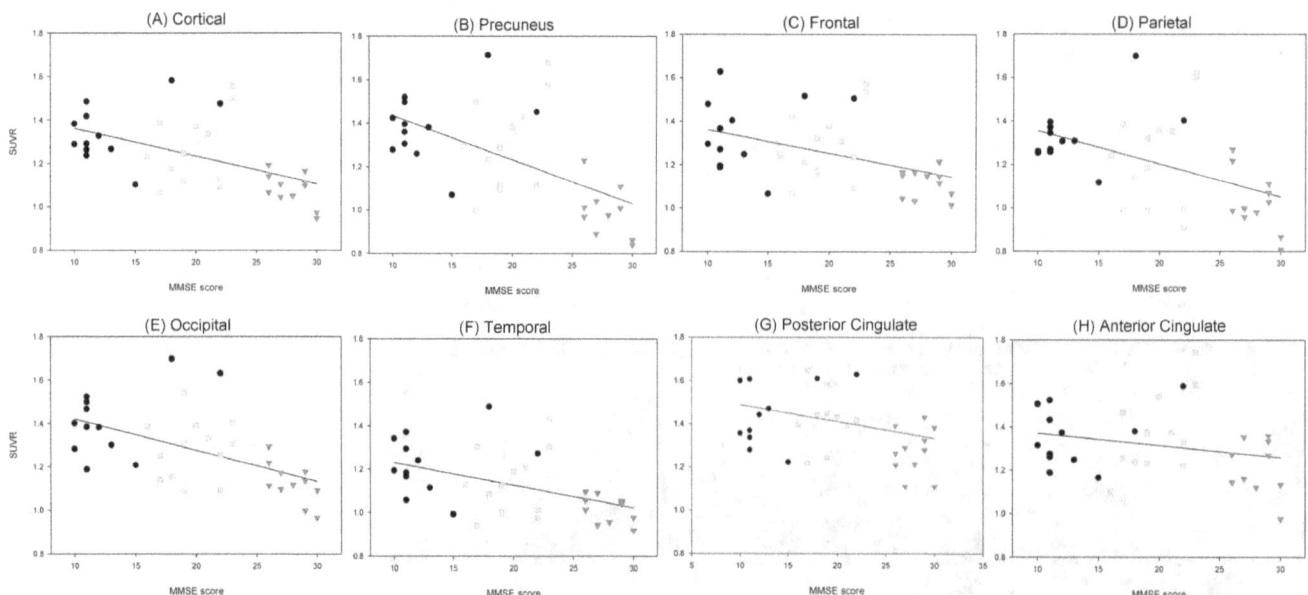

Figure 4. Relationship between MMSE scores and global and regional cortical [^{18}F]AV-45 retention. Results of the negative regressions between MMSE scores and global and regional cortical [^{18}F]AV-45 SUVRs among the cognitive normal, amnestic mild cognitive impairment, and Alzheimer's disease subjects with age and years of education as covariates.
doi:10.1371/journal.pone.0058974.g004

regions as compared to the Japanese elderly normal subjects on the florbetaben PET [31]. To our knowledge, this is the first [^{18}F]AV-45 PET study to compare the amyloid loads among CN, aMCI, and AD subjects in vivo in an Eastern population. We found that the [^{18}F]AV-45 SUVR was markedly increased in aMCI and AD subjects compared to CN subjects, regardless of whether it was measured with the VOI or SPM methods. In addition, we also applied the ROC method to determine the threshold for global cortical amyloid positivity, which was 1.178 with a sensitivity of 92% and a specificity of 91%, respectively. Our findings are concordant with those of Fleisher et al [33]. They applied the data from another post-mortem study to determine the [^{18}F]AV-45 threshold for amyloid positivity, and the pathology-based threshold was 1.17, which is similar to our clinical diagnosis-based threshold of 1.178.

At present, the diagnosis of AD is mainly based on clinical manifestations, brain structure imaging, laboratory study, and neuropsychological assessment. Around 10–20% of clinically diagnosed AD patients do not have amyloid plaques on post-mortem pathological examination [34,35]. In our study, the positivity of amyloidosis in the CN, aMCI, and AD groups was 9%, 62%, and 92%, respectively. The positivity for amyloidosis in AD patients (92%) is relatively high compared to the 80.9% observed by Fleisher et al [33]. One of the reasons is that our AD subjects had a relatively low cognitive performance and education attainment. Besides, the average disease duration was 5.9±2.2 years. Interestingly, 1 of the 12 AD patients (8%) had a relatively low global cortical SUVR, with a level similar to that of the CN subjects in our study, despite the fact that the patient exhibited a typical presentation of AD and fulfilled the most widely applied NINCDS-ADRDA criteria. However, the criteria may still allow a degree of uncertainty given the fact of the lack of pathological findings. On the other hand, PET radiotracers may fail to bind amyloid plaques because different fibrillary amyloid aggregate forms may have different affinities for amyloid radiotracers [36,37].

The accumulation of amyloid plaques is a relentless process with a stereotypic progression pattern in the disease course of AD. In our study, the distribution of [^{18}F]AV-45 uptake in the aMCI group was intermediate between that of the CN and AD groups. Comparing the regional [^{18}F]AV-45 SUVRs between aMCI and CN subjects, a higher [^{18}F]AV-45 SUVR was noted over the precuneus, frontal, occipital and posterior cingulate areas. These findings were similar with the report from Kempainen et al that aMCI patients had higher [^{11}C]PIB retention in the frontal, parietal, temporal, and posterior cingulate areas under SPM analysis [38]. Furthermore, the averaged [^{18}F]AV-45 SUVR distribution pattern in aMCI subjects positive for amyloidosis was more like Stage B by the Braak and Braak's amyloid deposition category, while the distribution pattern in aMCI subjects negative for amyloidosis was more like Stage A (Figure 2) [26]. Additionally, a more widely spread [^{18}F]AV-45 uptake was noted over the frontal, temporal, and parietal areas in AD subjects than aMCI subjects in SPM analysis, which are concordant with those of the previous [^{18}F]AV-45 and [^{11}C]PIB studies [19,39,40]. Although the [^{18}F]AV-45 distribution among the CN, aMCI and AD groups could mirror the pathological staging, its association with cognitive decline needs to be followed up in further cohort studies.

The deposition of amyloid plaques has been reported to occur at least 10 years prior to the clinical diagnosis of AD; about 21% of non-demented elderly have amyloid pathology [41]. However, the positivity of cerebral amyloidosis was relatively low in our CN group. Age is associated with amyloid load, and the relatively

young age in our CN group may contribute to the low positivity [42].

Mild cognitive impairment is a transitional state between normal cognition and AD; it can be present years before the diagnosis of AD. The amyloid load in subjects with MCI is correlated with the rate of conversion from MCI to AD, suggesting that it is a prognostic marker in MCI subjects [27]. However, many clinical and genetic factors, such as age, APOE4 allele carrier, and cerebral atrophy severity, may also influence the amyloid load in MCI subjects [17,42,43]. Therefore, the distribution of amyloid load in MCI subjects could be diverse, and a great overlap with CN and AD groups can be expected [33,44]. In our study, AD subjects tended to have a higher global cortical [^{18}F]AV-45 SUVR (1.34±0.13) than aMCI patients (1.27±0.16) with an effect size of 0.45, but the sample size in this study is not large enough to differentiate the 2 groups based on the VOI analysis. Nonetheless, a more extensive [^{18}F]AV-45 retention could be noted over the frontal, parietal, temporal and occipital areas under the voxelwise SPM analysis. On the other hand, amyloid deposition is an early change in the pathogenesis of AD. Rather than the cortical amyloid load, the downstream pathway such as synaptic dysfunction and brain structure change may play a more important role in determining the cognitive declines from MCI to AD [2,27], and the application of multimodal neuro-chemical and imaging biomarkers should be considered to early identify predementia and even preclinical asymptomatic stages of AD [45].

Alzheimer's disease is characteristic of progressive amyloid plaques accumulation accompanied with cognitive decline. Roe et al found that mean cortical [^{11}C]PIB binding potential was not only related to MMSE scores, but also the cognitive measures associated with executive functions among AD and CN subjects [46]. However, they didn't correlate the regional cortical [^{11}C]PIB binding potential with the various cognitive measures. In the study by Barthel et al, both the frontal and total brain amyloid volumes on [^{18}F]AV-1 PET were negatively correlated with MMSE scores among AD and CN subjects [47]. These findings are consistent with our study results that there was a negative correlation between MMSE scores and [^{18}F]AV-45 SUVRs of various cortical regions, especially over the frontal, temporal and precuneus areas even after controlling for age and years of education. The presence of negative correlation between MMSE scores and the SUVRs of different amyloid radiotracers on PET may support the cascade hypothesis that amyloid plaque accumulation plays a pivotal role in the AD pathophysiological process [48].

There were several limitations in the current study. Correcting partial volume effect (PVE) is important for VOI-based analysis and in particular, for amyloid imaging. Therefore, the first limitation in this study is that no PVE correction was performed. The use of binary gray matter mask in this work is to avoid extracting activity from both CSF and white matter regions by confining VOI quantification only to gray matter region. To improve quantification accuracy in small VOIs, PVE correction should be included as a future work. Second, the sample size in our study is relatively small, and the results are not generalizable to the Chinese population. In addition, a cutoff value of 1.178 for neocortical [^{18}F]AV-45 uptake was derived to differentiate Chinese AD from CN subjects, and its application to predict the conversion to AD from CN or aMCI subjects has to be verified in a longitudinal cohort study.

Conclusions

The findings from our study show that [^{18}F]AV-45 PET can be applied in vivo to differentiate the cerebral amyloid burden among CN, aMCI, and AD subjects using continuous or binary measurements, and [^{18}F]AV-45 SUVR is associated with MMSE scores. The clinical diagnosis-based threshold for cerebral amyloidosis derived from AD patients is similar to the pathology-based threshold. Therefore, [^{18}F]AV-45 PET is a potential biomarker for AD in multicenter monitoring and treatment trials.

Supporting Information

Table S1 Comparing [^{18}F]AV-45 uptake between Alzheimer's disease (AD) patients and amnestic mild cognitive impairment (aMCI) patients. The locations and values of the most significant increased [^{18}F]AV-45 uptake in AD patients than aMCI patients, p<0.01 (unc.), extent voxels = 100. (DOC)

Table S2 Comparing [^{18}F]AV-45 uptake between amnestic mild cognitive impairment (aMCI) patients and cognitively normal (CN) subjects. The locations and values of the most significant increased [^{18}F]AV-45 uptake in aMCI patients than CN subjects, p<0.01 (unc.), extent voxels = 100. (DOC)

Table S3 Comparing [^{18}F]AV-45 uptake between Alzheimer's disease (AD) patients and cognitively normal (CN) subjects. The locations and values of the most significant increased [^{18}F]AV-45 uptake in AD patients than CN subjects, p<0.01 (unc.), extent voxels = 100. (DOC)

Acknowledgments

We would like to thank Ko-Ting Chao and Yu-Chen Hsieh for their technical assistance. We also thank Avid Radiopharmaceuticals, Inc. (Philadelphia, PA, USA) for providing the precursor for the preparation of [^{18}F]AV-45.

Author Contributions

Conceived and designed the experiments: KLH MPK TCY CCH. Performed the experiments: KLH KJL HCK WCH WLC TCY CCH. Analyzed the data: KLH KJL ITH MPK SPW CJH YYW TCY CCH. Contributed reagents/materials/analysis tools: KLH KJH ITH TCY CCH. Wrote the paper: KLH KJL MPK YYW TCY CCH.

References

1. Löppönen M, Räihä I, Isoaho R, Vahlberg T, Kivelä SL (2003) Diagnosing cognitive impairment and dementia in primary health care – a more active approach is needed. Age Ageing 32: 606–612.
2. Sperling RA, Aisen PS, Beckett LA, Bennett DA, Craft S, et al. (2011) Toward defining the preclinical stages of Alzheimer's disease: recommendations from the National Institute on Aging-Alzheimer's Association workgroups on diagnostic guidelines for Alzheimer's disease. Alzheimer's Dement 7: 280–292.
3. Klunk WE, Wang Y, Huang GF, Debnath ML, Holt DP, et al. (2001) Uncharged thioflavin-T derivatives bind to amyloid-beta protein with high affinity and readily enter the brain. Life Sci 69: 1471–1484.
4. Ono M, Cheng Y, Kimura H, Cui M, Kagawa S, et al. (2011) Novel 18F-labeled benzofuran derivatives with improved properties for positron emission tomography (PET) imaging of β-Amyloid plaques in Alzheimer's brains. J Med Chem 54: 2971–2979.
5. Kudo Y, Okamura N, Furumoto S, Tashiro M, Furukawa K, et al. (2007) 2-(2-[2-dimethylaminothiazol-5-yl]ethenyl)-6- (2-[fluoro]ethoxy) benzoxazole: a Novel PET agent for in vivo detection of dense amyloid plaques in Alzheimer's disease patients. J Nucl Med 48: 553–561.
6. Seneca N, Cai L, Liow JS, Zoghbi SS, Gladding RL, et al. (2007) Brain and whole-body imaging in nonhuman primates with [11C]MeS-IMPY, a candidate radioligand for β-amyloid plaques. Nucl Med Biol 34: 681–689.
7. Shoghi-Jadid K, Barrio JR, Kepe V, Wu HM, Small GW, et al. (2005) Imaging β-amyloid fibrils in Alzheimer's disease: a critical analysis through simulation of amyloid fibril polymerization. Nucl Med Biol 32: 337–351.
8. Lin KJ, Hsu WC, Hsiao IT, Wey SP, Jin LW, et al. (2010) Whole-body biodistribution and brain PET imaging with [18F]AV-45, a novel amyloid imaging agent - a pilot study. Nucl Med Biol 37: 497–508.
9. Rowe CC, Ackerman U, Browne W, Mulligan R, Pike KL, et al. (2008) Imaging of amyloid beta in Alzheimer's disease with 18F-BAY94-9172, a novel PET tracer: proof of mechanism. Lancet Neurol 7: 129–135.
10. Koole M, Lewis DM, Buckley C, Nelissen N, Vandenbulcke M, et al. (2009) Whole-body biodistribution and radiation dosimetry of 18F-GE067: a radioligand for in vivo brain amyloid imaging. J Nucl Med 50: 818–822.
11. Jagust WJ, Bandy D, Chen K, Foster NL, Landau SM, et al. (2010) The Alzheimer's Disease Neuroimaging Initiative positron emission tomography core. Alzheimer's Dement 6: 221–229.
12. Clark CM, Schneider JA, Bedell BJ, Beach TG, Bilker WB, et al. (2011) Use of Florbetapir-PET for Imaging β-Amyloid Pathology. JAMA 305: 275–283.
13. Petersen RC, Doody R, Kurz A, Mohs RC, Morris JC, et al. (2001) Current concepts in mild cognitive impairment. Arch Neurol 58: 1985–1992.
14. American Psychiatric Association (1994) Diagnostic and statistical manual of mental disorders, DSM-IV. Washington, DC: American Psychiatric Association.
15. McKhann G, Drachman D, Folstein M, Katzman R, Price D, et al. (1984) Clinical diagnosis of Alzheimer's disease. Neurology 34: 939.
16. Folstein MF, Folstein SE, McHugh PR (1975) Mini-mental state: a practical method for grading the cognitive state of patients for the clinician. J Psychiat Res 12: 189–198.
17. Wang PN, Hong CJ, Lin KN, Liu HC, Chen WT (2011) APOE ε4 increases the risk of progression from amnestic mild cognitive impairment to Alzheimer's disease among ethnic Chinese in Taiwan. J Neurol Neurosurg Psychiatry 82: 165–169.
18. Yao CH, Lin KJ, Weng CC, Hsiao IT, Ting YS, et al. (2010) GMP-compliant automated synthesis of [(18)F]AV-45 (Florbetapir F 18) for imaging beta-amyloid plaques in human brain. Appl Radiat Isot 68: 2293–2297.
19. Wong DF, Rosenberg PB, Zhou Y, Kumar A, Raymont V, et al. (2010) In vivo imaging of amyloid deposition in Alzheimer disease using the radioligand 18F-AV-45 (Florbetapir F 18). J Nucl Med 51: 913–920.
20. Hsiao IT, Huang CC, Hsieh CJ, Hsu WC, Wey SP, et al. (2012) Correlation of early-phase 18F-florbetapir (AV-45/Amyvid) PET images to FDG images: preliminary studies. Eur J Nucl Med Mol Imaging 39: 613–620.
21. Tzourio-Mazoyer N, Landeau B, Papathanassiou D, Crivello F, Etard O, et al. (2002) Automated anatomical labeling of activations in SPM using a macroscopic anatomical parcellation of the MNI MRI single-subject brain. NeuroImage 15: 273–289.
22. Huang KL, Lin KJ, Ho MY, Chang YJ, Chang CH, et al. (2012) Amyloid deposition after cerebral hypoperfusion: evidenced on [18F]AV-45 positron emission tomography. J Neurol Sci 319: 124–129.
23. Hsieh CJ, Fan L, Lin KJ, Hsiao IT, Huang CC, et al. (2011) Precise F-18 florbetapir (AV-45) PET image spatial normalization using early-phase image template. J Nucl Med 52: 549.
24. Ashburner J, Friston KJ (2005) Unified segmentation. NeuroImage 26: 839–851.
25. Juh R, Kim J, Moon D, Choe B, Suh T (2004) Different metabolic patterns analysis of Parkinsonism on the 18F-FDG PET. European Journal of Radiology 51: 223–233.
26. Braak H, Braak E (1997) Frequency of Stages of Alzheimer-Related Lesions in Different Age Categories. Neurobiol Aging 18: 351–357.
27. Okello A, Koivunen J, Edison P, Archer HA, Turkheimer FE, et al. (2009) Conversion of amyloid positive and negative MCI to AD over 3 years: an 11C-PIB PET study. Neurology 73: 754–760.
28. Small GW (2006) Diagnostic issues in dementia: neuroimaging as a surrogate marker of disease. J Geriatr Psychiatry Neurol 19: 180–185.
29. Herholz K, Ebmeier K (2011) Clinical amyloid imaging in Alzheimer's disease. The Lancet Neurology 10: 667–670.
30. Hatashita S, Yamasaki H (2010) Clinically different stages of Alzheimer's disease associated by amyloid deposition with [11C]-PIB PET imaging. J Alzheimers Dis 21: 995–1003.
31. Barthel H, Senda M, Yamane T, Patt M, Sattler B, et al. (2010) Phase 1 trials on florbetaben brain PET in elderly normal controls. J Nucl Med 51: 385.
32. Senda M, Yamane T, Sasaki M, Shimizu K, Barthel H, et al. (2010) Ethnic comparability of safety and pharmacokinetics of florbetaben (BAY 94-9172) in normal Caucasian and Asian subjects. J Nucl Med 51: 1754.
33. Fleisher AS, Chen K, Liu X, Roontiva A, Thiyyagura P, et al. (2011) Using positron emission tomography and florbetapir F 18 to image cortical amyloid in patients with mild cognitive impairment or dementia due to Alzheimer disease. Arch Neurol 68: 1404–1411.
34. Jobst KA, Barnetson LPD, Shepstone BJ (1998) Accurate prediction of histologically confirmed Alzheimer's disease and the differential diagnosis of dementia: the use of NINCDS-ADRDA and DSM-III-R criteria, SPECT, X-Ray CT, and Apo E4 in medial temporal lobe dementias. Int Psychogeriatr 10: 271–302.

35. Ranginwala NA, Hynan LS, Weiner MF, White CLI (2008) Clinical criteria for the diagnosis of Alzheimer disease: still good after all these years. Am J Geriatr Psychiatry 16: 384-388.

36. LeVine III H, Walker LC (2010) Molecular polymorphism of Aβ in Alzheimer's disease. Neurobiol Aging 31: 542–548.

37. Lockhart A, Lamb JR, Osredkar T, Sue LI, Joyce JN, et al. (2007) PIB is a non-specific imaging marker of amyloid-beta (Aβ) peptide-related cerebral amyloid-osis. Brain 130: 2607–2615.

38. Kemppainen NM, Aalto S, Wilson IA, Nagren K, Helin S, et al. (2007) PET amyloid ligand [11C]PIB uptake is increased in mild cognitive impairment. Neurology 68: 1603–1606.

39. Forsberg A, Engler H, Almkvist O, Blomquist G, Hagman G, et al. (2008) PET imaging of amyloid deposition in patients with mild cognitive impairment. Neurobiol Aging 29: 1456–1465.

40. Rowe CC, Ng S, Ackermann U, Gong SJ, Pike K, et al. (2007) Imaging beta-amyloid burden in aging and dementia. Neurology 68: 1718–1725.

41. Aizenstein HJ, Nebes RD, Saxton JA, Price JC, Mathis CA, et al. (2008) Frequent amyloid deposition without significant cognitive impairment among the elderly. Arch Neurol 65: 1509–1517.

42. Rowe CC, Ellis KA, Rimajova M, Bourgeat P, Pike KE, et al. (2010) Amyloid imaging results from the Australian Imaging, Biomarkers and Lifestyle (AIBL) study of aging. Neurobiol Aging 31: 1275–1283.

43. Chetelat G, Villemagne VL, Bourgeat P, Pike KE, Jones G, et al. (2010) Relationship between atrophy and beta-amyloid deposition in Alzheimer disease. Ann Neurol 67: 317–324.

44. Jack CR Jr, Lowe VJ, Weigand SD, Wiste HJ, Senjem ML, et al. (2009) Serial PIB and MRI in normal, mild cognitive impairment and Alzheimer's disease: implications for sequence of pathological events in Alzheimer's disease. Brain 132: 1355–1365.

45. Teipel SJ, Sabri O, Grothe M, Barthel H, Prvulovic D, et al. (2013) Perspectives for Multimodal Neurochemical and Imaging Biomarkers in Alzheimer's Disease. J Alzheimers Dis 33: S329–S347.

46. Roe CM, Mintun MA, D'Angelo G, Xiong C, Grant EA, et al. (2008) Alzheimer Disease and Cognitive Reserve: Variation of Education Effect With Carbon 11-Labeled Pittsburgh Compound B Uptake. Arch Neurol 65: 1467–1471.

47. Barthel H, Luthardt J, Becker G, Patt M, Hammerstein E, et al. (2011) Individualized quantification of brain β-amyloid burden: results of a proof of mechanism phase 0 florbetaben PET trial in patients with Alzheimer's disease and healthy controls. Eur J Nucl Med Mol Imaging 38: 1702–1714.

48. Jack Jr CR, Knopman DS, Jagust WJ, Shaw LM, Aisen PS, et al. (2010) Hypothetical model of dynamic biomarkers of the Alzheimer's pathological cascade. The Lancet Neurology 9: 119–128.

Multi-Method Analysis of MRI Images in Early Diagnostics of Alzheimer's Disease

Robin Wolz[1,9], Valtteri Julkunen[2,9], Juha Koikkalainen[3], Eini Niskanen[2,4], Dong Ping Zhang[1], Daniel Rueckert[1], Hilkka Soininen[2,5], Jyrki Lötjönen[3]*, the Alzheimer's Disease Neuroimaging Initiative[¶]

1 Biomedical Image Analysis Group, Department of Computing, Imperial College London, London, United Kingdom, 2 Department of Neurology, Kuopio University Hospital, Kuopio, Finland, 3 Knowledge Intensive Services, VTT Technical Research Centre of Finland, Tampere, Finland, 4 Department of Applied Physics, University of Eastern Finland, Kuopio, Finland, 5 Institute of Clinical Medicine, Neurology, University of Eastern Finland, Kuopio, Finland

Abstract

The role of structural brain magnetic resonance imaging (MRI) is becoming more and more emphasized in the early diagnostics of Alzheimer's disease (AD). This study aimed to assess the improvement in classification accuracy that can be achieved by combining features from different structural MRI analysis techniques. Automatically estimated MR features used are hippocampal volume, tensor-based morphometry, cortical thickness and a novel technique based on manifold learning. Baseline MRIs acquired from all 834 subjects (231 healthy controls (HC), 238 stable mild cognitive impairment (S-MCI), 167 MCI to AD progressors (P-MCI), 198 AD) from the Alzheimer's Disease Neuroimaging Initiative (ADNI) database were used for evaluation. We compared the classification accuracy achieved with linear discriminant analysis (LDA) and support vector machines (SVM). The best results achieved with individual features are 90% sensitivity and 84% specificity (HC/AD classification), 64%/66% (S-MCI/P-MCI) and 82%/76% (HC/P-MCI) with the LDA classifier. The combination of all features improved these results to 93% sensitivity and 85% specificity (HC/AD), 67%/69% (S-MCI/P-MCI) and 86%/82% (HC/P-MCI). Compared with previously published results in the ADNI database using individual MR-based features, the presented results show that a comprehensive analysis of MRI images combining multiple features improves classification accuracy and predictive power in detecting early AD. The most stable and reliable classification was achieved when combining all available features.

Citation: Wolz R, Julkunen V, Koikkalainen J, Niskanen E, Zhang DP, et al. (2011) Multi-Method Analysis of MRI Images in Early Diagnostics of Alzheimer's Disease. PLoS ONE 6(10): e25446. doi:10.1371/journal.pone.0025446

Editor: Celia Oreja-Guevara, University Hospital La Paz, Spain

Received July 12, 2011; **Accepted** September 5, 2011; **Published** October 13, 2011

Funding: This project is partially funded under the 7th Framework Programme by the European Commission (http://cordis.europa.eu/ist/). Data collection and sharing for this project was funded by the Alzheimer's Disease Neuroimaging Initiative (ADNI; Principal Investigator: Michael Weiner; NIH grant U01 AG024904). ADNI is funded by the National Institute on Aging, the National Institute of Biomedical Imaging and Bioengineering (NIBIB), and through generous contributions from the following: Pzer Inc., Wyeth Research, Bristol-Myers Squibb, Eli Lilly and Company, GlaxoSmithKline, Merck & Co. Inc., AstraZeneca AB, Novartis Pharmaceuticals Corporation, Alzheimer's Association, Eisai Global Clinical Development, Elan Corporation, plc, Forest Laboratories, and the Institute for the Study of Aging, with participation from the U.S. Food and Drug Administration. Industry partnerships are coordinated through the Foundation for the National Institutes of Health. The grantee organization is the Northern California Institute for Research and Education, and the study is coordinated by the Alzheimer's Disease Cooperative Study at the University of California San Diego. ADNI data are disseminated by the Laboratory of Neuro Imaging at the University of California Los Angeles. Data used in the preparation of this article were obtained from the ADNI database (www.loni.ucla.edu/ADNI). As such, the investigators within the ADNI contributed to the design and implementation of ADNI and/or provided data but did not participate in analysis or writing of this report. ADNI investigators include (complete listing available at http://adni.loni.ucla.edu/wp-content/uploads/how_to_apply/ADNI_Authorship_List.pdf).

Competing Interests: The authors have declared that no competing interests exist.

* E-mail: jyrki.lotjonen@vtt.fi

[9] These authors contributed equally to this work.

[¶] For information on the Alzheimer's Disease Neuroimaging Initiative please see the Acknowledgments section.

Introduction

Alzheimer's disease (AD) is the most common cause of dementia globally and one of the major healthcare issues of the future. It has been estimated that during the next four decades the prevalence of AD will quadruple from 27 to 106 million by which time 1 in 85 persons worldwide will be living with the disease [1]. Even a modest delay of one year in disease onset and progression could reduce the number of cases by 9 million [1]. Interventions are postulated to be most effective when directed at patients at the earliest stages of the disease, which underlines the importance of early diagnosis of AD [2]. Mild cognitive impairment (MCI) is a heterogeneous syndrome that increases the risk of developing AD markedly [3]. However, not all MCI subjects convert to AD and some may even return to normal cognition [4].

The search for reliable biomarkers of AD-type pathology and predictors of disease progression among MCI subjects is ongoing. AD is characterized by neurofibrillary tangles and amyloid plaques in the brain [5]. Degenerative changes in the human neurotransmitter system lead to atrophy in selected brain regions [6]. The most promising candidate biomarkers are the ones derived from structural and functional neuroimaging as well as those measured in cerebrospinal fluid (CSF) and plasma [7]. Amyloid-based measures like the CSF-peptide $A\beta_{42}$ and the uptake of the PiB tracer on positron emission imaging (PET) show the earliest AD-type changes [7]. However, there is evidence that the number of amyloid plaques reach their saturation levels already by the time patients have clinically apparent symptoms of cognitive impairment [8,9], whereas atrophy, neuronal loss, synaptic loss, and the number of tangles increase with severity of illness [10]. These findings suggest that, although amyloid-based biomarkers may be used as longitudinal markers of AD type pathology, they seem to offer only limited insight into which MCI subjects will most likely convert to AD in the near future. In a recently published dynamic model of biomarker behavior in the AD spectrum, biomarkers based on structural magnetic resonance imaging (MRI) have been shown to be correlated with a progression from MCI to AD [11]. Such biomarkers could therefore improve the accuracy of early AD diagnostics and reduce especially the amount of false positive diagnoses. Besides providing chance for a more focused and earlier intervention, structural MRI biomarkers of AD could also aid the development of new disease-modifying drugs by acting as surrogate markers of disease progression, reduce the number of subjects needed to detect significant drug effect and provide quantitative measures of treatment benefits [12].

It has been shown that the early diagnostics of AD can be improved by using multiple different biomarkers simultaneously. Usually these studies have combined MRI-based markers with biomarkers based on positron emission tomography (PET) [13,14], cerebrospinal fluid (CSF) [15,16] or both [17–19]. Achieved results vary from no additional benefit [15,17] to significant improvement [13,14,16,20]. However, availability of all three biomarkers (CSF, PET, MRI) is not very common in clinical practice since obtaining all measures is laborious for the patient and clinician, induces delays and increases the costs of the diagnosis significantly. Furthermore, measurements obtained from CSF and PET are considered invasive. Recent studies focusing on only structural MRI have reached correct classification accuracys (CCR) of 76–94% in identifying healthy controls (HC) from patients with AD and 64–82% in predicting which MCI subjects will convert to AD in the imminent future [21–27]. The high variation in these results can be attributed to differences in study populations as well as evaluation designs. With the Alzheimer's Disease Neuroimaging Study (ADNI) [28], a large multi-center study on MR imaging in AD has been established that is available to the wider research community. Based on a large sub-group of ADNI subjects, Cuingnet et al. [29] presented a comparison of ten MRI-based feature extraction methods and their ability to discriminate between clinically relevant subject groups. The ten methods evaluated comprise five voxel-based methods, three methods based on cortical thickness and two methods based on the hippocampus. Best sensitivity/specificity values reported are 81%/95% for AD vs HC, 70%/61% for S-MCI vs P-MCI and 73%/85% for HC vs P-MCI.

In this paper we use the ADNI database to evaluate the ability of the combination of different MR-based features to increase classification accuracy. We evaluate the power of hippocampal volume (HV), cortical thickness (CTH), tensor-based morphometry (TBM) and features extracted from a recently proposed manifold-based learning (MBL) framework to discriminate healthy controls from subjects with AD and to predict conversion from MCI to AD. For evaluation we used all 834 ADNI baseline images that were available from the ADNI webpage. Compared to previous work this paper aims at establishing the improvement in accuracy and stability that can be achieved by combining more than one MR-based feature. To the best of our knowledge it is the first comprehensive study that analyzes MRI-derived features for the full ADNI dataset. For direct comparison with the work by Cuingnet et al. [29] we also evaluated all results on the subset used in their work.

To test the influence of the classification method used, we utilized both support vector machines (SVMs) and a linear discriminant analys (LDA) to evaluate classification accuracy (CCR), sensitivity (SEN) and specificity (SPE) in each experiment.

Materials and Methods

Subjects

In the ADNI study, brain MR images were acquired at regular intervals after an initial baseline scan from approximately 200 cognitively normal older subjects (HC), 400 subjects with mild cognitive impairment (MCI), and 200 subjects with early AD. Detailled inclusion/exclusion criteria used for the different subject groups in ADNI are defined in [30]. The AD group has scores between 20–26 (inclusive) on the Mini-Mental State Examination (MMSE) [31], and a Clinical Dementia Rating (CDR) [32] of 0.5 or 1.0. Furthermore, these subjects fulfil the NINCDS/ADRDA criteria for probable AD [33]. MCI subjects included have MMSE scores between 24–30 (inclusive), a memory complaint, have objective memory loss measured by education adjusted scores on Wechsler Memory Scale Logical Memory II, a CDR of 0.5, absence of significant levels of impairment in other cognitive domains, essentially preserved activities of daily living, and an absence of dementia [30]. Healthy subjects have MMSE scores between 24–30 (inclusive), a CDR of 0, are non-depressed, non MCI, and nondemented. A more detailed description of the ADNI study is given in Appendix S1.

All 834 ADNI subjects (231 HC, 238 S-MCI, 167 P-MCI, 198 AD) for which a 1.5T T1-weighted MRI scan at baseline was available were included in this study. 167 subjects in the MCI group converted to AD as of July 2011. We therefore independently analysed progressive MCI (P-MCI) subjects and subjects with a stable diagnosis of MCI (S-MCI).

Table 1 shows the demographics for the 834 study subjects. Statistically significant differences in the demographics and clinical variables between the study groups were assessed using Student's unpaired t-test. In this work, the difference was considered statistically significant if $p < 0.05$ if not stated otherwise. There were more men than women in all other groups besides the AD group. MMSE scores were significantly different in the pairwise comparisons between all study groups. CDR scores of the HC and AD groups are significantly different to the ones of the two MCI groups. Healthy subjects had a significantly lower Geriatric Depression Scale (GDS) compared to all other groups. Compared to all other groups, AD subjects had significantly shorter education

MRI Acquisition

Standard 1.5T screening/baseline T1-weighted images obtained using volumetric 3D MPRAGE protocol with resolutions

Table 1. Subjects.

Group	HC	S-MCI	P-MCI	AD
N	231	238	167	198
Men	52%	66%	62%	52%
Age	76.02 (5.0)	74.85 (7.8)	74.6 (7.0)	75.68 (7.7)
MMSE	29.1* (1.0)	27.3* (1.8)	26.6* (1.7)	23.3* (2.0)
CDR	0 (0)	0.49 (0.05)	0.50 (0)	0.75 (0.25)
GDS	0.83* (1.14)	1.60 (1.42)	1.53 (1.30)	1.67 (1.42)
Education	16.0 (2.8)	15.6 (3.1)	15.7 (2.9)	14.7* (3.1)
APOE4 status ($\varepsilon 3\varepsilon 4/\varepsilon 4\varepsilon 4$)	23%/2%	31%/8%	50%/16%	42%/18%
Months to conversion			18.2 (10.1)	

*means statistically significant different from all other groups.
doi:10.1371/journal.pone.0025446.t001

ranging from 0.9 mm × 0.9 mm × 1.20 mm to 1.3 mm × 1.3 mm × 1.20 mm were included from the ADNI database. For detailed information of the MRI protocols and preprocessing steps see [34].

Feature extraction

All fully automated feature extraction methods described below were applied to images that were preprocessed by the ADNI pipeline.

Hippocampal volume. Baseline hippocampal volumes were measured using an approach based on fast and robust multi-atlas segmentation [35,36]. In this approach, multi-atlas label propagation is applied in combination with atlas selection to obtain the hippocampus segmentation. A set of hippocampus atlases is selected from a pool of atlas images according to image similarity with the query image. After registering all atlases to the query image, a spatial prior is generated from the multiple label maps. This spatial prior is then used to obtain a final segmentation based on an expectation maximization (EM) segmentation algorithm [37].

Cortical thickness. CTH is measured in the baseline T1-weighted structural MR images by using an automated computational surface-based method developed at the McConnell Brain Imaging Centre, Montreal Neurological Institute, McGill University, Montreal, Canada (http://www2.bic.mni.mcgill.ca/) [38]. Individual MRI volumes were registered to standard space using the ICBM152 template [39]. Intensity non-uniformities were corrected [40] before the final brain mask was calculated [41]. Tissues were segmented into white matter (WM), grey matter (GM) and cerebrospinal fluid (CSF) using the INSECT-algorithm [42] and the magnitude of PVE was estimated by using the trimmed minimum covariance determinant (TMCD) method [43]. The brains were divided automatically into two separate hemispheres and the inner and outer surfaces of the cortex were extracted according to intersections between WM and GM (white matter surface, WMS) as well as GM and CSF (grey matter surface, GMS) using the Constrained Laplacian-Based Automated Segmentation with Proximities (CLASP) algorithm [44]. The inner surface was first formed by deforming an ellipsoid polygon mesh to the shape of the WMS. GMS was obtained by further expanding the inner surface. Each polygon mesh surface consisted of 81,920 polygons and 40,962 nodes per hemisphere. The thickness of the cortex was defined at each linked node as the distance between the two concentrically linked polygon meshes on the WMS and the GMS. This t-link metric has been proven to be the simplest yet most precise way to determine cortical thickness [38]. Although MR images were transformed to standard space to allow for group analysis, thickness calculations were performed in each subject's native space. Finally, cortical thickness maps were smoothed with a 20 mm FWHM diffusion smoothing kernel to improve the signal-to-noise ratio and statistical power [45]. The described toolbox did not achieve satisfactory results on some study subjects because of i) failure in tissue segmentation and brain masking (48 subjects) and ii) failure in partial volume effect estimation (59 subjects). As a result the pipeline crashed and CTH measures were not obtained for 76 subjects (24 control, 35 MCI, 17 AD). Also the cortical model of 31 subjects (10 control, 13 MCI, 8 AD) was completely deformed and thus unusable. For these 107 subjects the CTH features were considered as missing values. CTH features used in the classification experiments are introduced below.

Tensor-based morphometry. The TBM analysis was performed using a multi-template approach [46,47]. In TBM, a template image is non-rigidly registered to a study image, and, typically, the determinant of the Jacobian matrix ('the Jacobian') of the deformation is used to measure the voxel-level morphometry.

Instead of using just one template image, we used 30 randomly selected images (10 controls, 10 MCIs, and 10 ADs) from the ADNI database as template images. The template images were used also in the classification analysis to maximize the number of subjects. Each template image was registered to a study image, and Jacobian maps were computed for each template image. To combine the results of multiple templates, all template images were registered to the mean anatomical template generated from the 30 images, and all the results were normalized to this reference space [47]. The combination of the results was performed by averaging the ROI-wise feature values of all the templates as described in detail below.

Manifold-based learning. In this machine learning approach, non-linear dimensionality reduction with Laplacian eigenmaps [48] is used to learn features to discriminate between different subject groups. Laplacian eigenmaps estimates the low-dimensional representation of a set of input images based on a similarity graph that is defined with pairwise image similarities [48]. The hypothesis is that such a low-dimensional representation captures the variability in the dataset in a more compact way than pairwise image similarities directly. We estimate pairwise image similarities from the intensity appearance in a region around hippocampus and amygdala since both structures are known to be affected by AD in an early stage. All images are aligned in a template space using a coarse non-rigid registration (10 mm B-spline control-point spacing, [49]). Such a coarse non-rigid alignment ensures that corresponding brain structures are aligned but still allows to measure subject-specific differences. After performing dimensionality reduction, the first 20 dimensions of the resulting manifold are used as features to perform classification with the different methods used. More details on the theory and application of this manifold learning approach can be found in [20,50]. Figure 1 exemplarily shows a 2D embedding of a set of ADNI images acquired from healthy controls and subjects with AD. It can be seen that even two embedding dimensions give a relatively good separation between both groups. In our experiments we used a higher dimensional space allowing better discrimination.

ROI-wise features for CTH and TBM

Both CTH and TBM analyses produce local (point-wise) information, either on cortical thickness or the volume. Thus, the number of original features is enormous, and to make the classification more efficient and robust, the number of features has to be reduced. We evaluated both features in a statistical region of interest (ROI) defined as detailed in Appendix S2. Figures 2 and 3 show t-values for statistically significant differences between study groups for TBM and CTH respectively. A detailed description of the definition of these statistical ROIs is given in Appendix S2.

Study design

Table 2 presents an overview on the features calculated for all 834 available ADNI baseline images. All feature values were corrected for age and gender using a linear regression model where control subjects were used as the training set, i.e., the normal, not disease-related, age and gender related differences in the classification features were removed. Feature selection was then carried out on the corrected feature sets using stepwise regression [51].

We used two subsets to perform classification:

I.   All 834 available baseline images described in the subjects section

II. 509 baseline images used by Cuingnet et al. [29] and detailed in their publication.

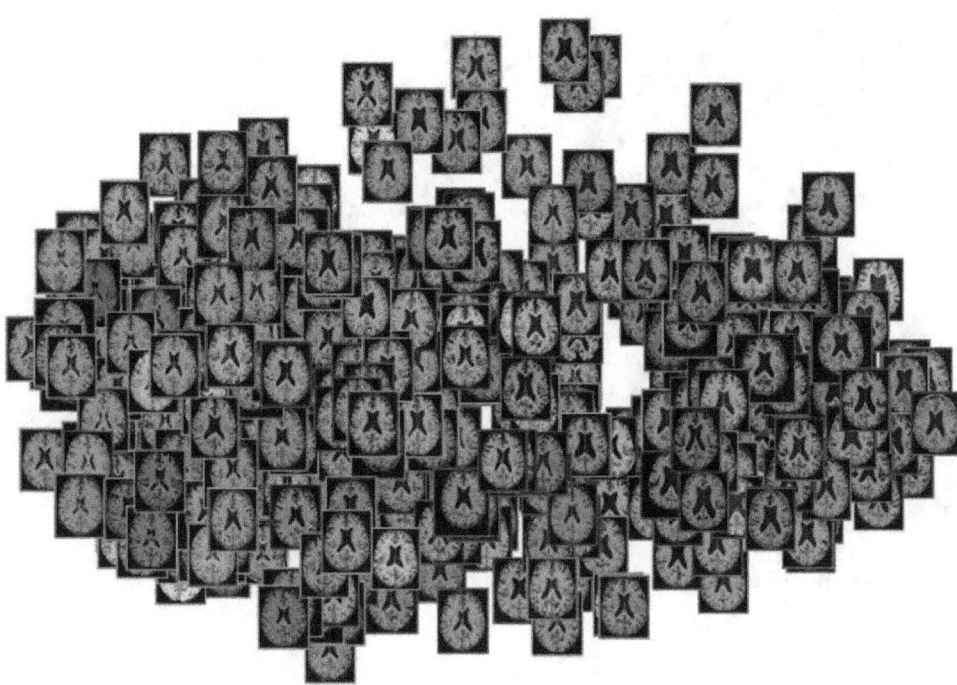

Figure 1. 2D manifold embedding of a set of images acquired from healthy controls (red) and subjects with AD (blue).
doi:10.1371/journal.pone.0025446.g001

The following sections describe the definition of the statistical ROIs and evaluation strategy used for the two datasets respectively.

Dataset I. In order to perform the study using cross-validation in the full dataset, it was divided into three equally sized parts. One part was used to perform the statistical tests for the CTH and TBM features, and the remaining two parts were used to evaluate the classification accuracy. This was repeated three times so that each part was once used to perform the statistical tests. Afterwards, the results of the three repetitions were averaged. The classification accuracy was evaluated using leave-N-out cross validation on those subjects not included in the statistical tests. Five percent of the evaluation subjects were regarded as the test set, and the remaining 95% of the subjects were used to train a classifier which was then applied to the test set. This was repeated table-1-caption100 times, each time selecting randomly the test set subjects. Finally, the results of the 100 repetitions were averaged.

Consequently, in overall, the classification evaluation was performed using 300 (3×100) repetitions, and the results presented in this paper are the average values of all these classifications.

Dataset II. Statistical ROIs for CTH and TBM feature extraction were calculated from the 325 baseline images that are not part of dataset II. In order to allow direct comparison of classification accuracy with the work by Cuingnet et al. [29], separate training and testing sets for the different comparisons were defined using the exact sub-groups reported in their manuscript. Around 50% of all subjects are used to train the different types of classifiers and the reported results are based on classifying the remaining subjects.

Classification methods

We used two different widely used methods to perform classification based on individual features and their combination:

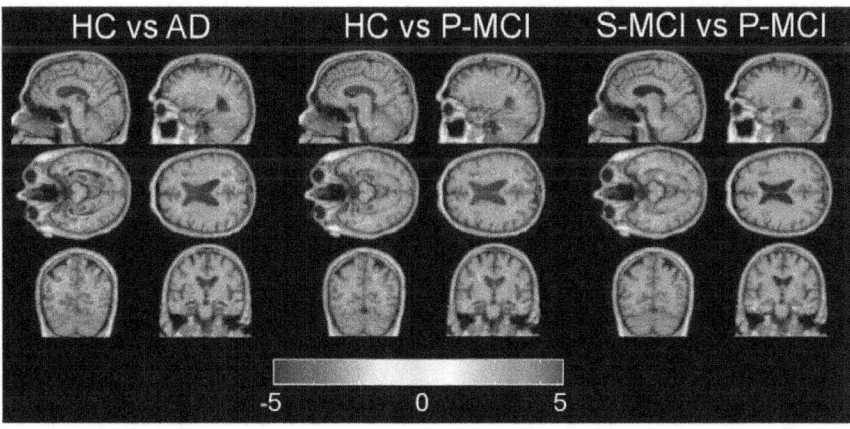

Figure 2. Results for voxelwise t-tests for statistically significant group differences with features extracted from TBM.
doi:10.1371/journal.pone.0025446.g002

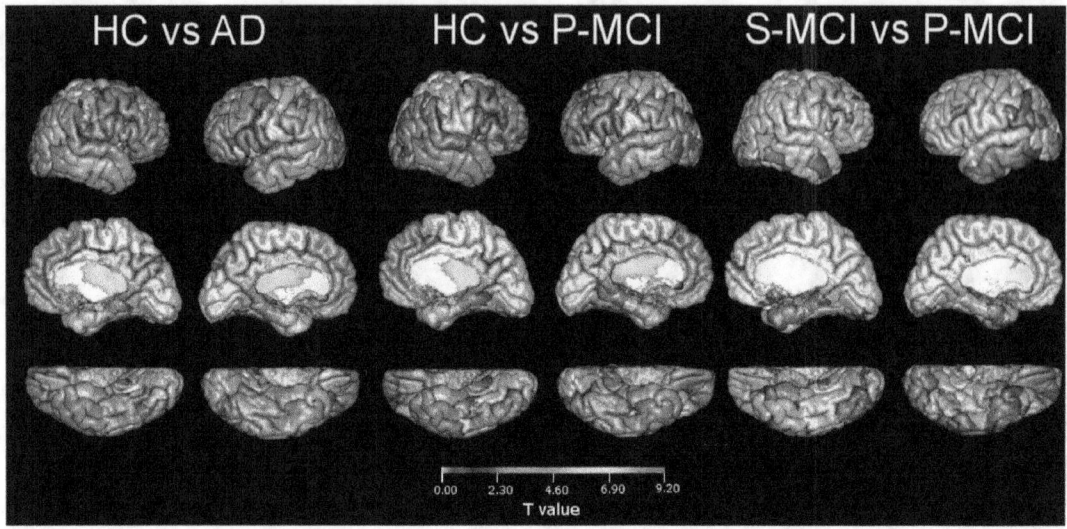

Figure 3. Results for t-tests for statistically significant group differences based on cortical thickness measurements.
doi:10.1371/journal.pone.0025446.g003

Linear discriminant analysis (LDA). Linear discriminant analysis (LDA) is a widely used technique to find a linear combination of features to best separate several classes [52]. In this work we used LDA as implemented in the *classify* function in Matlab with a multivariate normal density model with uninformative priors (p = 0.5).

Support vector machines (SVM). Support vector machines use training data to find a separating hyperplane in the n-dimensional training space that best separates two subject groups [53]. Test subjects are then classified according to their position relative to the defined hyperplane in the n-dimensional feature space. We used the libSVM library to perform the analysis. The radial basis function kernel was selected based on the guidelines provided by the libSVM library (Software available 2.3.2011 at http://www.csie.ntu.edu.tw/cjlin/libsvm).

Results

We used both classification methods to measure classification accuracy based on individual features as well as the combination of all features. The results for the comparisons HC vs AD, HC vs P-MCI and S-MCI vs P-MCI in the full ADNI database are presented in Tables 3, 4 and 5 respectively. Presented are classification accuracy (CCR), sensitivity (SEN) and specificity (SPE). Furthermore, the 95% confidence interval for the classification accuracy is estimated based on the multiple classification runs. Statistically

significant improvements achieved when combining all features are marked with † (p < 0.0001). To test for significance, unpaired t-tests were carried out between distribution estimates for the corresponding classification rates based on the multiple runs. All estimated distributions passed a normality test using a Kolmogorov-Smirnov test at $\alpha = 0.05$.

For direct comparison with work presented by Cuingnet et al. [29], we performed classification based on the training- and testing sets defined in their manuscript as described above. S-MCI and P-MCI groups are defined in the same way as in the original publication. Sensitivity and specificity values for the classification in all three clinical pairings are reported in Table 6. Following the clear advantage for LDA in the performance on the full dataset, we only report results with this classifier for dataset II.

Discussion

In this study we assessed the automatic diagnostic capabilities of 4 structural MRI features (MBL, HC, CTH, TBM) separately and combined in 834 baseline images acquired in the ADNI study. When applied separately, TBM provided the overall best results, closely followed by MBL. Combining all features improved the results in all study experiments. Our results show how a combination of different MRI-based features can improve results based on only one measurement, resulting in a more powerful and stable classifier. The most significant improvement of the combination

Table 2. Features used in the study.

Method	No of features	Description
Hippocampal volume (HV)	1	total volume of left and right hippopcampus
Cortical thickness	9 (HC vs AD)	average cortical thickness within a ROI defined based on group-level statistical analysis
(CTH)	7 (HC vs P-MCI)	
	8 (S-MCI vs P-MCI)	
Tensor-based morphometry (TBM)	84	average Jacobian of atrophic voxels within a ROI, weighted based on voxel-wise p-values
Manifold-based learning (MBL)	20	coordinates of a subject in a low-dimensional manifold space learned from pairwise image similarities

doi:10.1371/journal.pone.0025446.t002

Table 3. Classification results for HC vs AD.

Feature	LDA			SVM		
	CCR [95% CI]	SEN	SPE	CCR [95% CI]	SEN	SPE
MBL	85† [64 100]	87	83	85 [64 100]	87	83
HV	81† [57 100]	81	79	81† [57 100]	84	77
CTH	81† [64 100]	89	71	82† [57 100]	90	73
TBM	87† [71 100]	90	84	87 [71 100]	89	84
All	89 [71 100]	93	85	86 [71 100]	94	78

†means statistically significant different from the combined results with p < 0.0001. CCR = Correct classification rate, SEN = Sensitivity, SPE = Specificity.
doi:10.1371/journal.pone.0025446.t003

Table 5. Classification results for S-MCI vs P-MCI.

Feature	LDA			SVM		
	CCR [95% CI]	SEN	SPE	CCR [95% CI]	SEN	SPE
MBL	65† [36 86]	64	66	65† [43 86]	77	48
HV	65† [36 86]	63	67	62 [36 86]	83	33
CTH	56† [29 86]	63	45	59 [36 79]	96	03
TBM	64† [36 86]	65	62	64† [36 86]	77	44
All	68 [43 93]	67	69	60 [36 86]	92	14

†means statistically significant different from the combined results with p < 0.0001.
doi:10.1371/journal.pone.0025446.t005

over the best individual feature can be observed for HC vs P-MCI with 5% units followed by 3 and 2% units for S-MCI vs P-MCI and HC vs AD, respectively. These improvements lead to 20, 12 and 9 subjects more being correctly classified respectively when using the combined feature set as compared to the best single feature for every comparison. Comparing two classification approaches based on LDA and SVMs resulted in a clear advantage of the former.

Several studies reported classification results using single MRI methods for the HC/AD classification (Table 7). Liu et al. [24] reported SEN/SPE of 92/90 in the classification of HC/AD subjects using regional cortical volumes in the AddNeuroMed dataset. McEvoy et al. [26] report a CCR of 89 on images from the ADNI database using features from cortical thickness and structural volumes. Vemuri et al. [54] present a SEN/SPE of 86/86 on 380 subjects using the STAND score. In our study the results obtained with single methods are lower (71–90) but almost identical when the methods were combined. It should be noted, however, that Liu and colleagues did not use cross-validation or separate training/testing sets when producing the results which could lead to overestimation of the results in a dataset outside the study cohort. Gerardin et al. [23] acquired a high SEN/SPE of 96/92 by using hippocampal shape analysis, but the number of subjects (25 HC, 23 AD) was quite low in order to produce results with good generalizability. Westman et al. [55] reported a CCR of 82 for HC vs AD classification and 73 for HC vs P-MCI classification by using various regional brain volumes. Our results are substantially more accurate, the group sizes are larger and clinical follow-up time is one year longer. Chupin et al. [21] reported SEN/SPE of 75/77 (hippocampal volume) and Querbes et al. [27] a CCR of 85 (cortical thickness), both lower than the

results acquired with the combination of features or TBM features independently in our study.

Varying results concerning AD prediction (S-MCI/P-MCI classification using baseline measurements) have been published (Table 7): Querbes et al. [27] reported a CCR of 73, Liu et al. [25] a SEN/SPE of 76/68, Chupin et al. [21] reported a SEN/SPE of 60/65 and Davatzikos et al. [15] SEN/SPE of 95/38. Our results with separate and combined baseline features lie in the range of these results (SEN/SPE 63/67, 64/66 and 67/69 when using HV, MBL and the combined features, respectively).

There can be several explanations for the variation in the reported results. A majority of the studies in this field have used different statistical methods and MRI feature extraction strategies on different datasets, which makes a comparison of the results complicated. Also the variation in the size of the study samples and the use (or ignoring) of cross-validation or separate training/testing sets are important factors, which both have crucial impact on the reliability and generalizability of the results. In Lötjönen et al. [36], we demonstrated that choosing from a population of 350 cases several times 2/3 for the training set and 1/3 for the test set and using hippocampus volume as a classification feature can lead to any classification accuracy between 53% and 77%. This observation is also confirmed by the high confidence intervals for the classification accuracies reported in Tables 3, 4 and 5. This shows that a fair comparison of methods based on the classification accuracy is difficult if not exactly the same data and classification approaches are used. Furthermore, since the ADNI study is still ongoing, several subjects labeled as S-MCI will progress in the future to the P-MCI group.

A recent study with a subset of ADNI subjects assessed the classification performance of several structural MRI methods in experiments comparable to our investigation [29]. Reported

Table 4. Classification results for HC vs P-MCI.

Feature	LDA			SVM		
	CCR [95% CI]	SEN	SPE	CCR [95% CI]	SEN	SPE
MBL	78† [54 100]	81	75	77† [54 92]	84	69
HV	76† [54 92]	77	76	78 [54 92]	83	71
CTH	77† [54 100]	85	65	77 [54 100]	89	62
TBM	79† [62 100]	82	76	80† [62 100]	85	74
All	84 [62 100]	86	82	82 [62 100]	93	67

†means statistically significant different from the combined results with p < 0.0001.
doi:10.1371/journal.pone.0025446.t004

Table 6. Classification results based on a subset of ADNI that was previously used for classification by Cuingnet et al. [29].

Feature	HC vs AD		HC vs P-MCI		S-MCI vs P-MCI	
	SEN	SPE	SEN	SPE	SEN	SPE
MBL	90	74	84	92	55	76
HV	80	69	75	76	63	70
CTH	85	75	86	59	72	35
TBM	93	76	90	84	63	59
All	94	76	94	89	69	54

doi:10.1371/journal.pone.0025446.t006

Table 7. Classification results of healthy control (HC), mild cognitive impairment (MCI) and Alzheimer's disease subjects reported in the recent literature.

Study	N	Features	HC vs AD			HC vs P-MCI			S-MCI vs P-MCI		
			CCR	SEN	SPE	CCR	SEN	SPE	CCR	SEN	SPE
Liu et al. [24]	333	Cortical volumes	91	92	90	-	-	-	-	-	-
Gerardin et al. [23]*	70	Hippocampus shape	94	96	92	-	-	-	-	-	-
Chupin et al. [21]*	605	Hippocampus volume	76	75	77	-	-	-	64	60	65
Querbes et al. [27]*	382	Cortical thickness	85	-	-	-	-	-	73	75	68
Liu et al. [25]	312	Amygdala/caudate volumes	-	-	-	-	-	-	69	76	68
Davatzikos et al. [15]*	356	SPARE-AD index	-	-	-	-	-	-	56	95	38
Cuingnet et al. [29]*	509	Various	-	81	95	-	73	85	-	62	69
Hinrichs et al. [14]*	159	MRI & PET	81	-	-	60	92	14	-	-	-
Westman et al. [55]	351	Various volumes	82	-	-	73	-	-	-	-	-
McEvoy et al. [26]*	398	Cortical thickness/various volumes	89	83	93	-	-	-	-	-	-
Vemuri et al. [54]	380	STAND score	-	86	86	-	-	-	-	-	-

N = Number of study subjects,
* = ADNI dataset.
doi:10.1371/journal.pone.0025446.t007

SEN/SPE lie in the ranges 59/81–81/95 (HC vs AD) and 70/73–73/85 (HC vs P-MCI). While most methods tested did not exceed the accuracy of a random classifier for the discrimination between S-MCI and P-MCI, the best results reported for this task were a SEN/SPE of 62/69 when using hippocampal volume. To allow a direct comparison of the results reported by Cuingnet et al. [29], we evaluated our features on the exact same training- and testing sets used in their paper. This direct comparison shows that our results compare favourably to other, established methods in neuroimaging. For HC vs AD classification, individual features in our study give more sensitive but less specific results than most methods in the previous publication. Combining all features gives an overall better classification accuracy than the majority of previously tested methods. Our results on the combined feature set furthermore outperform the majority of methods tested by Cuingnet et al. [29] when predicting MCI conversion as well as all methods for the classification between HC and P-MCI. A significant difference in classification accuracy can be observed between the full ADNI dataset and this smaller subset used for comparison with previous work. Reasons may include a strict separation into trainin- and testing sets which may result in less generalisability as well as the shorter follow-up period that was considered to define progression to AD.

Some studies have also combined different biomarkers (CSF, MRI, PET) with the idea of measuring different aspects of AD pathology and thus improve the classification accuracy. Hinrichs et al. [14] improved their HC/AD classification CCR by a few % units to 81 by combining MRI and PET. Eckerström et al. [16] studied the separation of a unified HC/S-MCI group from P-MCI group with CSF proteins and manual hippocampal volumes. They found CSF to be superior to MRI (SEN/SPE of 95/79 vs 86/66) while the combination performed best (SEN/SPE 90/91). However, it should be noted that the study sample in that particular study was small (a total of 68 subjects) and neither cross-validation or separate training/testing sets were used in order to ensure good generalizability of the results. In Kohannim et al. [17], the improvement from using multiple biomarkers was not significant and Davatzikos et al. [15] reported marginal improvements which, however, may be related to the fact that results with only one biomarker were not very good to begin with.

Considering solely the classification accuracies of the present study and those reported in literature, it seems questionable if the collection of several biomarkers is worth the effort and resource. A combination of different features extracted from a single MRI seems to provide results that are comparable or better than those obtained with other or multiple biomarkers. In a clinical point of view, this is interesting since it means that a single MRI scan provides not only aid to differential diagnostics of cognitive impairment, but also reliably describes a persons phase in the HC/AD continuum. MRI is also widely available, non-invasive and often useful in the differential diagnostics of memory problems thus making it a compelling option as the first biomarker that would be obtained from a patient with mild memory problems. However, a comprehensive differential diagnostics between AD and non-AD cognitive impairments will still require assessment of various different biomarkers. Also, it should be noted that the computational techniques used in this paper are not widely available in the clinical environment and thus limit their usage in the clinical work at present.

Strengths of the presented study are i) the use of multiple features extracted from one imaging modality, ii) large groups, iii) rigorous validation process of the results using cross-validation, and iv) results comparable or better than the ones published so far.

Our study has also some limitations that should be mentioned. The results are obtained from a single (although collected from multiple sites) cohort and should be also validated in other cohorts. A longer clinical follow-up time would be needed to see if the classification results of S-MCI/P-MCI experiment changed when more of the MCI subjects converted to AD. Furthermore, the ADNI study does not provide postmortem pathological confirmation of the clinical status. With this limitation, individual subjects might be wrongly categorized. Although a rigorous validation process was used, optimally we need to establish standardized cut-offs that would be well generalizable to other cohorts outside ADNI. That is, however, beyond the possibilities of this study and will require vast standardization and validation procedures. Also, the CTH pipeline had problems especially with severely atrophied brains or MRI scans with poor image quality. A more robust pipeline would be desirable in order to guarantee a more reliable feature extraction.

Supporting Information

Appendix S1 The Alzheimer's Disease Neuroimaging Initiative. (DOCX)

Appendix S2 ROI-wise features for CTH and TBM. (DOCX)

Acknowledgments

Data used in the preparation of this article were obtained from the ADNI database (www.loni.ucla.edu/ADNI). As such, the investigators within the ADNI contributed to the design and implementation of ADNI and/or provided data but did not participate in analysis or writing of this report. ADNI investigators include (complete listing available at http://adni.loni.ucla.edu/wp-content/uploads/how_to_apply/ADNI_Authorship_List.pdf).

Author Contributions

Conceived and designed the experiments: RW VJ JK DR HS JL. Performed the experiments: RW VJ JK EN DPZ. Analyzed the data: RW VJ JK. Contributed reagents/materials/analysis tools: RW JK DR JL. Wrote the paper: RW VJ.

References

1. Brookmeyer R, Johnson E, Ziegler-Graham K, Arrighi HM (2007) Forecasting the global burden of Alzheimer's disease. Alzheimer's and Dementia 3: 186–191.
2. Cummings J, Doody R, Clark C (2007) Disease-modifying therapies for alzheimer disease: challenges to early intervention. Neurology 69: 1622–1634.
3. Petersen R (2001) Practice parameter: early detection of dementia: mild cognitive impairment (an evidence-based review). Neurology 56: 1133.
4. Gauthier S, Reisberg B, Zaudig M, Petersen R, Ritchie K, et al. (2006) Mild cognitive impairment. Lancet 367: 1262–1270.
5. Braak H, Braak E (1991) Neuropathological stageing of Alzheimer-related changes. Acta Neuropathologica 82: 239–259.
6. Wenk G (2003) Neuropathologic changes in alzheimer's disease. Journal of Clinical Psychiatry 64 Suppl 9.
7. Hampel H, Brger K, Teipel SJ, Bokde AL, Zetterberg H, et al. (2008) Core candidate neurochemical and imaging biomarkers of alzheimer's disease. Alzheimer's and Dementia 4: 38–48.
8. Hyman BT, Marzloff K, Arriagada PV (1993) The lack of accumulation of senile plaques or amyloid burden in Alzheimer's disease suggests a dynamic balance between amyloid deposition and resolution. J Neuropathol Exp Neurol 52: 594–600.
9. Gmez-Isla T, Hollister R, West H, Mui S, Growdon J, et al. (1997) Neuronal loss correlates with but exceeds neurofibrillary tangles in alzheimer's disease. Ann Neurol 41: 17–24.
10. Ingelsson M, Fukumoto H, Newell KL, Growdon JH, Hedley-Whyte ET, et al. (2004) Early abeta accumulation and progressive synaptic loss, gliosis, and tangle formation in ad brain. Neurology 62: 925–31.
11. Jack C, Jr., Knopman D, Jagust W, Shaw L, Aisen P, et al. (2010) Hypothetical model of dynamic biomarkers of the alzheimer's pathological cascade. Lancet Neurology 27: 685–691.
12. Hampel H, Frank R, Broich K, Teipel S, Katz J, abd Hardy RG, et al. (2010) Biomarkers for alzheimer's disease: academic, industry and regulatory perspectives. NatRevDrug Discov 9: 560–574.
13. Fan Y, Resnick SM, Wu X, Davatzikos C (2008) Structural and functional biomarkers of prodromal alzheimer's disease: A high-dimensional pattern classification study. NeuroImage 41: 277–285.
14. Hinrichs C, Singh V, Xu G, Johnson S (2009) Mkl for robust multi-modality ad classification. In: MICCAI (II) Springer, volume 5762 of Lecture Notes in Computer Science. pp 786–794.
15. Davatzikos C, Bhatt P, Shaw LM, Batmanghelich KN, Trojanowski JQ (2010) Prediction of MCI to AD conversion, via MRI, CSF biomarkers, and pattern classification. Neurobiology of Aging In Press, Corrected Proof: -.
16. Eckerstrom C, Andreasson U, Olsson E, Rolstad S, Blennow K, et al. (2010) Combination of hippocampal volume and cerebrospinal uid biomarkers improves predictive value in mild cognitive impairment. Dement Geriatr Cogn Disord 29: 294–300.
17. Kohannim O, Hua X, Hibar DP, Lee S, Chou YY, et al. (2010) Boosting power for clinical trials using classifiers based on multiple biomarkers. Neurobiology of Aging 31: 1429–1442.
18. Landau S, Harvey D, Madison C, Reiman E, Foster N, et al. (2010) Comparing predictors of conversion and decline in mild cognitive impairment. Neurology 75: 230–8.
19. Walhovd KB, Fjell AM, Brewer J, McEvoy LK, Fennema-Notestine C, et al. (2010) Combining MR Imaging, Positron-Emission Tomography, and CSF Biomarkers in the Diagnosis and Prognosis of Alzheimer Disease. American Journal of Neuroradiology 31: 347–354+.
20. Wolz R, Aljabar P, Hajnal JV, Lotjonen J, Rueckert D (2011) Manifold learning combining imaging with non-imaging information. In: IEEE International Symposium on Biomedical Imaging. pp 960–963.
21. Chupin M, Hammers A, Liu R, Colliot O, Burdett J, et al. (2009) Automatic segmentation of the hippocampus and the amygdala driven by hybrid constraints: Method and validation. NeuroImage 46: 749–761.
22. Devanand DP, Pradhaban G, Liu X, Khandji A, De Santi S, et al. (2007) Hippocampal and entorhinal atrophy in mild cognitive impairment - Prediction of Alzheimer disease. Neurology 68: 828–836+.
23. Gerardin E, Chetelat G, Chupin M, Cuingnet R, Desgranges B, et al. (2009) Multidimensional classification of hippocampal shape features discriminates Alzheimer's disease and mild cognitive impairment from normal aging. NeuroImage 47: 1476–1486.
24. Liu Y, Paajanen T, Zhang Y, Westman E, Wahlund LO, et al. (2009) Combination analysis of neuropsychological tests and structural MRI measures in differentiating AD, MCI and control groups–The AddNeuroMed study. Neurobiology of Aging In Press, Corrected Proof: -.
25. Liu Y, Paajanen T, Zhang Y, Westman E, Wahlund LO, et al. (2010) Analysis of regional MRI volumes and thicknesses as predictors of conversion from mild cognitive impairment to Alzheimer's disease. Neurobiology of Aging 31: 1375–1385.
26. McEvoy L, Fennema-Notestine C, JC R, Hagler D, Holland D, et al. (2009) Alzheimer disease: quantitative structural neuroimaging for detection and prediction of clinical and structural changes in mild cognitive impairment. Radiology 251: 1950–205.
27. Querbes O, Aubry F, Pariente J, Lotterie JA, Dmonet JF, et al. (2009) Early diagnosis of alzheimer's disease using cortical thickness: impact of cognitive reserve. Brain 132: 2036–2047.
28. Mueller SG, Weiner MW, Thal LJ, Petersen RC, Jack C, et al. (2005) The Alzheimer's Disease Neuroimaging Initiative. Neuroimaging Clinics of North America 15: 869–877.
29. Cuingnet R, Gerardin E, Tessieras J, Auzias G, Lehricy S, et al. (2010) Automatic classification of patients with Alzheimer's disease from structural MRI: A comparison of ten methods using the ADNI database. NeuroImage In Press, Corrected Proof: -.
30. Petersen RC, Aisen PS, Beckett LA, Donohue MC, Gamst AC, et al. (2010) Alzheimer's Disease Neuroimaging Initiative (ADNI): clinical characterization. Neurology 74: 201–209.
31. Folstein MF, Folstein SE, McHugh PR (1975) Mini-mental state: A practical method for grading the cognitive state of patients for the clinician. Journal of Psychiatric Research 12(3): 189–198.
32. Morris J (1993) The Clinical Dementia Rating (CDR): current version and scoring rules. Neurology 43: 2412–2414.
33. McKhann G, Drachman D, Folstein M, Katzman R, Price D, et al. (1984) Clinical diagnosis of alzheimer's disease: report of the nincds-adrda work group under the auspices of department of health and human services task force on alzheimer's disease. Neurology 34: 939–944.
34. Jack CR, Jr., Bernstein MA, Fox NC, Thompson P, Alexander G, et al. (2008) The Alzheimer's disease neuroimaging initiative (ADNI): MRI methods. Journal of Magnetic Resonance Imaging 27: 685–691.
35. Lotjonen JM, Wolz R, Koikkalainen JR, Thurfjell L, Waldemar G, et al. (2010) Fast and robust multi-atlas segmentation of brain magnetic resonance images. NeuroImage 49: 2352–2365.
36. Lotjonen J, Wolz R, Koikkalainen J, Julkunen V, Thurfjell L, et al. (2011) Fast and robust extraction of hippocampus from mr images for diagnostics of alzheimer's disease. NeuroImage 56: 185–196.
37. Van Leemput K, Maes F, Vandermeulen D, Suetens P (1999) Automated model-based tissue classification of MR images of the brain. IEEE Transactions on Medical Imaging 18: 897–908.
38. Lerch J, Evans A (2005) Cortical thickness analysis examined through power analysis and a population simulation. NeuroImage 24: 163–173.
39. Mazziotta J, Toga A, Evans A, Fox P, Lancaster J, et al. (2001) A probabilistic atlas and reference system for the human brain: International Consortium for Brain Mapping (ICBM). Philos Trans R Soc Lond B Biol Sci 356: 1293–1322.
40. Sled JG, Zijdenbos AP, Evans AC (1998) A nonparametric method for automatic correction of intensity nonuniformity in MRI data. IEEE Transactions on Medical Imaging 17: 87–97.
41. Smith SM (2002) Fast robust automated brain extraction. Hum Brain Mapp 17: 143–155.
42. Zijdenbos AP, Forghani R, Evans AC (1998) Automatic quantification of MS lesions in 3D MRI brain data sets: Validation of INSECT. In: III WMM, Colchester ACF, Delp SL, eds. MICCAI Springer, volume 1496 of Lecture Notes in Computer Science. pp 439–448.
43. Tohka J, Zijdenbos A, Evans A (2004) Fast and robust parameter estimation for statistical partial volume models in brain mri. NeuroImage 23: 84–97.
44. Kim JS, Singh V, Lee JK, Lerch J, Ad-Dab'bagh Y, et al. (2005) Automated 3-d extraction and evaluation of the inner and outer cortical surfaces using a laplacian map and partial volume effect classification. NeuroImage 27: 210–221.
45. Chung M, Taylor J (2004) Diffusion smoothing on brain surface via finite element method. In: ISBI IEEE. pp 432–435.

46. Brun CC, Lepor N, Pennec X, Lee AD, Barysheva M, et al. (2009) Mapping the regional inuence of genetics on brain structure variability – a tensor-based morphometry study. NeuroImage 48: 37–49.

47. Koikkalainen J, Lotjonen J, Thurfjell L, Rueckert D, Waldemar G, et al. (2011) Multi-template tensor-based morphometry: Application to analysis of alzheimer's disease. NeuroImage 56: 1134–1144.

48. Belkin M, Niyogi P (2003) Laplacian eigenmaps for dimensionality reduction and data representation. Neural Computation 15: 1373–1396.

49. Rueckert D, Sonoda LI, Hayes C, Hill DLG, Leach MO, et al. (1999) Nonrigid registration using free-form deformations: Application to breast MR images. IEEE Transactions on Medical Imaging 18: 712–721.

50. Wolz R, Heckemann RA, Aljabar P, Hajnal JV, Hammers A, et al. (2010) Measurement of hippocampal atrophy using 4D graph-cut segmentation: Application to ADNI. NeuroImage 52: 1009–1018.

51. Draper NR, Smith H (1998) Applied Regression Analysis (Wiley Series in Probability and Statistics). Wiley.

52. Krzanowski WJ (1988) Principles of Multivariate Analysis: A User's Perspective Oxford University Press.

53. Cortes C, Vapnik V (1995) Support-vector networks. Machine Learning 20: 273–297.

54. Vemuri P, Gunter JL, Senjem ML, Whitwell JL, Kantarci K, et al. (2008) Alzheimer's disease diagnosis in individual subjects using structural mr images: Validation studies. NeuroImage 39: 1186–1197.

55. Westman E, Simmons A, Zhang Y, Muehlboeck JS, Tunnard C, et al. (2011) Multivariate analysis of mri data for alzheimer's disease, mild cognitive impairment and healthy controls. NeuroImage 54: 1178–1187.

Combined Evaluation of FDG-PET and MRI Improves Detection and Differentiation of Dementia

Juergen Dukart[1]*, Karsten Mueller[1], Annette Horstmann[1], Henryk Barthel[3], Harald E. Möller[1], Arno Villringer[1,2], Osama Sabri[3], Matthias L. Schroeter[1,2]

1 Max Planck Institute for Human Cognitive and Brain Sciences, Leipzig, Germany, 2 Day Clinic of Cognitive Neurology, University of Leipzig, Leipzig, Germany, 3 Department of Nuclear Medicine, University of Leipzig, Leipzig, Germany

Abstract

Introduction: Various biomarkers have been reported in recent literature regarding imaging abnormalities in different types of dementia. These biomarkers have helped to significantly improve early detection and also differentiation of various dementia syndromes. In this study, we systematically applied whole-brain and region-of-interest (ROI) based support vector machine classification separately and on combined information from different imaging modalities to improve the detection and differentiation of different types of dementia.

Methods: Patients with clinically diagnosed Alzheimer's disease (AD: n = 21), with frontotemporal lobar degeneration (FTLD: n = 14) and control subjects (n = 13) underwent both [F18]fluorodeoxyglucose positron emission tomography (FDG-PET) scanning and magnetic resonance imaging (MRI), together with clinical and behavioral assessment. FDG-PET and MRI data were commonly processed to get a precise overlap of all regions in both modalities. Support vector machine classification was applied with varying parameters separately for both modalities and to combined information obtained from MR and FDG-PET images. ROIs were extracted from comprehensive systematic and quantitative meta-analyses investigating both disorders.

Results: Using single-modality whole-brain and ROI information FDG-PET provided highest accuracy rates for both, detection and differentiation of AD and FTLD compared to structural information from MRI. The ROI-based multimodal classification, combining FDG-PET and MRI information, was highly superior to the unimodal approach and to the whole-brain pattern classification. With this method, accuracy rate of up to 92% for the differentiation of the three groups and an accuracy of 94% for the differentiation of AD and FTLD patients was obtained.

Conclusion: Accuracy rate obtained using combined information from both imaging modalities is the highest reported up to now for differentiation of both types of dementia. Our results indicate a substantial gain in accuracy using combined FDG-PET and MRI information and suggest the incorporation of such approaches to clinical diagnosis and to differential diagnostic procedures of neurodegenerative disorders.

Citation: Dukart J, Mueller K, Horstmann A, Barthel H, Möller HE, et al. (2011) Combined Evaluation of FDG-PET and MRI Improves Detection and Differentiation of Dementia. PLoS ONE 6(3): e18111. doi:10.1371/journal.pone.0018111

Editor: Wang Zhan, University of California, San Francisco, United States of America

Received August 30, 2010; **Accepted** February 25, 2011; **Published** March 23, 2011

Funding: The work was funded by the Max Planck Society. The funders had no role in study design, data collection and analysis, decision to publish, or preparation of the manuscript.

Competing Interests: The authors have declared that no competing interests exist.

* E-mail: dukart@cbs.mpg.de

Introduction

In recent research, various biomarkers have been reported to differentiate between early stages of dementia and healthy control subjects or between different types of neurodegenerative disorders, suggesting an integration of these would improve diagnostic accuracy of dementia [1]–[9].

For the detection of dementia, accuracy rates significantly above 90% have recently been reported using univariate and multivariate statistical approaches in magnetic resonance imaging (MRI) and [F18]fluorodeoxyglucose positron emission tomography (FDG-PET) [1],[10]–[14]. However, the differentiation of the two most common types of dementia, namely Alzheimer's disease (AD) and frontotemporal lobar degeneration (FTLD), is still

problematic. For this differentiation, accuracy rates ranging between 84 and 89% are still in need of improvement, especially due to a substantially lower sensitivity compared with specificity of actual methods [10],[12],[15]. Nevertheless, the use of biomarkers has significantly helped to improve diagnostic accuracy compared with diagnoses based solely on clinical and neuropsychological evaluation [16],[17]. For these reasons, recent studies have suggested to incorporate imaging findings into criteria for diagnosis of dementia [17],[18].

For AD patients imaging studies have shown reduced glucose consumption mainly in parietotemporal and posterior cingulate cortices [9],[20],[21] and structural changes in the hippocampus and entorhinal area relative to healthy controls [9],[21],[22]. In FTLD patients, atrophy and reduced metabolic rate for glucose have been reported to be predominately located in the medial thalamus, amygdala and in frontotemporal and anterior cingulate cortices [4],[8],[20],[21],[23].

For multivariate differentiation of different types of dementia support vector machine classification (SVM) is used based on whole-brain voxel information [10] or most frequently on ROI values [6],[12]–[13],[24]–[26]. A major problem of the ROI-based approach is the limited generalizability of the trained classifier, because the ROIs are selected based on features showing a between-group differentiation in the same groups in a univariate analysis. Although ROIs selected with this method provide a good discrimination between groups used in these specific studies, they might show significantly reduced discrimination power when applied to new data sets. This could be the case if the selected regions just detect differences between groups, which are not necessarily attributed to the specific neurodegenerative disorder. Furthermore, AD and FTLD patients have been shown to develop a differential regional pattern of glucose hypometabolism and atrophy [21],[27]. However, the previously proposed approaches only used single modality information for the classification algorithms loosing this way the differential information which various biomarkers might provide for a better detection and differentiation of dementia syndromes.

Here, we apply SVM as the most frequently used multivariate approach to evaluate its contribution for detection and differentiation of dementia in multimodal imaging. To increase the validity of our method we apply SVM classification on data extracted from ROIs based on disorder-specific metabolic reductions and atrophy reported in comprehensive meta-analyses investigating AD and FTLD. This method allows a better generalization of our classification algorithms to other clinical centers and ensures that only disorder-specific changes are used for SVM based discrimination. We hypothesize that common use of different imaging modalities might substantially improve early detection and differentiation of dementia.

Methods

Ethics Statement

The research protocol was approved by the Ethics Committee of the University of Leipzig, and was in accordance with the latest version of the Declaration of Helsinki. Informed consent was obtained from all subjects.

Subjects

We analyzed FDG-PET and T1-weighted MRI data of 21 patients (Table 1) with an early stage of probable AD, 14 patients with an early stage of FTLD and 13 control subjects. Patients were recruited from the Day Clinic of Cognitive Neurology at the University of Leipzig. Probable AD was diagnosed according to NINCDS-ADRDA criteria [28]. Although all AD subjects also fulfilled the revised NINCDS-ADRDA criteria suggested by Dubois et al. [17] the fulfillment of the original McKhann criteria was sufficient for the inclusion into the study. Diagnosis of FTLD was based on criteria suggested by Neary et al. [29]. The control group included subjects who visited the Day Clinic with subjective cognitive complaints, which were not objectively confirmed by a comprehensive neuropsychological and clinical evaluation. FDG-PET and MRI for these subjects was conducted for diagnostic reasons within the clinical assessment. This control group was chosen because, in clinical practice, it is crucial to discriminate between these subjects showing a normal age-related decrease in cognitive performance and patients with an early stage of dementia. Patients were excluded if structural imaging revealed

Table 1. Subject group characteristics.

	Controls	AD	FTLD	ANOVA (df,F,P)
Number	13	21	14	–
Male/Female	7/6	9/12	7/7	–
Age (years)	53.9±6.0	61.1±6.7	60.8±6.4	2, 5.76, 0.006
CDR (score)	0.23±0.26	0.71±0.25	0.82±0.42	2, 13.93, 0.000
MMSE (score)	n.a.	23.2±3.9	24.4±4.2	–
Education (years)	12.3±3.1	10.7±3.1	11.6±3.8	2,1.02,0.368

Mean ± standard deviation. AD Alzheimer's disease, ANOVA analysis of variance, CDR Clinical Dementia Rating Scale, FTLD frontotemporal lobar degeneration, MMSE Mini Mental State Examination, n.a. not available.
doi:10.1371/journal.pone.0018111.t001

lesions due to stroke, traumatic head injury, brain tumor or inflammatory diseases.

Data acquisition

MRI data. For each subject, a high-resolution T1-weighted MRI scan was obtained, consisting of 128 sagittal slices adjusted to AC-PC line and a with slice thickness of 1.5 mm and pixel size of 1×1 mm^2. MRI was performed on two different 3T scanners (MedSpec 30/100, Bruker Biospin, Ettlingen Germany and Magnetom Trio, Siemens, Erlangen, Germany) using two different T1-weighted sequences (MDEFT or MP-RAGE with TR = 1300 ms, TI = 650 ms, TE = 3.93 ms or TE = 10 ms; FOV 25×25 cm^2; matrix = 256×256 voxels). On the MedSpec scanner, only the MDEFT-sequence and on the Magnetom Trio scanner, either MDEFT or MP-RAGE sequences were used. The distribution of scanner types and sequences used to obtain the MRI data was random across subjects and did not differ significantly in its distribution between the groups nor for scanner type nor for sequence.

PET data. Each subject also underwent FDG-PET imaging either a few a weeks before or after the MRI scan. All PET data were acquired on a Siemens ECAT EXACT HR+ scanner (CTI/Siemens, Knoxville, TN, USA) under a standard resting condition in 2-dimensional (2D) mode. The 2D acquisition mode was used because it allows a better quantification of the PET data due to lower scatter radiation. Sixty-three slices were simultaneously collected with an axial resolution of 5 mm full width at half maximum (FWHM) and in-plane resolution of 4.6 mm. After correction for attenuation, scatter, decay and scanner-specific dead-time, images were reconstructed by filtered back-projection using a Hann-filter of 4.9 mm FWHM. The 63 transaxial slices obtained had a matrix of 128×128 voxels with an edge length of 2.45 mm.

Image processing and statistical analysis

The procedure described below has been specifically designed for this study, aiming at a most accurate co-processing of FDG-PET and MRI data to obtain a more precise between subject anatomical overlap (Figure 1). All image-processing steps were carried out using the SPM5 software package (Statistical Parametric Mapping software: http://www.fil.ion.ucl.ac.uk/spm/) implemented in Matlab 7.7 (MathWorks Inc., Sherborn, MA). SVM classification was conducted with the LIBSVM software [30] using the Matlab interface.

MR images. The MR images were first interpolated to get an isotropic resolution of $1\times1\times1$ mm^3. The resultant MR images

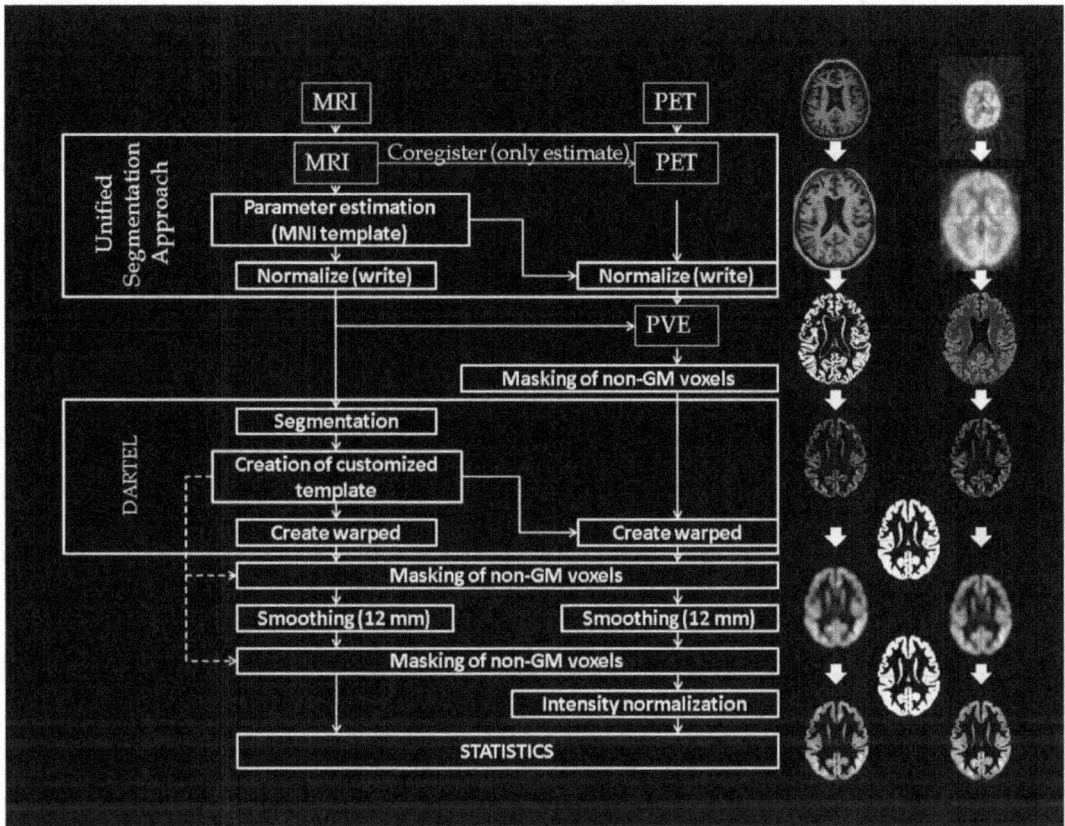

Figure 1. Schematic representation of the procedure for FDG-PET and MRI data handling and processing steps. FDG-PET [F18]fluorodeoxyglucose positron emission tomography, MRI magnetic resonance imaging, MNI Montreal Neurological Institute, PVE partial volume effect correction.
doi:10.1371/journal.pone.0018111.g001

were coregistered on their respective FDG-PET images and bias corrected for inhomogeneity artifacts using the Unified Segmentation Approach described in detail by Ashburner and Friston [31]. This specific method performs a better coregistration of images from different modalities and allows a more accurate segmentation due to the bias correction. A further reason to use this approach was that the straightforward coregistration implemented in the PVElab software described later sometimes failed. We used this software for automatic partial volume correction of the FDG-PET images. The coregistered MR images were processed using the DARTEL (Diffeomorphic Anatomical Registration Through Exponentiated Lie algebra) approach [32] to enable a more accurate spatial normalization. This approach registers all gray matter (GM) and white matter (WM) images to an averaged-size template created from all subjects used in this study and modulates the images to preserve the total amount of signal from each region in the images. Subsequently, the images were smoothed using a Gaussian kernel of 12 mm FWHM. This smoothing factor, although higher then usual MR kernels, was selected based on extensive tests, because it allows the optimal coevaluation with lower resolution FDG-PET images.

FDG-PET data. Within the common registration with MRI data using the Unified Segmentation Approach described above, PET images were interpolated to the same voxel size as the MR images, namely $1 \times 1 \times 1$ mm^3. This processing does not introduce any additional noise into the PET images. However, in our experience, it substantially improves the subsequent partial volume effect (PVE) correction of voxels representing GM intensities using

the modified Müller-Gärtner method [33],[34]. Due to the interpolation, they are exactly overlaid with the MR tissue class images of the same subject obtained from the segmentation step in the PVE approach. Thus, the within-voxel correction is done only for those voxels directly overlaying the GM structures in the MR images. Instead of smoothing the MR data to the resolution of PET data and thus loosing the exact quantitative and qualitative information of GM distribution, which is usually done in the PVE correction, the interpolation of FDG-PET preserves this information. This allows a more accurate correction of atrophy effects onto glucose utilization. The subsequent PVE correction including all image processing steps was done by using the automatic algorithm implemented in the PVElab software package [35]. Because the modified Müller-Gärtner method sets all WM voxel values to the mean WM intensity value, these regions do not contain any further valuable regional information after the PVE correction. For this reason, all voxels belonging to WM were masked using the ImCalc function in the SPM5 software package by filtering this specific intensity in the whole image. After the PVE correction, the DARTEL flow fields calculated from the MR images were applied to their respective PET images to obtain an anatomically exact overlap between GM and PET images of all subjects with modulation to preserve the total amount of signal from each region. In the same way as the MR data, the PET data were smoothed by a Gaussian kernel of 12 mm FWHM. Finally, the FDG-PET data were intensity normalized using cerebellar ROIs to account for individual differences in global PET measures. This region has been shown to be least affected in mild to moderate stages of AD [36]. Additionally, normalization to this region improves the statistical discrimination between dementia patients and control subjects in comparison to other regions reported in the literature [37]–[39].

Masking. The MR and PET images obtained as described above were masked to avoid contamination by misclassified voxels. Voxels lying between WM and ventricular cerebrospinal fluid tend to be misclassified as GM voxels due to their similar intensity. The mask was obtained after extensive testing by excluding all voxels in the first and the last template created by the DARTEL approach with a probability of below 0.2 for belonging to GM and including only the voxels that exceed this threshold in both templates. This mask was applied twice: firstly prior to smoothing to avoid misclassification, and secondly, after the smoothing to avoid big edge effects. WM images were exclusively masked using the same mask to avoid overlaps between GM and WM voxels due to smoothing. The masked images were used for the subsequent SVM analysis of the data.

ROI extraction. ROI coordinates (Table 2) were extracted from two comprehensive, systematic and quantitative meta-analyses investigating biomarkers of AD and FTLD in MR and FDG-PET images. The meta-analyses included a total number of 1618 patients (AD/FTLD: 1351/267) and 1448 healthy control subjects (1097/351) [8],[9]. These meta-analyses extracted the prototypical networks of AD and FTLD by applying what is currently the most sophisticated and best-validated of coordinate-based voxel-wise meta-analyses, anatomical likelihood estimate. In the FTLD meta-analyses [8] only coordinates which are common to all subgroups of FTLD patients were used. In total, 10 regions from MRI and 6 regions from FDG-PET were used from the FTLD meta-analysis. From AD meta-analysis, 6 regions were used from both, MRI and FDG-PET. The AD meta-analysis also identified one additional region in the fornix which was differentiating between early-onset AD patients (age<65 years) and control subjects but not between late-onset AD patients and control subjects. This region was not included into the ROI-based classification to avoid a discrimination bias towards early-onset AD patients. Although unequal numbers of ROIs were used from both imaging modalities, this number is also a highly important information as it also provides a measurement for the amount of changes present in a specific modality. Because the coordinates in both meta-analyses were reported in the Talairach space, they were transformed to MNI space according to a formula proposed by Matthew Brett (published on the Internet: http://www.mrccbu.cam.ac.uk/Imaging/Common/mnispace.shtml). DARTEL preprocessed data are registered to an averaged size template created from all subjects in this study. To transform these data to the MNI space we normalized them to an a priori MNI template in SPM by using affine-only spatial normalization. Due to the affine-only transformation, our images still differed in shape from the MNI template, so some reported coordinates were slightly outside of the anatomic regions in our imaging data. In this case, the center coordinates for the ROIs were moved slightly towards the closest point of the corresponding anatomical region reported in the meta-analyses. ROIs were selected using the 3D fill tool in the MRIcron software package (http://www.sph.sc.edu/comd/rorden/mricron). Separate ROI masks were created for MR and FDG-PET images based on the origin of the peak values reported in the meta-analyses and using all regions reported for AD and FTLD in a single mask for each modality. Each ROI was restricted to a sphere with a radius of 5 mm around the reported coordinate (Figure 2). Additionally, to increase the signal-to-noise ratio, all zero voxels and edge voxels with an intensity deviation of 13 intensity units in the MRIcron 3D fill tool were excluded from the ROI. The edge voxel restriction excludes all voxels at the edge of the smoothed GM structures within the sphere. These voxels carry much

Table 2. Coordinates of ROIs used for SVM classification.

FTLD vs. Controls					
FDG-PET	**BA**	**Lat**	**x**	**y**	**z**
Pregenual anterior cingulate gyrus	24/32	L	−5	34	21
Lentiform nucleus; Caudate head		L	−20	3	−3
Medial thalamus		L	−2	−19	6
Anterior insula	15/16	L	−47	10	−7
Anterior medial frontal cortex	10	R	1	54	0
Amygdala		R	25	−2	−25
MRI	**BA**	**Lat**	**x**	**y**	**z**
Anterior medial frontal cortex	9	L	−5	49	25
Pregenual anterior cingulate gyrus	24/32	L	−5	34	21
Inferior frontal gyrus, pars opercularis	44	L	−54	11	20
Lentiform nucleus; Caudate head		L	−20	3	−3
Anterior insula	15/16	L	−47	10	−7
Subcallosal/septal area	25	L	−2	10	−10
Amygdala		R	25	−2	−25
Amygdala; Ento-and perirhinal cortex		L	−26	−5	−25
Temporal pole	38	L	−29	11	−43
Temporal pole	38	L	−47	8	−44
AD vs. Controls					
FDG-PET	**BA**	**Lat**	**x**	**y**	**z**
Angular gyrus	39	L	−38	−68	37
Angular gyrus	39	R	43	−68	33
Posterior superior temporal sulcus	21/22				
Anterior medial frontal cortex	9/10	R	1	31	31
Pregenual anterior cingulate gyrus	32				
Inferior precuneus	31	R	1	−36	27
Dorsal posterior cingulate cortex	23				
Posterior superior temporal sulcus	21/22	L	−51	−61	23
Middle inferior temporal sulcus	20/21	R	59	−31	−23
MRI	**BA**	**Lat**	**x**	**y**	**z**
Posterior insula	13	L	−38	−25	15
Medial thalamus		L	−5	−13	3
Hippocampal body/tail		R	31	−38	−6
Middle temporal gyrus/superior temporal sulcus	21/22	L	−63	−21	−5
Amygdala, anterior hippocampal formation, uncus, (trans-) entorhinal area	28/34	R	25	−8	−18
Amygdala, anterior hippocampal formation, uncus, (trans-) entorhinal area	28/34	L	−26	−8	−18

Coordinates are in MNI space (L left, R right). AD Alzheimer's disease, BA Brodmann area, FDG-PET [18F]fluorodeoxyglucose positron emission tomography, MRI magnetic resonance imaging, ROI region-of-interest, SVM support vector machine.
doi:10.1371/journal.pone.0018111.t002

less information due to their further distance from the GM structures in the unsmoothed data and so decrease the signal-to-noise ratio in the corresponding ROI.

SVM. Multivariate pattern classification, as described in Klöppel et al. [10], was performed with a linear kernel by identifying a separating hyperplane that maximizes the distance

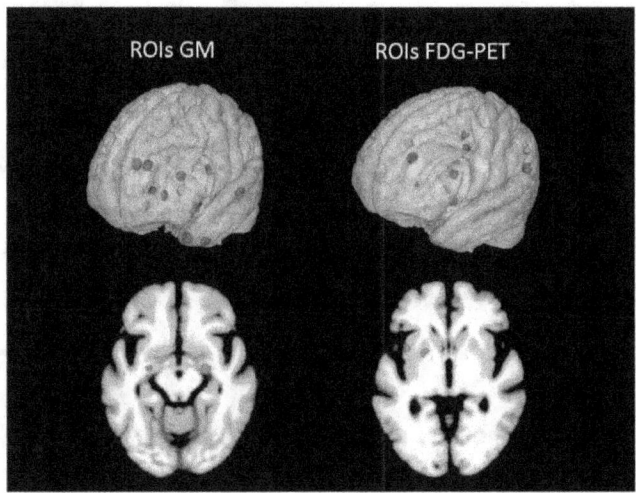

Figure 2. Regions of interest extracted from gray matter (left) and FDG-PET (right) data for AD and FTLD patients and used for support vector machine classification projected onto a glass brain (top) and onto an axial slice (bottom). AD Alzheimer's disease, FDG-PET [F18]fluorodeoxyglucose positron emission tomography, FTLD frontotemporal lobar degeneration, GM gray matter, ROIs regions of interest.

doi:10.1371/journal.pone.0018111.g002

between different clinical groups based on whole-brain or ROIs information. The cross-validation of the trained SVM was performed by using the leave-one-out method. This procedure iteratively leaves out the information of each subject and trains the model on the remaining subjects for subsequent class assignation of the person that was not included in the training procedure. This validation method enables the generalization of the trained SVM to data that have never been presented to the SVM algorithms previously. The reported accuracy is the percentage of subjects correctly assigned to the clinical diagnosis. Usually SVM classification is performed without smoothing of the data, because single voxels are assumed to contain information, for example, for prediction of future action based on functional MR images. However, in neurodegenerative disorders single voxels are unlikely to contain generalizable information due to a limited across-subject registration of MR and FDG-PET images. Although SVM classification based on unsmoothed data has been shown to differentiate reasonably between different groups (Klöppel et al., 2007), an additional smoothing should make this approach more reliable and generalizable to new data. To control for the effect of smoothing we ran the same whole-brain classification twice for GM, PET and for integration of GM and PET in the same vector with and without smoothing.

We performed the whole-brain SVM classification using GM, WM or FDG-PET images separately and by combining information from different modalities. For the SVM classification, all data of a subject are transformed into a vector, with information of an additional modality simply attached by extending the vector. Additionally, we repeated the whole-brain SVM classification by adding MR to FDG-PET information combining both modalities in a single image. ROI-based SVM classification was performed on data extracted from smoothed images separately for GM and FDG-PET images and also by integrating information from both modalities in a single vector. In order to reduce the number of voxels in the ROI-based classification, only nonzero voxels were included in the vector. This was done because otherwise the whole-brain SVM

classification is a highly memory-consuming approach. To ensure that our classification results were not based on factors randomly discriminating between groups, we reran the whole-brain and ROI-based classification for comparison 30 times by randomly assigning all subjects to the three groups independently from the clinical diagnosis and calculating the classification accuracy by using the leave-one-out procedure described above.

Statistical analysis. Group comparisons for age, education and CDR (Clinical Dementia Rating Scale) [40] were performed by conducting ANOVAs (analyses of variance). If an ANOVA revealed a significant between-group effect, a Bonferroni t-test was calculated with a significance threshold of $p<05$ (corrected for multiple comparisons, two-tailed). MMSE (Mini Mental State Examination) [41], was only present for 20 patients with AD and 11 patients with FTLD. MMSE scores of these two groups were compared to each other using an independent samples t-test. Group differences regarding sex were evaluated using a chi-square test for independent samples. The statistical analysis was performed with the commercial software package SPSS 17.0 (http://www.spss.com/statistics/).

Results

Clinical characteristics

The chi-square test for independent samples did not reveal any statistical differences in sex between the groups $[\chi^2(2)=0.42; p=0.809]$. The three groups did not differ in education (Table 1). CDR scores differed significantly in the three groups. The post-hoc test revealed no differences in the mean CDR scores between both groups of dementia patients $[t(33)=0.94;p=0.977]$. As expected, both early AD $[t(32)=5.36;p<0.001]$ and early FTLD $[t(25)=4.35;p<0.001]$ had significantly higher CDR scores compared to the control subjects. MMSE scores also did not differ between both groups of dementia patients indicating a similar severity of dementia syndrome $[t(29)=-81;p=0.95]$. The ANOVA also revealed a significant group difference in age. The two groups of dementia patients did not differ significantly in age $[t(33)=0.16;p=1.0]$. There was a minor but significant difference between AD patients and controls $[t(32)=3.18;p=008]$ and FTLD patients and controls $[t(25)=2.86; p=024]$.

SVM – Whole-brain analysis

Multivariate classification of the data using SVM at the whole-brain level revealed the best discrimination accuracy for all three groups using FDG-PET, with 81% (chance level 33%), in comparison to GM and WM information, with lowest accuracy using WM information on its own (Table 3). The combination of metabolism and GM values in a single image revealed a similar accuracy for differentiation of the three groups, with higher accuracy for differentiation between both types of dementia, however, with slightly lower discrimination between dementia patients and control subjects. Whole-brain SVM classification for the three groups without smoothing revealed lower accuracy rates in all classifications in comparison to differentiation based on smoothed images. The accuracy increase due to smoothing ranged between 2 (GM) and 6% (FDG-PET). Figure 3 displays regions that were most influential in making binary classification between the AD, FTLD and control subjects based on smoothed whole-brain information.

SVM – ROI analysis

Accuracy based on ROIs from both meta-analyses using only GM information was substantially lower for differentiation between AD and FTLD patients in comparison with whole-brain classification. However, it was comparable to the whole-brain

Table 3. Accuracy rates for whole-brain and ROI-based SVM classification for FDG-PET and MRI.

	AD, FTLD and Controls	AD vs FTLD	AD vs Controls	FTLD vs Controls
GM whole-brain	72.9%	80.0%	88.2%	77.8%
WM whole-brain	66.7%	74.3%	79.4%	77.8%
FDG-PET whole-brain	81.3%	82.9%	94.1%	92.6%
GM/ FDG-PET whole-brain	79.2%	82.9%	94.1%	88.9%
GM/WM/FDG-PET whole-brain	77.1%	82.9%	91.2%	85.2%
GM + FDG-PET whole-brain	81.3%	88.6%	91.2%	88.9%
GM ROIs	56.3%	60.0%	82.4%	85.2%
FDG-PET ROIs	75.0%	80.0%	94.1%	85.2%
GM/FDG-PET ROIs	91.7%	94.3%	100.0%	92.6%

Accuracy represents the percentage of subjects correctly assigned to the correct condition. AD Alzheimer's disease, FDG-PET [18F]fluorodeoxyglucose positron emission tomography, FTLD frontotemporal lobar degeneration, GM gray matter, MRI magnetic resonance imaging, ROI region-of-interest, SVM support vector machine, WM white matter.
doi:10.1371/journal.pone.0018111.t003

approach in differentiating between patients with both types of dementia and control subjects. ROIs extracted from FDG-PET data showed slightly lower discrimination accuracy compared to whole-brain information. The best accuracy rates of all SVM classifications were obtained using combined information extracted from FDG-PET and GM data. This approach resulted in a classification accuracy of 92% for the differentiation of all three groups and an accuracy rate of 94% for differentiation between AD and FTLD patients. Sensitivity of this ROI-based classification ranged between 85.7% for FTLD and 100% for AD and specificity of 100% for discrimination of both types of dementia from control subjects (Table 4).

The classification accuracy in the 30 trials randomly assigning all subjects to the three groups resulted in a mean accuracy rate of $34\pm7.7\%$ (mean $\pm$ standard deviation), ranging between 21 and 52% for the ROI-based SVM classification, and $33.7\pm8.2\%$ ranging between 12 and 50% for the whole-brain classification.

Discussion

In this study we performed a multimodal comparison and discrimination of dementia patients using FDG-PET and MRI. To enable a more accurate coevaluation of both imaging modalities, we developed a new preprocessing algorithm. This algorithm was designed to enable an accurate anatomical registration of both modalities. All processing steps were performed as far as possible simultaneously by applying the same deformations and preprocessing parameters to both modalities of the same subject. This procedure resulted in an accurate anatomical overlap of both imaging modalities and in an accurate between-subject registration, with both images having the same voxel size and approximately the same effective smoothness.

SVM

SVM classification is a very promising tool for detection and differentiation of different dementia syndromes, as has been shown

by previous studies [10],[12],[13],[24]. It not only captures univariate relationships of a single voxel across all subjects but is also able to detect multivariate relationships over a large group of information, as, for example, between different structures and modalities in the brain. Furthermore, this tool provides an easy way to use this information for classifying imaging data of new subjects to a specific condition.

Here, we systematically compared different information provided by FDG-PET and MRI to enable the most accurate detection and differentiation of dementia. The diagnosis was based on comprehensive clinical and neuropsychological testing. Although the data are not histopathologically confirmed to be sure of assigning them to the correct condition, generally higher conformity with the clinical diagnosis should also result in more accurate classification of histopathologically validated data.

The whole-brain SVM classification provided the most accurate classification using only FDG-PET information. GM and WM based classification accuracy was lower for all comparisons indicating a lower sensitivity for detection of dementia-relevant information. Nonetheless, classification based on GM, WM and FDG-PET separately or combining them revealed a discrimination accuracy which was above chance level for the correct categorization of the three groups. All classification results substantially exceeded the best classification accuracy obtained by randomly assigning all subjects to different groups. Additionally, smoothing of the data improved the classification accuracy in both imaging modalities as expected.

However, in whole-brain classification noise is introduced by using a great deal of information for classification that does not differentiate between the groups. Recent comprehensive meta-analyses identified the "prototypical" networks for both disorders in both modalities using VBM [8],[9]. The involved regions have been shown to be affected in AD and FTLD patients most consistently in all studies investigating these disorders. By using this information, we ruled out the possibility that our classification results are dependent to our group of patients. Although this

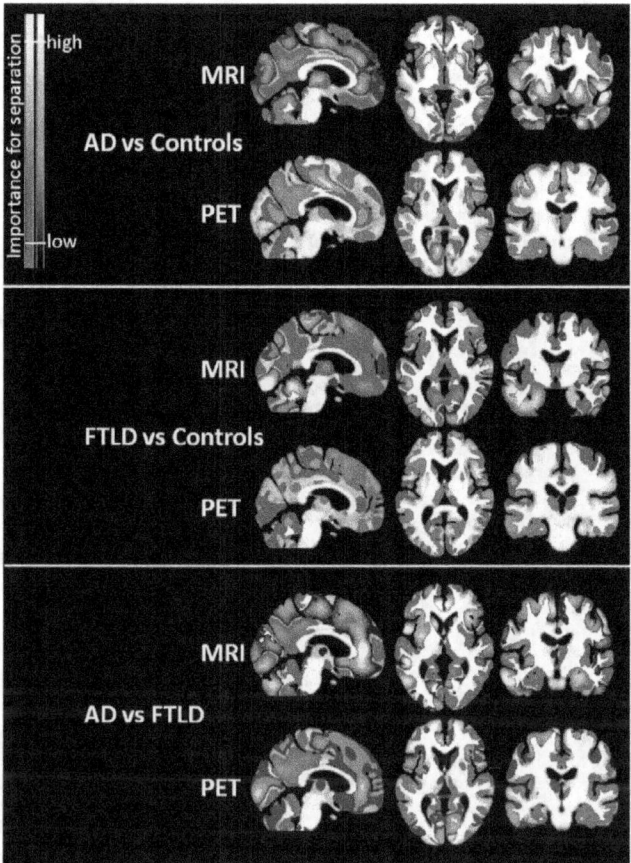

Figure 3. Weights of voxels most relevant for classification of both groups of patients and control subjects in FDG-PET and MRI after SVM training. Weights are relative, and have no applicable units. AD and FTLD vs Controls: Blue and light blue indicate decreased gray matter intensity (upper row) or reduced metabolic rate (lower row) that increase the likelihood of classification into a dementia group. Red and yellow indicate the opposite. AD vs FTLD: Blue and light blue indicate decreased gray matter intensity (upper row) or reduced metabolic rate (lower row) that increase the likelihood of classification into the AD group. Red and yellow indicate the opposite. Regions with bright colors (yellow and light blue) have a higher importance for separation than regions with dark colors (blue and red). AD Alzheimer's disease, FTLD frontotemporal lobar degeneration. MRI magnetic resonance imaging, PET positron emission tomography. doi:10.1371/journal.pone.0018111.g003

method provides lower accuracy rates for GM or FDG-PET information on their own, it shows a significantly higher discrimination rate by combining both information modalities into a single vector. This ROI-based discrimination is superior to

Table 4. Differentiation rates for combined region-of-interest information from FDG-PET and MRI.

	Accuracy	Sensitivity	Specificity
AD vs FTLD	94.3%	95.2%*	92.9%
AD vs Controls	100.0%	100.0%	100.0%
FTLD vs Controls	92.6%	85.7%	100.0%

*Considering a correctly identified AD as a true positive. AD Alzheimer's disease, FDG-PET [18F]fluorodeoxyglucose positron emission tomography, FTLD frontotemporal lobar degeneration, MRI magnetic resonance imaging.
doi:10.1371/journal.pone.0018111.t004

whole-brain classification with the highest accuracy gain for the differentiation of both types of dementia, which, with 94%, is the highest differentiation rate reported up to now. Accordingly, we suggest this method as a diagnostic standard for the classification of dementia syndromes.

Nonetheless, some limitations should be considered regarding the results of the present study. First of all, the number of subjects used for classification is too low to allow a generalizable conclusion for patients from other clinical centers. This is especially a problem because the accuracy of the clinical diagnosis for specific dementia syndromes, which was used here for validation, strongly varies between different clinical centers. Therefore, in a future work this approach should be validated using a larger and more generalizable dataset like the data provided by the Alzheimer's disease Neuroimaging Initiative (ADNI: www.adni-info.org). A further limitation of the present work is the significantly younger age of the control group in comparison to the patient cohort. However, this aspect might only have contributed to the discrimination between dementia patients and control subjects but not to the high classification accuracy of AD and FTLD patients as these were very similar in their age range. If age contributed to the classification accuracy there should be lower classification accuracy for young dementia patients and older control subjects as they did not differ in age. For comparison of both types of dementia patients and control subjects the classification accuracy did not differ for younger and older dementia patients although half of the patients were in the same age range as the control group. In AD group all patients were classified correctly. In FTLD group one younger and one older patient were misclassified. Independently of age, all control subjects were classified correctly for both comparisons. These results indicate that the slight mean age differences is not the decisive factor for the high discrimination accuracy using combined information from FDG-PET and MRI. Furthermore, if age still slightly contributed to the high discrimination of dementia patients and control subjects this contribution was also present in all other single modality and multimodal whole-brain and ROI-based SVM classifications applied in this study. Therefore, age cannot account for increased differentiation accuracies when combined ROI information from FDG-PET and MRI are used for differentiation of dementia patients and control subjects.

Another point is that subjects in the control group in our study reported subjective cognitive complaints which might have limited the interpretation of the results of our study. However, only subjects were included whose cognitive complaints were not confirmed by comprehensive neuropsychological evaluation. The CDR is a semi-structural interview and is highly dependent on the subjectively perceived memory impairment which resulted in a CDR score of 0.5 for these control subjects in our study. In recent literature it has been shown that the CDR stage of 0.5 has a poor discriminative value for healthy control subjects and subjects with Mild Cognitive Impairment (MCI) [42],[43]. Meguro et al. [42] have shown that about 30% of a normal population older then 65 got a CDR score of 0.5 while the prevalence of MCI in the same population was only about 5% which suggests that CDR score of 0.5 is not a good indicator of MCI. Due to the absence of any objective cognitive impairment in all neuropsychological tests for all subjects included in the control group in our study this group of subjects can be regarded as cognitively unimpaired.

Conclusion and perspectives

In our study, we investigated the advantages of SVM classification using combined information from FDG-PET and MRI to improve detection and differentiation of dementia.

Furthermore, based on affected regions reported in previous studies, investigating Alzheimer's disease and frontotemporal lobar degeneration with univariate approaches and summarized in two meta-analyses, we applied linear support vector machine classification algorithm using information from both imaging modalities. Combining region-of-interest information from FDG-PET and MRI resulted in a substantial gain in accuracy compared to whole-brain and to single modality classification for both detection and differentiation of Alzheimer's disease and frontotemporal lobar degeneration. Our results indicate that integration and combination of results from different imaging modalities might provide a new way to improve the diagnostic accuracy of these dementia disorders.

Author Contributions

Conceived and designed the experiments: JD KM AH HB HEM AV OS MLS. Performed the experiments: JD KM AH HB HEM AV OS MLS. Analyzed the data: JD KM AH HB HEM AV OS MLS. Contributed reagents/materials/analysis tools: JD KM AH HB HEM AV OS MLS. Wrote the paper: JD KM AH HB HEM AV OS MLS.

References

1. Hoffman JM, Welsh-Bohmer KA, Hanson M, Crain B, Hulette C, et al. (2000) FDG PET imaging in patients with pathologically verified dementia. J Nucl Med 41: 1920–1928.
2. Rosen HJ, Gorno-Tempini ML, Goldman WP, Perry RJ, Schuff N, et al. (2002) Patterns of brain atrophy in frontotemporal dementia and semantic dementia. Neurology 58: 198–208.
3. Diehl J, Grimmer T, Drzezga A, Riemenschneider M, Forstl H, et al. (2004) Cerebral metabolic patterns at early stages of frontotemporal dementia and semantic dementia. A PET study. Neurobiol Aging 25: 1051–1056.
4. Jeong Y, Cho SS, Park JM, Kang SJ, Lee JS, et al. (2005) 18F-FDG PET findings in frontotemporal dementia: an SPM analysis of 29 patients. J Nucl Med 46: 233–239.
5. Diehl-Schmid J, Grimmer T, Drzezga A, Bornschein S, Riemenschneider M, et al. (2007) Decline of cerebral glucose metabolism in frontotemporal dementia: a longitudinal 18F-FDG-PET-study. Neurobiol Aging 28: 42–50.
6. Fung G, Stoeckel J (2007) SVM feature selection for classification of SPECT images of Alzheimer's disease using spatial information. Knowledge and Information Systems 11: 243–258.
7. Sabri O, Kendziorra K, Wolf H, Gertz HJ, Brust P (2008) Acetylcholine receptors in dementia and mild cognitive impairment. Eur J Nucl Med Mol Imaging 35(Suppl 1): S30–45.
8. Schroeter ML, Raczka K, Neumann J, Yves von Cramon D (2007) Towards a nosology for frontotemporal lobar degenerations-a meta-analysis involving 267 subjects. Neuroimage 36: 497–510.
9. Schroeter ML, Stein T, Maslowski N, Neumann J (2009) Neural correlates of Alzheimer's disease and mild cognitive impairment: a systematic and quantitative meta-analysis involving 1351 patients. Neuroimage 47: 1196–1206.
10. Kloppel S, Stonnington CM, Chu C, Draganski B, Scahill RI, et al. (2008) Automatic classification of MR scans in Alzheimer's disease. Brain 131: 681–689.
11. Matsunari I, Samuraki M, Chen WP, Yanase D, Takeda N, et al. (2007) Comparison of 18F-FDG PET and optimized voxel-based morphometry for detection of Alzheimer's disease: aging effect on diagnostic performance. J Nucl Med 48: 1961–1970.
12. Davatzikos C, Resnick SM, Wu X, Parmpi P, Clark CM (2008) Individual patient diagnosis of AD and FTD via high-dimensional pattern classification of MRI. Neuroimage 41: 1220–1227.
13. Fan Y, Resnick SM, Wu X, Davatzikos C (2008) Structural and functional biomarkers of prodromal Alzheimer's disease: a high-dimensional pattern classification study. Neuroimage 41: 277–285.
14. Sadeghi N, Foster NL, Wang AY, Minoshima S, Lieberman AP, et al. (2008) Automatic classification of Alzheimer's disease vs. Frontotemporal dementia: A spatial decision tree approach with FDG-PET. 2008 Ieee International Symposium on Biomedical Imaging: From Nano to Macro Vols 1-4: 408–411.
15. Knopman DS, Boeve BF, Parisi JE, Dickson DW, Smith GE, et al. (2005) Antemortem diagnosis of frontotemporal lobar degeneration. Ann Neurol 57: 480–488.
16. Rascovsky K, Salmon DP, Ho GJ, Galasko D, Peavy GM, et al. (2002) Cognitive profiles differ in autopsy-confirmed frontotemporal dementia and AD. Neurology 58: 1801–1808.
17. Dubois B, Feldman HH, Jacova C, Dekosky ST, Barberger-Gateau P, et al. (2007) Research criteria for the diagnosis of Alzheimer's disease: revising the NINCDS-ADRDA criteria. Lancet Neurol 6: 734–746.
18. Kipps CM, Hodges JR, Fryer TD, Nestor PJ (2009) Combined magnetic resonance imaging and positron emission tomography brain imaging in behavioural variant frontotemporal degeneration: refining the clinical phenotype. Brain 132: 2566–2578.
19. Ishii K, Willoch F, Minoshima S, Drzezga A, Ficaro EP, et al. (2001) Statistical brain mapping of 18F-FDG PET in Alzheimer's disease: validation of anatomic standardization for atrophied brains. J Nucl Med 42: 548–557.
20. Ishii K, Sasaki H, Kono AK, Miyamoto N, Fukuda T, et al. (2005) Comparison of gray matter and metabolic reduction in mild Alzheimer's disease using FDG-PET and voxel-based morphometric MR studies. Eur J Nucl Med Mol Imaging 32: 959–963.
21. Kanda T, Ishii K, Uemura T, Miyamoto N, Yoshikawa T, et al. (2008) Comparison of grey matter and metabolic reductions in frontotemporal dementia using FDG-PET and voxel-based morphometric MR studies. Eur J Nucl Med Mol Imaging 35: 2227–2234.
22. van de Pol LA, Hensel A, van der Flier WM, Visser PJ, Pijnenburg YA, et al. (2006) Hippocampal atrophy on MRI in frontotemporal lobar degeneration and Alzheimer's disease. J Neurol Neurosurg Psychiatry 77: 439–442.
23. Schroeter ML, Raczka K, Neumann J, von Cramon DY (2008) Neural networks in dementia and frontotemporal dementia– –a meta-analysis. Neurobiol Aging 29: 418–426.
24. Chaves R, Ramirez J, Gorriz JM, Lopez M, Salas-Gonzalez D, et al. (2009) SVM-based computer-aided diagnosis of the Alzheimer's disease using t-test NMSE feature selection with feature correlation weighting. Neurosci Lett 461: 293–297.
25. Horn JF, Habert MO, Kas A, Malek Z, Maksud P, et al. (2009) Differential automatic diagnosis between Alzheimer's disease and frontotemporal dementia based on perfusion SPECT images. Artif Intell Med 47: 147–158.
26. Ramirez J, Gorriz JM, Salas-Gonzales D, Romero A, Lopez M, et al. (2009) Computer-aided diagnosis of Alzheimer's type dementia combining support vector machines and discriminant set of features. Information Sciences: doi:10.1016/j.ins.2009.05.012.
27. Rabinovici GD, Seeley WW, Kim EJ, Gorno-Tempini ML, Rascovsky K, et al. (2007) Distinct MRI atrophy patterns in autopsy-proven Alzheimer's disease and frontotemporal lobar degeneration. Am J Alzheimers Dis Other Demen 22: 474–488.
28. McKhann G, Drachman D, Folstein M, Katzman R, Price D, et al. (1984) Clinical diagnosis of Alzheimer's disease: report of the NINCDS-ADRDA Work Group under the auspices of Department of Health and Human Services Task Force on Alzheimer's Disease. Neurology 34: 939–944.
29. Neary D, Snowden JS, Gustafson L, Passant U, Stuss D, et al. (1998) Frontotemporal lobar degeneration: a consensus on clinical diagnostic criteria. Neurology 51: 1546–1554.
30. Chang CC, Lin CJ (2001) LIBSVM: a library for support vector machines. Software available at: http://www.csie.ntu.edu.tw/~cjlin/libsvm.
31. Ashburner J, Friston KJ (2005) Unified segmentation. Neuroimage 26: 839–851.
32. Ashburner J (2007) A fast diffeomorphic image registration algorithm. Neuroimage 38: 95–113.
33. Muller-Gartner HW, Links JM, Prince JL, Bryan RN, McVeigh E, et al. (1992) Measurement of radiotracer concentration in brain gray matter using positron emission tomography: MRI-based correction for partial volume effects. J Cereb Blood Flow Metab 12: 571–583.
34. Rousset OG, Ma Y, Evans AC (1998) Correction for partial volume effects in PET: principle and validation. J Nucl Med 39: 904–911.
35. Quarantelli M, Berkouk K, Prinster A, Landeau B, Svarer C, et al. (2004) Integrated software for the analysis of brain PET/SPECT studies with partial-volume-effect correction. J Nucl Med 45: 192–201.
36. Ishii K, Sasaki M, Kitagaki H, Yamaji S, Sakamoto S, et al. (1997) Reduction of cerebellar glucose metabolism in advanced Alzheimer's disease. J Nucl Med 38: 925–928.
37. Yakushev I, Landvogt C, Buchholz HG, Fellgiebel A, Hammers A, et al. (2008) Choice of reference area in studies of Alzheimer's disease using positron emission tomography with fluorodeoxyglucose-F18. Psychiatry Res 164: 143–153.
38. Yakushev I, Hammers A, Fellgiebel A, Schmidtmann I, Scheurich A, et al. (2009) SPM-based count normalization provides excellent discrimination of mild Alzheimer's disease and amnestic mild cognitive impairment from healthy aging. Neuroimage 44: 43–50.
39. Dukart J, Mueller K, Horstmann A, Vogt B, Frisch S, et al. (2010) Differential effects of global and cerebellar normalization on detection and differentiation of dementia in FDG-PET studies. Neuroimage 49: 1490–1495.
40. Morris JC (1993) The Clinical Dementia Rating (CDR): current version and scoring rules. Neurology 43: 2412–2414.
41. Folstein MF, Folstein SE, McHugh PR (1975) Mini-Mental State (a practical method for grading the state of patients for the clinician). Journal of Psychiatric Research 12: 189–198.
42. Meguro K, Ishii H, Yamaguchi S, Ishizaki J, Sato M, et al. (2004) Prevalence and cognitive performances of clinical dementia rating 0.5 and mild cognitive impairment in Japan. The Tajiri project. Alzheimer disease and associated disorders 18: 3–10.
43. Perneczky R, Wagenpfeil S, Komossa K, Grimmer T, Diehl J, et al. (2006) Mapping scores onto stages: mini-mental state examination and clinical dementia rating. The American journal of geriatric psychiatry: official journal of the American Association for Geriatric Psychiatry 14: 139–144.

Plasma Based Markers of [11C] PiB-PET Brain Amyloid Burden

Steven John Kiddle[1,2]*, Madhav Thambisetty[3], Andrew Simmons[1,2], Joanna Riddoch-Contreras[2], Abdul Hye[2], Eric Westman[1,2], Ian Pike[4], Malcolm Ward[4], Caroline Johnston[1,2], Michelle Katharine Lupton[2], Katie Lunnon[2], Hilkka Soininen[5], Iwona Kłoszewska[6], Magda Tsolaki[7], Bruno Vellas[8], Patrizia Mecocci[9], Simon Lovestone[1,2], Stephen Newhouse[1,2⑨], Richard Dobson[1,2⑨]*, for the Alzheimers Disease Neuroimaging Initiative

1 National Institute of Health Research Biomedical Research Centre for Mental Health, South London and Maudsley National Health Service Foundation Trust, London, United Kingdom, 2 King's College London, Institute of Psychiatry, London, United Kingdom, 3 Laboratory of Behavioral Neuroscience, National Institute on Aging, Baltimore, Maryland, United States of America, 4 Proteome Sciences plc, Cobham, Surrey, United Kingdom, 5 School of Neurology, University of Eastern Finland and University Hospital of Kuopio, Kuopio, Finland, 6 Department of Old Age Psychiatry and Psychotic Disorders, Medical University of Lodz, Lodz, Poland, 7 3rd Department of Neurology, "G. Papanicolaou" Hospital, Aristotle University of Thessaloniki, Thessaloniki, Greece, 8 Department of Geriatric Medicine, Grontople de Toulouse, Toulouse University Hospital, Toulouse, France, 9 Institute of Gerontology and Geriatrics, University of Perugia, Perugia, Italy

Abstract

Changes in brain amyloid burden have been shown to relate to Alzheimer's disease pathology, and are believed to precede the development of cognitive decline. There is thus a need for inexpensive and non-invasive screening methods that are able to accurately estimate brain amyloid burden as a marker of Alzheimer's disease. One potential method would involve using demographic information and measurements on plasma samples to establish biomarkers of brain amyloid burden; in this study data from the Alzheimer's Disease Neuroimaging Initiative was used to explore this possibility. Sixteen of the analytes on the Rules Based Medicine Human Discovery Multi-Analyte Profile 1.0 panel were found to associate with [11C]-PiB PET measurements. Some of these markers of brain amyloid burden were also found to associate with other AD related phenotypes. Thirteen of these markers of brain amyloid burden – c-peptide, fibrinogen, alpha-1-antitrypsin, pancreatic polypeptide, complement C3, vitronectin, cortisol, AXL receptor kinase, interleukin-3, interleukin-13, matrix metalloproteinase-9 total, apolipoprotein E and immunoglobulin E – were used along with co-variates in multiple linear regression, and were shown by cross-validation to explain $>30\%$ of the variance of brain amyloid burden. When a threshold was used to classify subjects as PiB positive, the regression model was found to predict actual PiB positive individuals with a sensitivity of 0.918 and a specificity of 0.545. The number of $APOE\ \epsilon\ 4$ alleles and plasma apolipoprotein E level were found to contribute most to this model, and the relationship between these variables and brain amyloid burden was explored.

Citation: Kiddle SJ, Thambisetty M, Simmons A, Riddoch-Contreras J, Hye A, et al. (2012) Plasma Based Markers of [11C] PiB-PET Brain Amyloid Burden. PLoS ONE 7(9): e44260. doi:10.1371/journal.pone.0044260

Editor: Ashley I. Bush, Mental Health Research Institute of Victoria, Australia

Received April 13, 2012; **Accepted** July 31, 2012; **Published** September 24, 2012

Funding: Alzheimer's Disease Neuroimaging Initiative (ADNI) data collection and sharing for this project was funded by the ADNI (National Institutes of Health Grant U01 AG024904). ADNI is funded by the National Institute on Aging, the National Institute of Biomedical Imaging and Bioengineering, and through generous contributions from the following: Abbott; Alzheimer's Association; Alzheimer's Drug Discovery Foundation; Amorfix Life Sciences Ltd.; AstraZeneca; Bayer HealthCare; BioClinica, Inc.; Biogen Idec Inc.; Bristol-Myers Squibb Company; Eisai Inc.; Elan Pharmaceuticals Inc.; Eli Lilly and Company; F. Hoffmann-La Roche Ltd and its affiliated company Genentech, Inc.; GE Healthcare; Innogenetics, N.V.; Janssen Alzheimer Immunotherapy Research & Development, LLC.; Johnson & Johnson Pharmaceutical Research & Development LLC.; Medpace, Inc.; Merck & Co., Inc.; Meso Scale Diagnostics, LLC.; Novartis Pharmaceuticals Corporation; Pfizer Inc.; Servier; Synarc Inc.; and Takeda Pharmaceutical Company. The Canadian Institutes of Health Research is providing funds to support ADNI clinical sites in Canada. Private sector contributions are facilitated by the Foundation for the National Institutes of Health (www.fnih.org). The grantee organization is the Northern California Institute for Research and Education, and the study is coordinated by the Alzheimer's Disease Cooperative Study at the University of California, San Diego. ADNI data are disseminated by the Laboratory for Neuro Imaging at the University of California, Los Angeles. This research was also supported by National Institutes of Health grants P30 AG010129 and K01 AG030514. This study was supported by InnoMed (Innovative Medicines in Europe www.imi.europa.eu/) an Integrated Project funded by the European Union of the Sixth Framework program priority FP6-2004-LIFESCIHEALTH-5, Life Sciences, Genomics and Biotechnology for Health. This study was also supported by funds from the National Institutes for Health Research Biomedical Research Centre for Mental Health at the South London and Maudsley National Health Service Foundation Trust and Institute of Psychiatry, King's College London. The funders had no role in study design, data collection and analysis, decision to publish, or preparation of the manuscript.

Competing Interests: Intellectual property has been registered on the use of plasma proteins for use as biomarkers for AD by King's College London and Proteome Sciences, with SL and M. Thambisetty named as inventors. IP and MW were full-time employees of Proteome Sciences, London, United Kingdom, at the time of their contribution to the work described in this manuscript. This does not alter the authors' adherence to all the PLOS ONE policies on sharing data and materials. Patent Title Methods and Compositions Relating to Alzheimer's Disease Subject Covers utility of around 30 proteins, specifically listing 16 in the Dependent claims for diagnosis of Alzheimer's disease Filing Proteome Sciences with King's Business United Kingdom Priority GB0421639.6 dated 29/09/2004 PCT Application PCT/GB2005/003756 dated 29/09/2005 Application in Europe, Japan, United States, Australia, and Canada, dated 15/03/2007 to 16/10/2007. In addition Alzheimer's Disease Neuroimaging Initiative recieved funding from: Abbott; Alzheimer's Association; Alzheimer's Drug Discovery Foundation; Amorfix Life Sciences Ltd.; AstraZeneca; Bayer HealthCare; BioClinica, Inc.; Biogen Idec Inc.; Bristol-Myers Squibb Company; Eisai Inc.; Elan Pharmaceuticals Inc.; Eli Lilly and Company; F. Hoffmann-La Roche Ltd and its affiliated company Genentech, Inc.; GE Healthcare; Innogenetics, N.V.; Janssen Alzheimer Immunotherapy Research & Development, LLC.; Johnson & Johnson Pharmaceutical Research & Development LLC.; Medpace, Inc.; Merck & Co., Inc.; Meso Scale Diagnostics, LLC.; Novartis Pharmaceuticals Corporation; Pfizer Inc.; Servier; Synarc Inc.; and Takeda Pharmaceutical Company. This does not alter the authors' adherence to all the PLOS ONE policies on sharing data and materials.

* E-mail: steven.kiddle@kcl.ac.uk (SJK); richard.j.dobson@kcl.ac.uk (RD)

⑨ These authors contributed equally to this work.

Introduction

The failure of several clinical trials targeting brain amyloid deposition in patients with Alzheimers disease (AD) has led to the suggestion that these agents may be useful if targeted at older individuals in pre-symptomatic stages of the disease [1,2]. Screening methods that accurately identify at-risk non-demented older individuals who are most likely to benefit from such treatments will therefore represent a major advance in our ability to effectively test these disease-modifying treatments [3]. If clinical trials of amyloid lowering interventions were successful in the pre-symptomatic stages of AD, then there would be a desire to identify non-demented elderly individuals with elevated brain amyloid burden who could potentially benefit from early intervention. However identifying suitable individuals poses a great challenge in terms of feasibility and cost. To date, the two methods that are most likely to be useful in estimating levels of brain amyloid burden are in vivo imaging with positron emission tomography (PET) using radioligands binding to fibrillar amyloid beta ($A\beta$), such as [^{11}C] Pittsburgh B compound (PiB), and assays of $A\beta$ levels in cerebrospinal fluid (CSF) [4,5]. However, both these methods have inherent drawbacks that limit their utility as screening tools, especially in resource-poor settings. While PET scanning is expensive and limited to specialised centres, lumbar puncture to obtain CSF is associated with some patient discomfort and is unlikely to be used in primary health care centres to routinely screen large numbers of elderly patients. An inexpensive, non-invasive screening method that accurately estimates brain amyloid burden would therefore fulfil a critical unmet need in the care of the elderly.

The identification of blood-based biomarkers associated with AD diagnosis [6–9] or distinct endophenotypes of AD pathology such as brain atrophy [10–12], hippocampal metabolite abnormalities [13] and amyloid burden [14], have previously been reported. In these studies, proteomic analyses were combined with neuroimaging methods to identify plasma signals associated with measures of AD pathology. In this study, a different strategy was used by examining the association between brain amyloid burden and a panel of 146 plasma analytes – proteins, complexes and metabolites – measured by Rules Based Medicine, Inc. (RBM) (Austin, TX) using the Human Discovery Multi-Analyte Profile (MAP) 1.0 panel and a Luminex 100 platform. Some of the analytes on this panel, such as apolipoprotein E (APOE) and

complement C3 have previously been shown to associate with brain amyloid burden [14,15], while others are associated with other diseases. These assays were performed in plasma samples that were collected from participants in the Alzheimers Disease Neuroimaging Initiative (ADNI; http://adni.loni.ucle.edu) study who also underwent [^{11}C]-PiB PET imaging for quantification of fibrillar brain amyloid burden. The main aim of this study was to ask whether concentrations of a panel of plasma proteins and metabolites might accurately reflect the extent of fibrillar amyloid in the brain. A secondary aim was to understand the relationship between the number of $APOE\ \epsilon\ 4$ alleles and plasma based markers of brain amyloid burden.

Results

RBM analytes associate with $A\beta$ levels in the brain

Levels of analytes measured by the RBM Human Discovery MAP 1.0 from ADNI plasma samples were compared to fibrillar amyloid in the RBM-PiB PET cohort (N = 71). Characteristics of this subcohort are summarised in Table 1 where it can be seen that brain amyloid burden was almost significantly different at the 0.05 level between diagnostic groups (Kruskal-Wallis (KW) χ^2 test p-value 0.055). The distribution of brain amyloid burden in the RBM-PiB PET cohort is shown in Figure S1. In the slightly larger ADNI-PiB PET cohort (i.e. all ADNI subjects with [^{11}C] PiB-PET scans performed at baseline), whose sample characteristics are shown in Table S1, brain amyloid burden was found to be significantly different across diagnostic groups (KW p-value 0.022).

The analytes most associated with brain amyloid burden in the RBM-PiB PET cohort, after taking into account co-variates (age, gender, years of education, number of $APOE\ \epsilon\ 4$ alleles and the number of days between [^{11}C]-PiB PET scan and plasma sample), are shown in Table 2.

Prediction of brain amyloid burden using plasma RBM analytes

To determine if a subset of the RBM panel was able to predict fibrillar amyloid levels in the brain, multiple linear regression was used. In this analysis the following subject co-variates were included: age at plasma sample, years of education, gender, the number of $APOE\ \epsilon\ 4$ alleles and the difference, in days, between plasma sampling and [^{11}C]-PiB PET scan date. Multiple linear

Table 1. Characteristics of the ADNI RBM-PiB PET cohort.

Characteristics	Diagnostic group (number of subjects)			
	Control (3)	MCI (52)	AD (16)	P-value
Subject age in years at time of plasma sample (Median [IQR])	77.4 [5.6]	75.4 [11.1]	72.3 [8.2]	0.290
Sex (Male/Female)	1/2	37/15	10/6	0.263
Years of education (Median [IQR])	13.0 [3.0]	16.0 [5.0]	16.0 [5.3]	0.398
Number of $APOE\ \epsilon\ 4$ alleles (0/1/2)	2/1/0	25/22/5	7/7/2	0.977
Days between [^{11}C]-PiB PET scan and plasma sample (Median [IQR])	5.0 [15.5]	23.5 [60.5]	21.5 [42.3]	0.288
Average PiB uptake (Median [IQR])	1.31 [0.108]	1.98 [0.723]	1.90 [0.438]	0.055

Characteristics of the ADNI RBM-PiB PET subcohort by diagnostic group. P-values were calculated for differences across diagnostic groups using a Kruskal-Wallis χ^2 test for continuous characteristics and simulated contingency p-values for categorical characteristics.
doi:10.1371/journal.pone.0044260.t001

Table 2. RBM analytes associated with brain amyloid burden.

RBM analyte	Gene name	Uniprot ID	Partial SRC with $A\beta$	P-value	Benjamini-Hochberg corrected p-value
C-peptide	INS	P01308	−0.310	0.010	0.351
Fibrinogen (α, β and γ)	FG(A/B/G)	P02671 P02675 P02679	−0.307	0.010	0.351
Alpha-1-antitrypsin	SERPINA1	P01009	−0.302	0.012	0.351
Pancreatic polypeptide	PPY	P01298	−0.296	0.014	0.351
Complement C3	C3	P01024	−0.296	0.014	0.351
Vitronectin	VTN	P04004	−0.295	0.014	0.351
von Willebrand factor	VWF	P04275	−0.287	0.017	0.363
Cortisol	(NA)	(NA)	0.271	0.025	0.412
Serum amyloid p-component	APCS	P02743	−0.268	0.027	0.412
AXL receptor tyrosine kinase	AXL	P30530	0.266	0.028	0.412
Interleukin-3	IL3	P08700	0.261	0.032	0.412
Interleukin-13	IL13	P35225	0.252	0.038	0.412
Matrix metalloproteinase-9 total	MMP9	P14780	−0.250	0.040	0.412
APOE	APOE	P02649	−0.248	0.042	0.412
Leptin	LEP	P41159	−0.248	0.042	0.412
Immunoglobulin E (IgE)	(NA)	(NA)	−0.243	0.046	0.424

Analytes with a partial SRC p-value of <0.05 are shown. Benjamini-Hochberg corrected p-values were calculated to take into account the comparisons against all RBM analytes.
doi:10.1371/journal.pone.0044260.t002

regression was applied to predict brain amyloid burden using these co-variates only, giving a leave one out (LOO) cross validation (CV) R^2 of 0.040. When brain amyloid burden was regressed to *just* the number of APOE ϵ 4 alleles this gave a LOO CV R^2 of 0.123. Then multiple linear regression was applied to predict brain amyloid burden from both RBM analytes and co-variates; the analysis was restricted to the 16 RBM analytes that had a partial Spearmans rank correlation (SRC) uncorrected p-value <0.05 (Table 2) resulting in a LOO CV R^2 of 0.276.

Overfitting was reduced by grouping correlated variables and selecting one RBM analyte to represent each group (Figure 1); first all the 16 RBM analytes were used, then analytes were removed from the model one by one, in the order determined by clustering, and LOO CV repeated. The order of analyte removal was: (1) von willebrand factor, (2) leptin, (3) serum amyloid p-component, (4) vitronectin, (5) interleukin-13, (6) component C3, (7) matrix metalloproteinase-9 total, (8) immunoglobulin E (IgE), (9) APOE, (10) pancreatic polypeptide, (11) alpha-1-antitrypsin, (12) interleukin-3, (13) cortisol, (14) fibrinogen and finally (15) AXL receptor tyrosine kinase.

The grouping that resulted in the highest LOO CV R^2 over all possible hierarchical clustering cut-offs was used (Figure 2). This was achieved when 13 RBM analytes were used: c-peptide, fibrinogen, alpha-1-antitrypsin, pancreatic polypeptide, complement C3, vitronectin, cortisol, AXL receptor tyrosine kinase, interleukin-3, interleukin-13, matrix metalloproteinase-9 total, APOE and IgE (LOO CV R^2 0.310, permutation test p-value 4×10^{-5}). The 13 RBM analyte and co-variate model is able to account for approximately a third of the variance of brain amyloid burden. The relative importance of variables to the model is shown in Figure 3; the number of APOE ϵ 4 alleles was seen to be the most important variable for the model, but RBM analytes contribute more to the model than years of education or age. The 71 subjects brain amyloid burden was then dichotomised into

either PiB positive (brain amyloid burden >1.5) or PiB negative (brain amyloid burden <1.5), based on a threshold used in relevant literature [16]. Similarly, the subjects LOO CV predicted brain amyloid burden, based on the 13 RBM and co-variate model, was dichotomised into either predicted PiB positive (predicted brain amyloid burden >1.5) or predicted PiB negative (predicted brain amyloid burden <1.5). For each subject the predicted and actual PiB classes (positive or negative) were compared; the predicted PiB classes identified actual PiB positive subjects with a sensitivity of 0.918 and a specificity of 0.545. It was also found that removing all co-variates, except the number of APOE ϵ 4 alleles, from the 13 RBM and co-variate regression model gave a similar but slightly improved predictive ability (LOO CV R^2 0.311).

Markers of brain amyloid burden associate with other measures of AD pathology

The 16 RBM analytes found to associate with brain amyloid burden in the ADNI RBM-PiB PET cohort were then tested for association with other phenotypes known to relate to AD pathology in the ADNI-RBM cohort (sample characteristics shown in Table S2). In this analysis age, gender, years of education and the number of APOE ϵ 4 alleles were included in partial correlation analysis. Subjects with missing values for a relevant comparison were excluded. First the level of the markers of brain amyloid burden were compared with the level of $A\beta_{1-42}$ in the CSF. Leptin was found to associate with CSF $A\beta_{1-42}$ (partial SRC 0.183, BH MTC p-value 0.0183). Additionally, when multiple testing was not taken into account, vitronectin was associated with CSF $A\beta_{1-42}$ (partial SRC 0.131, uncorrected p-value 2.07×10^{-2}).

Markers of brain amyloid burden were then compared to AD relevant brain regions as measured by structural magentic resonance imaging (sMRI). The volume of the left and right

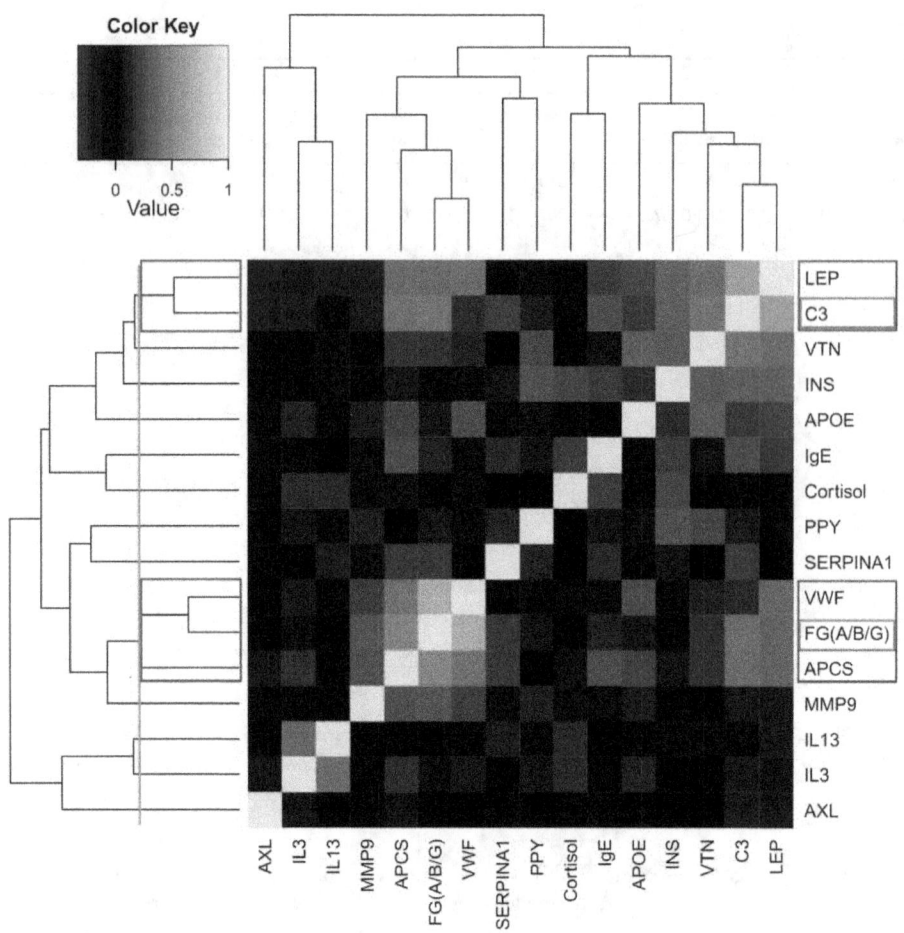

Figure 1. Analyte correlations. Heatmaps of partial SRC between RBM analytes significantly associated (p-value <0.05) with brain amyloid burden, taking into account: age, gender, years of education, number of *APOE* ϵ 4 alleles and the difference, in days, between plasma sampling and [^{11}C]-PiB PET scan date. RBM analytes have been ordered by hierarchical clustering, the final cut-off is shown in purple. Variables that have been grouped are shown in blue boxes, and the representative for each group is shown in a red box.
doi:10.1371/journal.pone.0044260.g001

hippocampi, and the thickness of the left and right entorhinal cortices were used, as these regions are known to be important in AD pathology [12]. Alpha-1-antitrypsin was found to associate at the 5% significance level with the thickness of both the left (partial SRC −0.132, BH MTC p-value 0.0289) and right (partial SRC −0.145, BH MTC p-value 9.82×10^{-3}) entorhinal cortices. Additionally, leptin was found to associate with the thickness of the right entorhinal cortex (partial SRC 0.124, BH MTC p-value 0.0264). Cortisol was found to associate at the 5% significance level with the volume of both the left (partial SRC −0.158, BH MTC p-value 2.71×10^{-3}) and right hippocampi (partial SRC −0.161, BH MTC p-value 2.07×10^{-3}).

Different cognitive tests, such as the Mini Mental State Exam (MMSE) and Alzheimer's Disease Assessment Scale-cognitive subscale (ADAS-cog) 13, assess different aspects of cognitive decline. The association between scores from these tests and levels of markers of brain amyloid burden was analysed; 4/16 of the markers of brain amyloid burden – alpha-1-antitrypsin (partial SRC −0.145, BH MTC p-value 3.02×10^{-3}), complement C3 (partial SRC −0.189, BH MTC p-value 9.46×10^{-5}), cortisol (partial SRC −0.162, BH MTC p-value 8.33×10^{-4}) and fibrinogen (partial SRC −0.130, BH MTC p-value 8.28×10^{-3}) – were found to associate with the total MMSE score at the 5%

level. In the same cohort (ADNI-RBM), three of these markers – alpha-1-antitrypsin (partial SRC 0.172, BH MTC p-value 0.0403), complement C3 (partial SRC 0.119, BH MTC p-value 0.0467) and fibrinogen (partial SRC 0.111, BH MTC p-value 6.34×10^{-4}) – were found to associate with the ADAS-cog 13 score at the 5% significance level.

Levels of the 16 markers of brain amyloid burden were then compared between different diagnostic groups (control, MCI and AD) in the various cohorts, to assess whether these markers were related to clinical diagnosis. It was found that half of the biomarkers of brain amyloid burden measured – APOE (BH MTC KW p-value 1.24×10^{-9}, AD/control median difference (MD) −0.143), complement C3 (BH MTC KW p-value 8.88×10^{-8}, MCI/control MD −0.0483), cortisol (BH MTC KW p-value 2.40×10^{-3}, AD/control MD 0.0366), interleukin-3 (BH MTC KW p-value 8.48×10^{-3}, AD/control MD −0.0670), leptin (BH MTC KW p-value 8.48×10^{-3}, AD/control MD −0.112), pancreatic polypeptide (BH MTC KW p-value 1.92×10^{-2}, AD/control MD 0.122), alpha-1-antitrypsin (BH MTC KW p-value 1.75×10^{-7}, AD/control MD 0.0300) and vitronectin (BH MTC KW p-value 5.50×10^{-3}, AD/control MD -0.0344) – significantly differ at the 5% level between diagnostic groups.

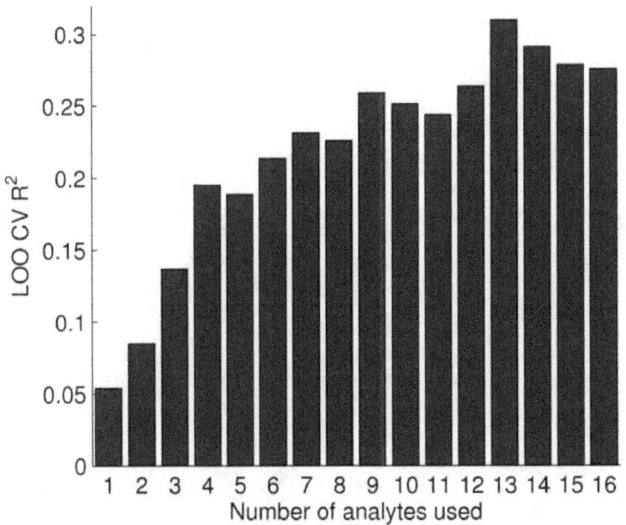

Figure 2. Cross validation of multiple linear regression. Barplot of the LOO CV R^2 of multiple linear regressions of brain amyloid burden against a range of RBM analytes and co-variates. Subsets of RBM analytes that associated with brain amyloid levels with a p-value <0.05 were used. Various subsets were chosen by hierarchical clustering at various cutoffs, with the analyte most associated with brain amyloid burden in each cluster chosen to represent that cluster. Age, gender, years of education, the number of *APOE* ϵ 4 alleles and the difference, in days, between plasma sampling and [^{11}C]-PiB PET scan were used as co-variates.
doi:10.1371/journal.pone.0044260.g002

The effect of *APOE* genotype on APOE level in plasma and brain amyloid burden

The number of *APOE* ϵ 4 alleles and the level of APOE in plasma were the two variables that contributed most to the regression model. A number of studies have shown that APOE level in plasma is affected by presence of *APOE* ϵ 4 alleles [14,15,17–19]. Additionally, Slooter et al., [17] have previously

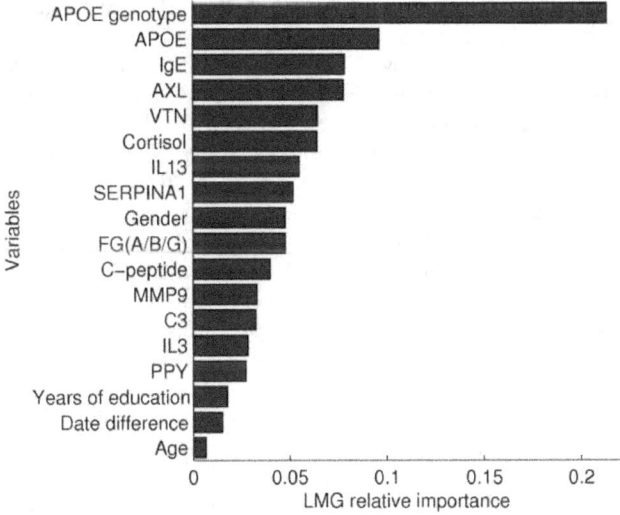

Figure 3. Relative importance in multiple linear regression. Relative importance of variables used in multiple linear regression assessed using the LMG relative importance score [51]. When all the data is used to fit the model it explains 62.0% of the variance of the brain amyloid burden, here the contribution of the variables used in this model are shown.
doi:10.1371/journal.pone.0044260.g003

shown that the difference in plasma APOE levels between AD and control subjects is largely driven by the *APOE* genotype, and so the interaction of these two variables was studied further. In the ADNI-RBM cohort the number of *APOE* ϵ 4 alleles was seen to have a negative effect on plasma APOE levels (KW p-value $<2.20\times10^{-16}$, Table 3). The negative effect of *APOE* genotype on plasma APOE levels in this ADNI subcohort was demonstrated recently using Analysis of Variance (ANOVA) [20]. The analysis presented here shows that this result holds when assumptions of normality are dropped. The negative effect of the number of *APOE* ϵ 4 alleles on plasma APOE levels observed fits with the findings of some literature [15,17,18], but is the opposite of the positive effect seen by both Evans et al. and Thambisetty et al. (2010) [14,19].

Given the discrepancy between this finding and those in two published studies, the relationship between the number of *APOE* ϵ 4 alleles and plasma APOE levels was studied in an independent cohort of 694 subjects (AddNeuroMed and King's Health Partners Dementia Case Register, ANM + KNPDCR). In the ANM + KHPDCR cohort the number of *APOE* ϵ 4 alleles was also seen to have a negative effect on plasma APOE levels (KW p-value $<2.20\times10^{-16}$, Table 3). Both studies that have found a positive relationship between *APOE* ϵ 4 alleles on plasma APOE levels have been conducted in cohorts of cognitively normal subjects [14,19], which may account for this inconsistency. However, a similar negative effect was found in the control subjects (who are cognitively normal) of the ANM + KHPDCR cohort (KW p-value 1.57×10^{-4}, Table 3). This suggests another factor, other than cognitive decline, is responsible for the discrepancies between these studies.

Given that the number of *APOE* ϵ 4 alleles affects both plasma APOE levels and brain amyloid burden, it is possible that the number of *APOE* ϵ 4 alleles confounds the association between plasma APOE levels and brain amyloid burden. To test this, partial correlation analysis was repeated excluding the number of *APOE* ϵ 4 alleles, this increased the correlation of plasma APOE level and brain amyloid burden (partial SRC −0.393, p-value 6.9×10^{-4}), which indicated that the association is indeed partly confounded by the number of *APOE* ϵ 4 alleles.

Discussion

In this study, fibrillar amyloid beta levels, in ADNI subjects, have been compared and related to the level of analytes on the RBM panel in plasma. Brain amyloid burden appears to be distributed bimodally in the RBM-PiB PET cohort, as has been previously reported for a larger ADNI subcohort by Ewers et al. [21]. Associations of C-peptide, fibrinogen, alpha-1-antitrypsin, pancreatic polypeptide, complement C3, vitronectin, von willebrand factor, cortisol, serum amyloid p-component, AXL receptor tyrosine kinase, interleukin-3, interleukin-13, matrix metallproteinase-9, APOE, leptin and immunoglobulin E with brain amyloid burden have been found in this study. Some of these markers of brain amyloid burden were also found to associate with other AD related phenotypes, such as CSF Aβ_{1-42}, MRI features, cognitive tests and diagnostic groups. In regression models it was found that models including both RBM analytes and co-variates performed better than those using only co-variate information, suggesting that the RBM panel of analytes can be used as markers of brain amyloid burden. Combining highly correlated variables was found to reduce overfitting and led to a set of 13 RBM analytes that together with co-variates could explain >30% of the variance of brain amyloid burden and predict PiB positive individuals with a high sensitivity. This result, and the increased predictive accuracy of the 13 RBM model in comparison to using

Table 3. The effect of *APOE* genotype on plasma APOE levels.

| Cohort | The plasma level in log µg/ml of APOE in subjects with n *APOE* ε 4 alleles (median [IQR]) | | | Kruskal-Wallis χ^2 P-value |
	n = 0	n = 1	n = 2	
ADNI-RBM	1.79 [0.200]	1.66 [0.203]	1.52 [0.233]	$<2.20 \times 10^{-16}$
ANM + KHPDCR	1.91 [9.75×10^{-2}]	1.88 [9.00×10^{-2}]	1.82 [7.00×10^{-2}]	$<2.20 \times 10^{-16}$
ANM + KHPDCR controls	1.9 [0.100]	1.88 [8.00×10^{-2}]	1.83 [3.00×10^{-2}]	1.57×10^{-4}

Level of plasma APOE stratified by the subjects number of *APOE* ε 4 alleles.
doi:10.1371/journal.pone.0044260.t003

only co-variates to predict fibrillar amyloid alone, indicate that these analytes reflect levels of fibrillar amyloid in the brain.

The potential of APOE level in plasma to be used as a biomarker for brain amyloid burden, previously shown in Thambisetty et al. (2010) [14], is given support by this study. However it should be noted that the association between plasma APOE level and brain amyloid burden was seen to be positive in that study and negative in this. This inconsistency may relate to differences between the cohorts, for example the BLSA cohort studied in Thambisetty et al. (2010) were selected to be cognitively normal. This fits with the recent finding that plasma level of APOE correlates negatively with brain amyloid burden in the Australian Imaging, Biomarker and Lifestyle Flagship Study of Ageing, which includes subjects suffering from AD [15]. Similarly, the effect of the presence of *APOE* ε 4 alleles on plasma APOE level in the study presented here was found to be the opposite of that found in both Thambisetty et al. (2010) and Evans et al. [14,19], however it is the same as that seen in Slooter et al., Siest et al. and Gupta et al. [15,17,18]. Additionally, this relation was replicated in an independent cohort (ANM + KHPDCR) and it's control subcohort. This latter finding suggests that the differences between the findings of these studies is not due to the subjects cognitive status. The factor/s responsible for these inconsistencies are not known, but the fact that strong associations are seen in all studies is encouraging.

While no association between the level of RBM analytes in plasma and brain amyloid burden was found to be significant at the 5% level after multiple testing corrections, it should be noted the cohort used (RBM-PiB PET) contained relatively few subjects and that many analytes that associated significantly at the uncorrected 0.05 level have known relations to AD pathology, for example levels of APOE and complement C3 in plasma have previously been found to associate with fibrillar amyloid levels in the Baltimore Longitudinal Study of Aging (BLSA) cohort [14]. In addition, some of these analytes were subsequently found to associate with surrogate phenotypes of AD pathology in the larger ADNI-RBM cohort, such as: diagnostic groups, MMSE score, ADAS-cog 13 score, CSF $A\beta_{1-42}$ level, and the thickness and/or volume of the entorhinal cortices. However, 7/16 of the markers of brain amyloid burden – c-peptide, von Willebrand factor, serum amyloid p-component, AXL receptor tyrosine kinase, interleukin-13, matrix metalloproteinase-9 total and IgE – were not found to associate with any of the surrogate phenotypes of AD pathology that were tested. It should be noted that 5 of the 7 are linked to AD in the literature (Table S3), only IgE and interleukin-13 have no prior reported association. Most of these surrogate phenotypes, except CSF $A\beta_{1-42}$, are believed to change at a later disease stage

than amyloid pathology, and so it is possible that the lack of association of some of the markers with, for example, diagnostic groups is due to the mixture of high and low brain amyloid burden control subjects used. However, the lack of association of the majority of the markers with CSF $A\beta_{1-42}$ levels is of greater concern because CSF $A\beta_{1-42}$ levels are strongly associated with brain amyloid burden [4,5]; this may indicate that we are over-fitting the available data and further highlights the need for datasets with larger sample sizes for future studies of markers of brain amyloid burden.

While half of the markers associated with diagnostic groups, 3/8 of these markers – alpha-1-antitrypsin, pancreatic polypeptide and interleukin-3 – had a median difference between AD (or MCI) and control subjects that was of the opposite sign to the partial SRC coefficient measuring their association with brain amyloid burden. This result is surprising as brain amyloid burden is positively associated with AD and MCI diagnosis groups. This discrepancy could relate to the delay between these disease stages, and may mean that the level of some of the markers in plasma changes during $A\beta$ deposition and then changes again, but in the opposite direction, before the onset of clinical symptoms. Similar u-shaped profiles, but between subjects in different diagnostic groups, have been observed (cross-sectionally) in the level of many leukocyte transcripts during AD progression [22].

Partial correlation showed that the number of *APOE* ε 4 alleles partly confounded the association between APOE level in plasma and brain amyloid burden; however, plasma APOE levels did help a regression model predict brain amyloid burden and so further study is required to get a clearer idea of the *APOE* ε 4 independent information conveyed by plasma APOE levels. This study has revealed many novel potential markers of brain amyloid burden, chosen to give *APOE* ε 4 independent information, as well as replicating findings from other studies. This will allow further validation work that can test the replicability and clinical utility of these markers.

In a previous study that used discovery proteomics to identify proteins associated with brain amyloid levels, Thambisetty et al. (2010) showed that levels of APOE and Complement C3 precursor in plasma were different between subjects with high and low brain amyloid burdens [14]. It was encouraging that both were seen to be associated with brain amyloid burden in this study as well. Complement C3 precursor has also been found to be associated with atrophy of hippocampal volume, another imaging marker of AD [11], and to have a role in plaque clearance in a mouse model [23]. It has also been found along with vitronectin to be at different levels in serum between control and AD subjects [6]. The level of fibrinogen gamma was also found to be associated with atrophy of hippocampal volume in Thambisetty et al. (2011) [11]. Fibrinogen alpha, beta and gamma are targeted by the same RBM analyte and were found to associate with brain amyloid burden in this study.

Of the 16 RBM analytes whose level in plasma associated with brain amyloid burden, many have known relationships with Alzheimer's disease. The levels of the following have previously been found to be different between control and AD subjects: alpha-1-antitrypsin [9,24], APOE [9], cortisol [9,25,26], interleukin-3 [27], matrix metalloproteinase-9 [9,28], pancreatic polypeptide [9,29], serum amyloid p-component [30] and von Willebrand factor [31]. Serum amyloid p-component [32] and insulin [33] have been shown to affect 'AD'-like pathology *in vitro*. Interleukin-3 [34] and leptin [35] have been found to affect the interaction of neurons and $A\beta$. Additionally, interleukin-13 has been found to be produced in microglia in response to $A\beta$ [36]. More recently, APOE and matrix metalloproteinase-9 have been shown to be involved together in the breakdown of the blood brain barrier, which can initiate neurodegeneration [37].

Given the relatively small number of subjects in this study it was not practical to separate the subjects into training and test sets, to assess the predictive accuracy of the regression model. Instead, k-fold cross-validation was used, allowing more of the subjects to be used for fitting the regression model. Generally it is advisable to use 10-fold cross-validation because it has been found to have a lower variance [38]. However, given the limited number of samples available, a leave one out cross-validation approach was used in this study to allow the maximal use of the subjects available. Given the limited number of subjects on which the model is based, it will be important in the future to study the ability of these biomarkers to predict brain amyloid burden in an independent cohort. Validation studies would benefit from greater numbers of subjects and better sampling strategies. For example, the distribution of brain amyloid burden in the RBM-PiB PET subcohort is affected by the sampling strategy applied to select control subjects for RBM measurements; only plasma of control subjects with high CSF $A\beta_{1-42}$ were selected, for reasons unrelated to the current study. This means that the resulting model may not extrapolate to cognitively normal subjects with high brain amyloid burden, this could be tested in a validation study. Additionally, the use of only three control subjects may make the regression model less likely to generalise to prediction of brain amyloid burden in early Alzheimer's disease.

In conclusion, analytes associating with brain amyloid burden have the potential to act as biomarkers of early AD-related pathology. In this study sixteen analytes were found to associate with brain amyloid burden, including two (APOE and complement C3) that had had already been shown to associate with brain amyloid burden in an independent cohort. Some of these analytes were also found to associate with other AD related phenotypes in a larger ADNI subcohort, such as: CSF $A\beta_{1-42}$, MRI features, cognitive scores and diagnostic groups. Some of these analytes were found to correlate highly with each other, and so a representative set of thirteen analytes – c-peptide, fibrinogen, alpha-1-antitrypsin, pancreatic polypeptide, complement C3, vitronectin, cortisol, AXL receptor kinase, interleukin-3, interleukin-13, matrix metalloproteinase-9 total, APOE and IgE – were used along with subject age, gender, years of education, the number of *APOE* ϵ 4 alleles and sampling dates to predict brain amyloid burden. The 13 analyte and co-variate model was found by cross-validation to account for >30% of the variance of brain amyloid burden, as opposed to ~ 4–13% using just co-variates alone, showing the potential of plasma analytes as markers of brain amyloid burden. The model was also able to predict PiB positive

individuals with a high sensitivity. The two variables with the largest contribution to the model were found to be the number of *APOE* ϵ 4 alleles and plasma APOE level. The association of plasma APOE level with brain amyloid burden was shown to be partly confounded by the number of *APOE* ϵ 4 alleles, highlighting the importance of novel biomarkers that are less confounded by the *APOE* genotype revealed by this study.

Materials and Methods

Ethics statement

Written informed consent was obtained from all participants in ADNI and the study was conducted with prior institutional ethics approval. Both ANM and KHPDCR were approved by the South London and Maudsley NHS Foundation Trust ethics committee. Ethics committee approval was also obtained at each of the participating centres in accordance with the Alzheimers Associations published recommendations [39].

ADNI Data

Data used in the preparation of this article were obtained from the ADNI database (adni.loni.ucla.edu). The ADNI was launched in 2003 by the National Institute on Aging (NIA), the National Institute of Biomedical Imaging and Bioengineering (NIBIB), the Food and Drug Administration (FDA), private pharmaceutical companies and non-profit organisations, as a $60 million, 5- year public-private partnership. The primary goal of ADNI has been to test whether serial magnetic resonance imaging (MRI), positron emission tomography (PET), other biological markers, and clinical and neuropsychological assessment can be combined to measure the progression of mild cognitive impairment (MCI) and early Alzheimers disease (AD). Determination of sensitive and specific markers of very early AD progression is intended to aid researchers and clinicians to develop new treatments and monitor their effectiveness, as well as lessen the time and cost of clinical trials.

The Principal Investigator of this initiative is Michael W. Weiner, MD, VA Medical Center and University of California San Francisco. ADNI is the result of efforts of many co-investigators from a broad range of academic institutions and private corporations, and subjects have been recruited from over 50 sites across the U.S. and Canada. The initial goal of ADNI was to recruit 800 adults, ages 55 to 90, to participate in the research, approximately 200 cognitively normal older individuals to be followed for 3 years, 400 people with MCI to be followed for 3 years and 200 people with early AD to be followed for 2 years. For up-to-date information, see www.adni-info.org.

Demographic (age, gender, years of education), genetic (number of *APOE* ϵ 4 alleles), diagnosis (control, MCI or AD at a given date) and analyte (metabolite/protein/complex) levels in plasma were compared with brain amyloid burden (or other markers of AD pathology such as: CSF $A\beta_{1-42}$ level, MRI features, cognitive scores or diagnostic groups). Diagnoses were recorded for each subject at each visit. Plasma and CSF were collected from fasted subjects using the procedures described previously [29,40]. Levels of 190 analytes were measured from subject plasma using the Rules Based Medicine (RBM, rulesbasedmedicine.com, Austin, TX) Human Discovery Multi-Analyte Profile (MAP) 1.0 panel and a Luminex 100 platform [41]. Measurements of 44 analytes were excluded on the basis of quality control, leaving 146 analytes in the subsequent analysis. The levels of all 146 analytes (except: apolipoprotein H, complement factor H, E selectin, epidermal growth factor, fibrinogen, interleukin-12 subunit p40, placenta growth factor, serum glutamic oxaloacetic transaminase and thrombopoietin) were log transformed to improve the fit of the levels to the normal distribution. Description of methods used to derive measurements of regional [11C] PiB-PET levels have been given in Jagust et al. (2010) and (2011) previously [16,42]. In this study a similar approach was taken by averaging over regional [11C] PiB-PET measurements in parietal, frontal, anterior cingulate and precuneus regions of interest, to derive a global measure of brain amyloid burden.

Data from either baseline or 12 months were used for these cohorts, as described above, chosen to increase the number of subjects with available data. Eighty four subjects (ADNI-PiB PET cohort) had a [11C] PiB-PET scan 12 months after baseline, the characteristics of this sample are shown in Table S1. Five hundred and sixty six subjects (ADNI-RBM cohort) had RBM analytes measured in plasma collected at baseline, the characteristics of this sample at baseline is shown in Table S2. Seventy one subjects (RBM-PiB PET cohort) had RBM analytes measured in plasma collected 12 months after baseline and a [11C] PiB-PET scan within a year of this, the characteristics of this sample at the date of plasma collection is shown in Table 1. Converters from control to MCI between plasma sample and [11C] PiB-PET scan date account for the discrepancy in diagnostic groups between the ADNI-PiB PET and RBM-PiB PET cohorts. Subject age was determined based on the same dates.

Sample characteristics of each cohort by diagnostic group were analysed in R [43]. Many continuous variables were not distributed normally, and so are described by median and interquartile range instead of mean and standard deviation, this was also the reason that non-parametric statistical tests were used. Continuous characteristics were tested for differences over diagnostic groups by the non-parametric Kruskal-Wallis χ^2 test, using kruskal.test in the R stats package. Discrete characteristics were tested for differences over diagnostic groups by simulated contingency table p-values, in the fisher.test function in the R stats package, using 2,000 Monte Carlo samples.

MRI scan analysis

Dicom format MRI data was downloaded from the ADNI website (www.loni.ucla.edu/ADNI). Data from 1.5 T scanners was used with data collected from a variety of MR-systems with protocols optimised for each type of scanner. The MRI protocol included a high resolution sagittal 3D T1-weighted MPRAGE volume (voxel size $1.1 \times 1.1 \times 1.2$ mm^3) acquired using a custom pulse sequence specifically designed for the ADNI study to ensure compatibility across scanners. Full brain and skull coverage was required for the MRI datasets and detailed quality control carried out on all MR images according to previously published quality control criteria [44,45].

We applied the Freesurfer pipeline (version 4.5.0) to the MRI images to produce regional cortical thickness and volumetric measures as previously described [46] to produce hippocampal and entorhinal cortex volumes, as well as entorhinal cortical thickness. All volumetric measures from each subject were normalised by the subjects intracranial volume. Cortical thickness measures were not normalised [47] and were used in their raw form.

Correlation analysis

R was used to analyse SRC and partial SRC, using cor.test in the stats package and pcor.test in the ppcor package [48] respectively. Partial correlations were used to take into account subjects: age, gender, years of education, number of *APOE* ε 4 alleles and the number of days separating the date of [11C]-PiB

PET scan and plasma sample. In the case of correlations between RBM analytes and CSF Aβ, ADAS-cog 13 or MRI features, subjects whose relevant data was missing were excluded. RBM analytes were clustered based upon (1 − their partial SRC) using the R function hclust in the stats package with default settings, and displayed using function heatmap.2 from the R gplots package [49].

Linear regression

Linear regression was performed using the lm function in the R stats package. This was appropriate because although many variables were not distributed normally, the residuals of the regression models used were approximately. Before regression, measurements of each RBM analyte were transformed to a standard deviation of one to allow each analyte to have equal influence on the model (but not transformed to a mean of zero, to make the analysis more comparable with that used in Thambisetty et al. (2010) [14]). LOO CV was performed by fitting linear regression models to the data, leaving out one subject at a time, and using the model to predict brain amyloid burden in that subject based on the fitted model. LOO CV R^2 was calculated as the square of the Pearson's correlation coefficient, calculated using cor.test, between the predicted and observed brain amyloid burden.

A cut-off of 1.5 was used to dichotomise brain amyloid burden in the RBM-PiB PET cohort as PiB positive (49 subjects) or negative (22 subjects), as previously suggested by Jagust et al. (2010) [16]. Predicted values were similarly dichotomised. Sensitivity and specificity of this prediction was calculated in R using epi.test in the epiR package [50].

Permutation tests were performed by permuting brain amyloid burden across subjects in the data, and re-calculating the LOO CV R^2 that was achieved by fitting the regression model to the resulting data. 100,000 permutations were used, and the number of cases in which the LOO CV R^2 exceeded that achieved with the original dataset was recorded. Relative importance was calculated using the LMG score [51], using the R package relaimpo [52].

Independent cohort data for validation of the effect of *APOE* ε 4 genotype on APOE level in plasma

EDTA plasma samples from fasted subjects were obtained from two independent cohorts: ANM a multicentre European study across six centres [53] and KHPDCR a UK based study. The combined cohort contained 269 control, 163 MCI and 262 AD subjects. *APOE* genotype was determined using DNA extracted from blood leukocytes by a standard phenol-chloroform extraction. The three main alleles *APOE* ε 2, *APOE* ε 3 and *APOE* ε 4 differ at two residues, so consist of a two single nucleotide polymorphism (SNP) haplotype. The SNPs rs429358 and rs7412 were genotyped and the allele inferred. SNPs were determined by allelic discrimination assays based on fluorogenic 5′ nuclease activity. TaqMan SNP genotyping assays were performed on an ABI Prism 7900HT and analyzed using SDS software, according to the manufacturer's instructions (Applied Biosystems, Warrington, UK). 199 control, 103 MCI and 120 AD subjects were found to have 0 *APOE* ε 4 alleles. 65 control, 56 MCI and 112 AD subjects were found to have 1 *APOE* ε 4 alleles. 5 control, 4 MCI and 30 AD subjects were found to have 2 *APOE* ε 4 alleles. The Human Neurodegenerative Panel 1 (7-plex) Cat. HNDG1-36K MILLIPLEX MAP multiplex panels, developed by Merck Millipore, was used to measure APOE level in plasma.

Supporting Information

Figure S1 Distribution of brain amyloid burden. A stacked histogram showing the distribution of brain amyloid burden for different diagnostic groups. Control (dark blue), MCI (green) and AD (red) represent subjects who remained in these diagnostic groups throughout follow up period. Control/MCI (light blue) and MCI/AD (orange) represents subjects whose diagnosis converted between these groups during the follow up period. Brain amyloid burden is in relative units.
(TIF)

Table S1 Characteristics of the ADNI-PiB PET cohort by diagnostic group. P-values were calculated when appropriate for differences across diagnostic groups, using a Kruskal-Wallis χ^2 test for continuous characteristics and simulated contingency table p-values for discrete characteristics.
(PDF)

Table S2 Characteristics of the ADNI-RBM cohort by diagnostic group. P-values were calculated when appropriate for differences across diagnostic groups, using a Kruskal-Wallis χ^2 test for continuous characteristics and simulated contingency table p-values for discrete characteristics.
(PDF)

Table S3 Association of markers with AD phenotypes. (PDF)

Acknowledgments

We are grateful to peer-reviewers, whose suggestions helped us to refine this manuscript.

Data used in preparation of this article were obtained from the Alzheimers Disease Neuroimaging Initiative (ADNI) database (adni.loni.ucla.edu). As such, the investigators within the ADNI contributed to the design and implementation of ADNI and/or provided data but did not participate in analysis or writing of this report. A complete listing of ADNI investigators can be found at: http://adni.loni.ucla.edu/wp-content/uploads/how_to_apply/ADNI_Acknowledgement_List.pdf.

Author Contributions

Conceived and designed the experiments: M. Thambisetty AS SL SN RD. Analyzed the data: SJK. Wrote the paper: SJK M. Thambisetty AS SN RD. APOE measurements in AddNeuroMed and DCR: JRC AH IP MW MKL KL. Input on image analysis: EW. Provided cluster computing support: CJ. AddNeuroMed clinical centre lead: HS IK M. Tsolaki BV PM.

References

1. Golde TE, Schneider LS, Koo EH (2008) Anti-Aβ therapeutics in Alzheimer's disease: the need for a paradigm shift. Neuron 69: 203–213.
2. Reiman EM, Langbaum JB, Fleisher AS, Caselli RJ, Chen K, et al. (2011) Alzheimer's Prevention Initiative: a plan to accelerate the evaluation of presymptomatic treatments. J Alzheimers Dis 26: 321–329.
3. Aisen PS, Andrieu S, Sampaio C, Carrillo M, Khachaturian ZS, et al. (2011) Report of the task force on designing clinical trials in early (predementia) AD. Neurology 76: 280–286.
4. Grimmer T, Riemenschneider M, Förstl H, Henriksen G, Klunk WE, et al. (2009) Beta amyloid in Alzheimer's disease: increased deposition in brain is reected in reduced concentration in cerebrospinal fluid. Biol Psychiatry 65: 927–934.
5. Koivunen J, Pirttilä T, Kemppainen N, Aalto S, Herukka SK, et al. (2008) PET amyloid ligand [11C] PIB uptake and cerebrospinal uid beta-amyloid in mild cognitive impairment. Dement Geriatr Cogn Disord 26: 378–383.
6. Zhang R, Barker L, Pinchev D, Marshall J, Rasamoelisolo M, et al. (2004) Mining biomarkers in human sera using proteomic tools. Proteomics 4: 244–256.
7. Hye A, Lynham S, Thambisetty M, Causevic M, Campbell J, et al. (2006) Proteome-based plasma biomarkers for Alzheimer's disease. Brain 129: 3042–3050.
8. Soares HD, Potter WZ, Pickering E, Kuhn M, Immermann FW, et al. (Ahead of print) Plasma biomarkers associated with the apolipoprotein e genotype and alzheimer disease. Arch Neurol.
9. Doecke JD, Laws SM, Faux NG, Wilson W, Burnham SC, et al. (Ahead of print) Blood-based protein biomarkers for diagnosis of Alzheimer disease. Arch Neurol.
10. Thambisetty M, Simmons A, Velayudhan L, Hye A, Campbell J, et al. (2010) Association of plasma clusterin concentration with severity, pathology, and progression in Alzheimer disease. Arch Gen Psychiatry 67: 739–748.
11. Thambisetty M, Simmons A, Hye A, Campbell J, Westman E, et al. (2011) Plasma biomarkers of brain atrophy in Alzheimer's disease. PloS one 6: e28527.
12. Thambisetty M, An Y, Kinsey A, Koka D, Saleem M, et al. (2012) Plasma clusterin concentration is associated with longitudinal brain atrophy in mild cognitive impairment. Neuroimage 59: 212–217.
13. Thambisetty M, Hye A, Foy C, Daly E, Glover A, et al. (2008) Proteome-based identification of plasma proteins associated with hippocampal metabolism in early Alzheimer's disease. J Neurol 255: 1712–1720.
14. Thambisetty M, Tripaldi R, Riddoch-Contreras J, Hye A, An Y, et al. (2010) Proteome-based plasma markers of brain amyloid-β deposition in non-demented older individuals. J Alzheimers Dis 22: 1099–1109.
15. Gupta VB, Laws SM, Villemagne VL, Ames D, Bush AI, et al. (2011) Plasma apolipoprotein E and Alzheimer disease risk: the AIBL study of aging. Neurology 76: 1091–1098.
16. Jagust WJ, Bandy D, Chen K, Foster NL, Landau SM, et al. (2010) The Alzheimer's Disease Neuroimaging Initiative positron emission tomography core. Alzheimers Dement 6: 221–229.
17. Slooter AJ, de Knijff P, Hofman A, Cruts M, Breteler MM, et al. (1998) Serum apolipoprotein E level is not increased in Alzheimer's disease: the Rotterdam study. Neurosci Lett 248: 21–24.
18. Siest G, Bertrand P, Qin B, Herbeth B, Serot JM, et al. (2000) Apolipoprotein E polymorphism and serum concentration in Alzheimer's disease in nine European centres: the ApoEurope study. Clin Chem Lab Med 38: 721–730.
19. Evans AE, Zhang W, Moreel JF, Bard JM, Ricard S, et al. (1993) Polymorphisms of the apolipoprotein B and E genes and their relationship to plasma lipid variables in healthy Chinese men. Hum Genet 92: 191–197.
20. Johnstone D, Milward EA, Berretta R, Moscato P, ADNI (2012) Multivariate protein signatures of pre-clinical Alzheimers disease in the Alzheimers Disease Neuroimaging Initiative (ADNI) plasma proteome dataset. PLoS one 7: e34341.
21. Ewers M, Insel P, Jagust WJ, Shaw L, Trojanowski JQ, et al. (2012) CSF Biomarker and PIBPET–Derived Beta-Amyloid Signature Predicts Metabolic, Gray Matter, and Cognitive Changes in Nondemented Subjects. Cerebral Cortex 22: 1993–2004.
22. Lunnon K, Ibrahim Z, Proitsi P, Lourdusamy A, Newhouse S, et al. (2012) Mitochondrial Dysfunction and Immune Activation are Detectable In Early Alzheimers Disease Blood. J Alz Dis 30: 685–710.
23. Maier M, Peng Y, Jiang L, Seabrook TJ, Carroll MC, et al. (2008) Complement C3 deficiency leads to accelerated amyloid β plaque deposition and neurodegeneration and modulation of the microglia/macrophage phenotype in amyloid precursor protein transgenic mice. J Neurosci 28: 6333–6341.
24. Wetterling T, Tegtmeyer KF (1994) Serum alpha 1-antitrypsin and alpha 2-macroglobulin in Alzheimer's and Binswanger's disease. Clin Investig 72: 196–199.
25. Bemelmans KJ, Noort A, Rijk RD, Middelkoop HAM, Kempen GMJV, et al. (2007) Plasma cortisol and norepinephrine in Alzheimer's disease: opposite relations with recall performance and stage of progression. Acta Neuropsychiatr 19: 231–237.
26. Lee BK, Glass TA, Wand GS, McAtee MJ, Bandeen-Roche K, et al. (2008) Apolipoprotein E genotype, cortisol, and cognitive function in community-dwelling older adults. Am J Psychiat 165: 1456–1464.
27. Ray S, Britschgi M, Herbert C, Takeda-Uchimura Y, Boxer A, et al. (2007) Classification and prediction of clinical Alzheimers diagnosis based on plasma signaling proteins. Nat Med 13: 1359–1362.
28. Lorenzl S, Albers DS, Relkin N, Ngyuen T, Hilgenberg SL, et al. (2003) Increased plasma levels of matrix metalloproteinase-9 in patients with Alzheimer's disease. Neurochem Int 43: 191–196.
29. O'Bryant SE, Xiao G, Barber R, Huebinger R, Wilhelmsen K, et al. (2011) A Blood-Based Screening Tool for Alzheimer's Disease That Spans Serum and Plasma: Findings from TARC and ADNI. PLoS one 6: e28092.
30. Nishiyama E, Iwamoto N, Kimura M, Arai H (1996) Serum amyloid P component level in Alzheimer's disease. Dementia 7: 256–259.
31. OBryant SE, Xiao G, Barber R, Reisch J, Doody R, et al. (2010) A serum protein-based algorithm for the detection of Alzheimer disease. Arch Neurol 67: 1077–1081.

32. Mold M, Shrive A (2012) Serum amyloid P component accelerates the formation and enhances the stability of amyloid fibrils in a physiologically significant under-saturated solution of amyloid-Aβ42. J Alzheimers Dis 29: 875–881.

33. de la Monte SM, Wands JR (2005) Review of insulin and insulin-like growth factor expression, signaling, and malfunction in the central nervous system: relevance to Alzheimer's disease. J Alzheimers Dis 7: 45–61.

34. Zambrano A, Otth C, Mujica L, Concha II, Maccioni RB (2007) Interleukin-3 prevents neuronal death induced by amyloid peptide. BMC Neurosci 8: 82.

35. Greco SJ, Sarkar S, Johnston JM, Tezapsidis N (2009) Leptin regulates tau phosphorylation and amyloid through AMPK in neuronal cells. Biochem Bioph Res Co 380: 98–104.

36. Szczepanik AM, Funes S, Petko W, Ringheim GE (2001) IL-4, IL-10 and IL-13 modulate Aβ(1-42)-induced cytokine and chemokine production in primary murine microglia and a human monocyte cell line. J Neuroimmunol 113: 49–62.

37. Bell RD, Winkler EA, Singh I, Sagare AP, Deane R, et al. (2012) Apolipoprotein E controls cerebrovascular integrity via cyclophilin A. Nature 485: 512–516.

38. Kohavi R (1995) A study of cross-validation and bootstrap for accuracy estimation and model selection. Proceedings of IJCAI'95 2: 1137–1143.

39. Alzheimers Association (2004) Research consent for cognitively impaired adults: recommendations for institutional review boards and investigators. Alzheimer Dis Assoc Disord 18: 171–175.

40. Vemuri P, Wiste HJ, Weigand SD, Shaw LM, Trojanowski JQ, et al. (2009) MRI and CSF biomarkers in normal, MCI, and AD subjects: diagnostic discrimination and cognitive correlations. Neurology 73: 287–297.

41. Trojanowski JQ, Vandeerstichele H, Korecka M, Clark CM, Aisen PS, et al. (2010) Update on the biomarker core of the Alzheimer's Disease Neuroimaging Initiative subjects. Alzheimers Dement 6: 230–238.

42. Jagust WJ, Landau SM, Shaw LM, Trojanowski JQ, Koeppe RA, et al. (2009) Relationships between biomarkers in aging and dementia. Neurology 73: 1193.

43. R Development Core Team (2011) R: A Language and Environment for Statistical Computing. R Foundation for Statistical Computing, Vienna, Austria. URL http://www.R-project.org. ISBN 3-900051-07-0.

44. Simmons A, Westman E, Muehlboeck S, Mecocci P, Vellas B, et al. (2009) MRI measures of Alzheimers disease and the AddNeuroMed study. Ann NY Acad Sci 1180: 47–55.

45. Simmons A, Westman E, Muehlboeck S, Mecocci P, Vellas B, et al. (2011) The AddNeuroMed framework for multi-centre MRI assessment of longitudinal changes in Alzheimers disease : experience from the first 24 months. Int J Ger Psych 26: 75–82.

46. Westman E, Muehlboeck JS, Simmons A (2012) Combining MRI and CSF measures for classification of Alzheimer's disease and prediction of mild cognitive impairment conversion. Neuroimage 62: 229–238.

47. Westman E, Aguilar C, Muehlboeck JS, Simmons A (In press) Regional magnetic resonance imaging measures for multivariate analysis in Alzheimers disease and mild cognitive impairment. Brain Topogr DOI: 10.1007/s10548-012-0246-x.

48. Kim S (2011) ppcor: Partial and Semi-partial (Part) correlation. The Comprehensive R Archive Network website. URL http://CRAN.R-project.org/package=ppcor. Accessed 2012 August 17. R package version 0.9-38.

49. Warnes GR, Bolker B, Bonebakker L, Gentleman R, Huber W, et al. (2011) gplots: Various R programming tools for plotting data. The Comprehensive R Archive Network website. URL http://CRAN.R-project.org/package=gplots. Accessed 2012 August 17. R package version 0.9-38.

50. Stevenson M, Nunes T, Sanchez J, Thornton R, Reiczigel J, et al. (2012) epiR: An R package for the analysis of epidemiological data. The Comprehensive R Archive Network website. URL http://CRAN.R-project.org/package=epiR. Accessed 2012 August 17. R package version 0.9-38.

51. Lindeman RH, Merenda PF, Gold RZ (1980) Introduction to Bivariate and Multivariate Analysis. Scott Foreman, Glenview, IL, 120–127.

52. Grömping U (2006) Relative importance for linear regression in R: the package relaimpo. J Stat Softw 17: 1–27.

53. Lovestone S, Francis P, Kloszewska I, Meccoci P, Simmons A, et al. (2009) AddNeuroMed – the European collaboration for the discovery of novel biomarkers for Alzheimer's disease. Ann NY Acad Sci 1180: 36–46.

Generative FDG-PET and MRI Model of Aging and Disease Progression in Alzheimer's Disease

Juergen Dukart[1,2]*, Ferath Kherif[1], Karsten Mueller[2], Stanislaw Adaszewski[1], Matthias L. Schroeter[2,3,4,5], Richard S. J. Frackowiak[1], Bogdan Draganski[1,2], for the Alzheimer's Disease Neuroimaging Initiative[¶]

1 LREN, Département des Neurosciences Cliniques, CHUV, Université de Lausanne, Lausanne, Switzerland, 2 Max-Planck-Institute for Human Cognitive and Brain Sciences, Leipzig, Germany, 3 Day Clinic of Cognitive Neurology, University of Leipzig, Leipzig, Germany, 4 LIFE - Leipzig Research Center for Civilization Diseases, University of Leipzig, Leipzig, Germany, 5 Consortium for Frontotemporal Lobar Degeneration, Leipzig, Germany

Abstract

The failure of current strategies to provide an explanation for controversial findings on the pattern of pathophysiological changes in Alzheimer's Disease (AD) motivates the necessity to develop new integrative approaches based on multi-modal neuroimaging data that captures various aspects of disease pathology. Previous studies using [18F]fluorodeoxyglucose positron emission tomography (FDG-PET) and structural magnetic resonance imaging (sMRI) report controversial results about time-line, spatial extent and magnitude of glucose hypometabolism and atrophy in AD that depend on clinical and demographic characteristics of the studied populations. Here, we provide and validate at a group level a generative anatomical model of glucose hypo-metabolism and atrophy progression in AD based on FDG-PET and sMRI data of 80 patients and 79 healthy controls to describe expected age and symptom severity related changes in AD relative to a baseline provided by healthy aging. We demonstrate a high level of anatomical accuracy for both modalities yielding strongly age- and symptom-severity- dependant glucose hypometabolism in temporal, parietal and precuneal regions and a more extensive network of atrophy in hippocampal, temporal, parietal, occipital and posterior caudate regions. The model suggests greater and more consistent changes in FDG-PET compared to sMRI at earlier and the inversion of this pattern at more advanced AD stages. Our model describes, integrates and predicts characteristic patterns of AD related pathology, uncontaminated by normal age effects, derived from multi-modal data. It further provides an integrative explanation for findings suggesting a dissociation between early- and late-onset AD. The generative model offers a basis for further development of individualized biomarkers allowing accurate early diagnosis and treatment evaluation.

Citation: Dukart J, Kherif F, Mueller K, Adaszewski S, Schroeter ML, et al. (2013) Generative FDG-PET and MRI Model of Aging and Disease Progression in Alzheimer's Disease. PLoS Comput Biol 9(4): e1002987. doi:10.1371/journal.pcbi.1002987

Editor: Olaf Sporns, Indiana University, United States of America

Received December 11, 2012; **Accepted** January 27, 2013; **Published** April 4, 2013

Funding: JD is supported by the Synapsy NCCR of the Swiss National Science Foundation (http://www.nccr-synapsy.ch/). BD is supported by the Swiss National Science Foundation (grant 320030_135679 and NCCR Synapsy), Foundation Parkinson Switzerland, Foundation Synapsys, Novartis Foundation for medical–biological research and Deutsche Forschungsgemeinschaft (Kfo 247). FK is supported by the Velux Stiftung. MLS is supported by the German Federal Ministry of Education and Research (BMBF; German FTLD consortium, www.ftld.de/) and LIFE - Leipzig Research Center for Civilization Diseases at the University of Leipzig (http://life.uni-leipzig.de/). LIFE is funded by means of the European Union, by the European Regional Development Fund (ERFD) and by means of the Free State of Saxony within the framework of the excellence initiative. Data collection and sharing for this project was funded by the Alzheimer's Disease Neuroimaging Initiative (ADNI, adni.loni.ucla.edu) (National Institutes of Health Grant U01 AG024904). ADNI is funded by the National Institute on Aging, the National Institute of Biomedical Imaging and Bioengineering, and through generous contributions from the following: Abbott, AstraZeneca AB, Bayer Schering Pharma AG, Bristol-Myers Squibb, Eisai Global Clinical Development, Elan Corporation, Genentech, GE Healthcare, GlaxoSmithKline, Innogenetics, Johnson and Johnson, Eli Lilly and Co., Medpace, Inc., Merck and Co., Inc., Novartis AG, Pfizer Inc, F. Hoffman-La Roche, Schering-Plough, Synarc, Inc., as well as non-profit partners the Alzheimer's Association and Alzheimer's Drug Discovery Foundation, with participation from the U.S. Food and Drug Administration. Private sector contributions to ADNI are facilitated by the Foundation for the National Institutes of Health (www.fnih.org). The grantee organization is the Northern California Institute for Research and Education, and the study is coordinated by the Alzheimer's Disease Cooperative Study at the University of California, San Diego. ADNI data are disseminated by the Laboratory for Neuro Imaging at the University of California, Los Angeles. This research was also supported by NIH grants P30 AG010129, K01 AG030514, and the Dana Foundation. The funders had no role in study design, data collection and analysis, decision to publish, or preparation of the manuscript.

Competing Interests: The authors have declared that no competing interests exist.

* E-mail: dukart@cbs.mpg.de

¶ Please see the acknowledgments for further details of the Alzheimer's Disease Neuroimaging Initiative.

Introduction

Neuroimaging studies using [18F]fluorodeoxyglucose positron emission tomography (FDG-PET) and structural magnetic resonance imaging (sMRI) provide substantial evidence of high sensitivity for early detection and progression assessment in Alzheimer's disease (AD) at a group and single subject level [1–11]. However, among these studies there are a number of discordant results in terms of spatial characteristics and magnitude of glucose hypometabolism and atrophy [12–14]. The supposition that age- and symptom severity-related variability are the main cause for these discrepancies has motivated researchers to adopt analytical strategies that split disease populations into subgroups depending on age- or symptom-severity (e.g. early- and late-onset AD) [12–14].

The question that needs to be answered is whether age and symptom severity indeed account for most of these discrepancies. In other words, what are the relative contributions of age and

Author Summary

Establishing an accurate diagnosis of Alzheimer's disease has been a major challenge in the past decades. With an increasing amount of studies aiming at detection and validation of imaging biomarkers for this disease, many apparently controversial findings have been reported over the time. The failure of current strategies to provide a consistent explanation for these differential findings motivates the necessity to develop new integrative approaches based on multi-modal data that capture various aspects of disease pathology. In our study we propose such a generative model providing a comprehensive approach towards integration of previously published differential findings in early- and late-onset AD. We believe that our analytical strategy not only provides the link between imaging biomarkers and clinical phenotype considering the effects of aging, but could also lead to new areas of research in terms of creation of new, individualized biomarkers for a more accurate diagnosis of Alzheimer's disease.

disease to the anatomical patterns of abnormality of structure and function? Investigation of these relationships may also provide clues to another long-time controversy – can the observed differences between young and aged AD patients be regarded as a continuum or is there a clear separation into two cohorts dependent on separate pathological mechanisms?

Recent studies have suggested that AD related brain changes may be similar to those associated with healthy aging. If so, this could explain age overestimation determined from sMR images from AD patients [15] and inaccuracies obtained with automated classification-based computer diagnostics in the eldest healthy controls and youngest AD patients [11]. However, these effects can also be explained in a more simple way by the applied methodology. Both AD and healthy aging have been linked to a decrease in grey matter (GM) volume in extensive networks covering substantial parts of the brain [16–18]. Partial overlaps between these networks are therefore very likely and also occur in some key regions for AD including the hippocampus and parietal cortices. A statistical classification/prediction model trained either for prediction of age or AD would therefore consider these regions as important for separation/prediction. An older healthy control would therefore have a higher probability to be misclassified as AD when applying a classifier trained on younger AD subjects. In contrast, age prediction in an AD patient using a model built on healthy controls would result in an age overestimation in this patient due to the partially overlapping network of reductions in GM volume. Both predictions are fully in line with previous findings [15,19].

Another controversially discussed issue is the relative capability and sensitivity of FDG-PET and sMRI to detect AD related pathology. Recent studies provided evidence for the superiority of each of the two imaging modalities as compared to the other to detect AD related pathology [10,20]. However, none of these findings can be interpreted without serious methodical considerations. Both studies restricted their analyses to univariate region-of-interest statistics to determine the power of each modality to discriminate between AD patients and control subjects. Although this approach provides a good estimation of the differential pathology in the region mostly affected by the disease, it does not at all reflect the whole pattern of AD related pathology over the whole brain. Yet, exactly this whole-brain pattern is crucial for detection and differentiation of AD from healthy aging and other neurodegenerative processes. A second methodological limitation of previous studies is related to pre-processing of FDG-PET data. These data are strongly affected by the underlying atrophy pattern. A reduction in grey matter volume in a specific region would therefore also lead to a reduction of the observed metabolic signal due to increased contribution of other tissue types. This effect is commonly known as partial volume effect (PVE) [21]. If not accounted for, this effect strongly restricts the interpretation of the observed FDG-PET signal due to a high susceptibility to the underlying atrophy. A correction for this effect is therefore necessary to enable a valid interpretation of the independent contribution of both imaging modalities to detection of AD related pathology.

To address these issues and questions we generate group level anatomical models of pathophysiological changes observed in AD using FDG-PET and sMRI data. In these models we account for PVE and integrate disease-, age- and symptom severity-associated changes in AD patients. We further dissociate them from healthy aging related changes using a combination of voxel-based general linear models (GLMs). We additionally assume that AD-induced changes are added to changes observed in healthy aging. We use the models to generate age- and symptom severity- specific whole-brain patterns of glucose hypometabolism and atrophy. To validate the obtained model and to address the questions described above, we contrapose the models' predictions in terms of anatomical plausibility to findings reported in previous studies investigating age- and AD-related changes. Thereby, we aim to provide at a group level an integrative explanation for the controversial findings described above regarding spatial characteristics and magnitude of glucose hypometabolism and atrophy in AD. We further make conclusions on the relative capability of FDG-PET and sMRI to predict AD related pathology at a group level.

We hypothesize, on the basis of the above considerations [12–14] that a generative model predicting age and symptom severity contributions to disease pathology based on data from two imaging modalities – FDG-PET and sMRI – would provide a robust and accurate differential pattern of glucose hypometabolism and atrophy at different ages in AD patients. We expect stronger changes in glucose metabolic compared to anatomical data in earlier disease stages, in accordance with a recently proposed model, which suggests that functional impairment precedes structural changes in AD [22]. We also hypothesize that patterns of brain atrophy associated with healthy aging would overlap those associated with disease progression yet also show a clearly distinguishable anatomical distribution pattern.

Methods

Subjects

To derive a generative model of age and symptom severity related changes, we extracted from the Alzheimer's disease Neuroimaging Initiative (ADNI) database (www.adni-info.org) sMRI and FDG-PET data from multiple centres of 80 patients with a clinical diagnosis of AD and 79 healthy controls (Table 1). A full list of subject and scan IDs used in this study is provided at the following location: http://www.unil.ch/webdav/site/lren/shared/Juergen/Overview_patandcon_MRIandPETdate.xlsx. For all subjects, follow-up evaluations were available for up to 5 years after initial examination. Control subjects and AD patient groups were matched for gender and age. A diagnosis of AD was based on NINCDS/ARDRA criteria [23]. Exclusion criteria for the ADNI data included the presence of any significant neurological disease other than AD, history of head trauma followed by persistent neurological deficits or structural brain abnormalities, psychotic features, agitation or behavioural problems within the previous three months or a history of alcohol or substance abuse. For most subjects, multiple follow-up FDG-PET and sMRI scans were available. Only data from the first examination date were used for analysis. The study was conducted according to the Declaration of Helsinki. Written informed consent was obtained from all participants before protocol-specific procedures were performed. Data used in the preparation of this article were obtained from the Alzheimer's Disease Neuroimaging Initiative (ADNI) database (adni.loni.ucla.edu).

The ADNI was launched in 2003 by the National Institute on Aging (NIA), the National Institute of Biomedical Imaging and Bioengineering (NIBIB), the Food and Drug Administration (FDA), private pharmaceutical companies and non-profit organizations, as a $60 million, 5- year public-private partnership. The primary goal of ADNI has been to test whether serial magnetic resonance imaging (MRI), positron emission tomography (PET), other biological markers, and clinical and neuropsychological assessment can be combined to measure the progression of mild cognitive impairment (MCI) and early Alzheimer's disease (AD). Determination of sensitive and specific markers of very early AD progression is intended to aid researchers and clinicians to develop new treatments and monitor their effectiveness, as well as lessen the time and cost of clinical trials. The Principal Investigator of this initiative is Michael W. Weiner, MD, VA Medical Center and University of California – San Francisco. ADNI is the result of efforts of many co-investigators from a broad range of academic institutions and private corporations, and subjects have been recruited from over 50 sites across the U.S. and Canada. The initial goal of ADNI was to recruit 800 adults, ages 55 to 90, to participate in the research, approximately 200 cognitively normal older individuals to be followed for 3 years, 400 people with MCI to be followed for 3 years and 200 people with early AD to be followed for 2 years." For up-to-date information, see www.adni-info.org.

sMRI data

The sMRI dataset included standard T1-weighted images obtained with different scanner types using a 3D MP-RAGE (magnetization-prepared 180 degrees radio-frequency pulses and rapid gradient-echo) sequence varying in TR and TE (repetition and echo time) with an in-plane resolution of 1.25×1.25 mm and 1.2 mm slice thickness acquired at 1.5T magnetic field strength. All raw data were pre-processed to correct for distortion and B1 non-uniformity as described on the ADNI webpage (http://www.loni.ucla.edu/ADNI/Data/ADNI_Data.shtml).

Table 1. Subject group characteristics.

	Controls	AD	T-test (df,t,p)
Number	79	80	-
Male/Female	41/38	40/40	-
Age (years)	75.8±4.9	75.7±7.0	157,0.1,.887
Age range (years)	62–87	55–88	-
MMSE (score)	28.7±1.6	23.6±2.2	157,16.6,<.001

Mean ± standard deviation. AD Alzheimer's disease, con converters, MMSE Mini Mental State Examination, noncon non-converters.
doi:10.1371/journal.pcbi.1002987.t001

FDG-PET data

We analysed FDG-PET data for subjects who also underwent sMRI scans. FDG-PET data were acquired with different PET-scanner types according to one of three different protocols: 1) dynamic: a 30 min six-frame acquisition (6 five-minute frames), with scanning from 30 to 60 min post FDG injection; 2) static: a single-frame, 30 min acquisition with scanning 30–60 min post injection; and 3) quantitative: a 60 min dynamic protocol consisting of 33 frames, with scanning beginning at injection and continuing for 60 min. The majority of the scans in the ADNI study were acquired with the first acquisition protocol. Images further differed in resolution, orientation, voxel and image dimensions and count statistics. The frames from 30 to 60 minutes post injection were spatially realigned to minimize inter-frame motion artefacts and a mean image of these frames was calculated for each subject. These mean images were used for further analysis.

Image pre-processing

All data processing steps were carried out using the SPM5 software package (Statistical Parametric Mapping software: http://www.fil.ion.ucl.ac.uk/spm/) implemented in Matlab 7.7 (MathWorks Inc., Sherborn, MA). The same pre-processing algorithm was used for sMRI and FDG-PET data, as described elsewhere [11]. This procedure includes co-registration and interpolation of both FDG-PET and sMR images to an isotropic resolution of $1 \times 1 \times 1$ mm^3, bias correction for inhomogeneity artefacts for sMRI data, segmentation of sMRI data into different tissue classes (only the grey matter tissue class is used for further analyses), and masking of non-GM voxels in FDG-PET data. PVE correction using the modified Müller-Gärtner method [21,24] was in the PVElab software package [25] that is compatible with SPM5 only. This procedure uses the segmented sMR images to account for PVE and for potential atrophy effects in FDG-PET. DARTEL (Diffeomorphic Anatomical Registration using Exponentiated Lie algebra) based on grey matter tissue probability maps was used for spatial normalization of data to an average size template created from all study participants [26]. Structural MR images were additionally modulated to preserve the total amount of signal from each region. The same deformation matrices used to normalise sMRI scans to a template were used to co-register the FDG-PET images. After spatial normalization anatomical regions of all subjects were located at same location in the images. Smoothing with a Gaussian kernel of 12 mm FWHM (full width at half maximum) accounted for minor misalignment errors.. FDG-PET data were intensity normalized to cerebellar mean [27] and masked to avoid big edge effects. The cerebellar region was chosen for intensity normalization of FDG-PET as it has been shown to be a region of choice for intensity normalization which is unaffected in healthy aging and early stages of AD when correcting for PVE caused by atrophy [27–29].

FDG-PET and sMRI models of healthy aging and AD

All statistical analyses were also carried out using the SPM5 software package and Matlab 7.7. The effect of aging in healthy control subjects was estimated separately for FDG-PET and sMRI with voxel-wise linear regressions. To obtain the healthy aging component of our generative model we used the beta coefficients of aging in healthy controls to simulate voxel-wise changes in both imaging modalities for the age range 50 to 80 years (Figure 1a). The estimated values at 50 years were used as a 100% baseline. Estimated age-related changes for the whole age range for both FDG-PET and sMRI were expressed as percent decreases relative to this baseline.

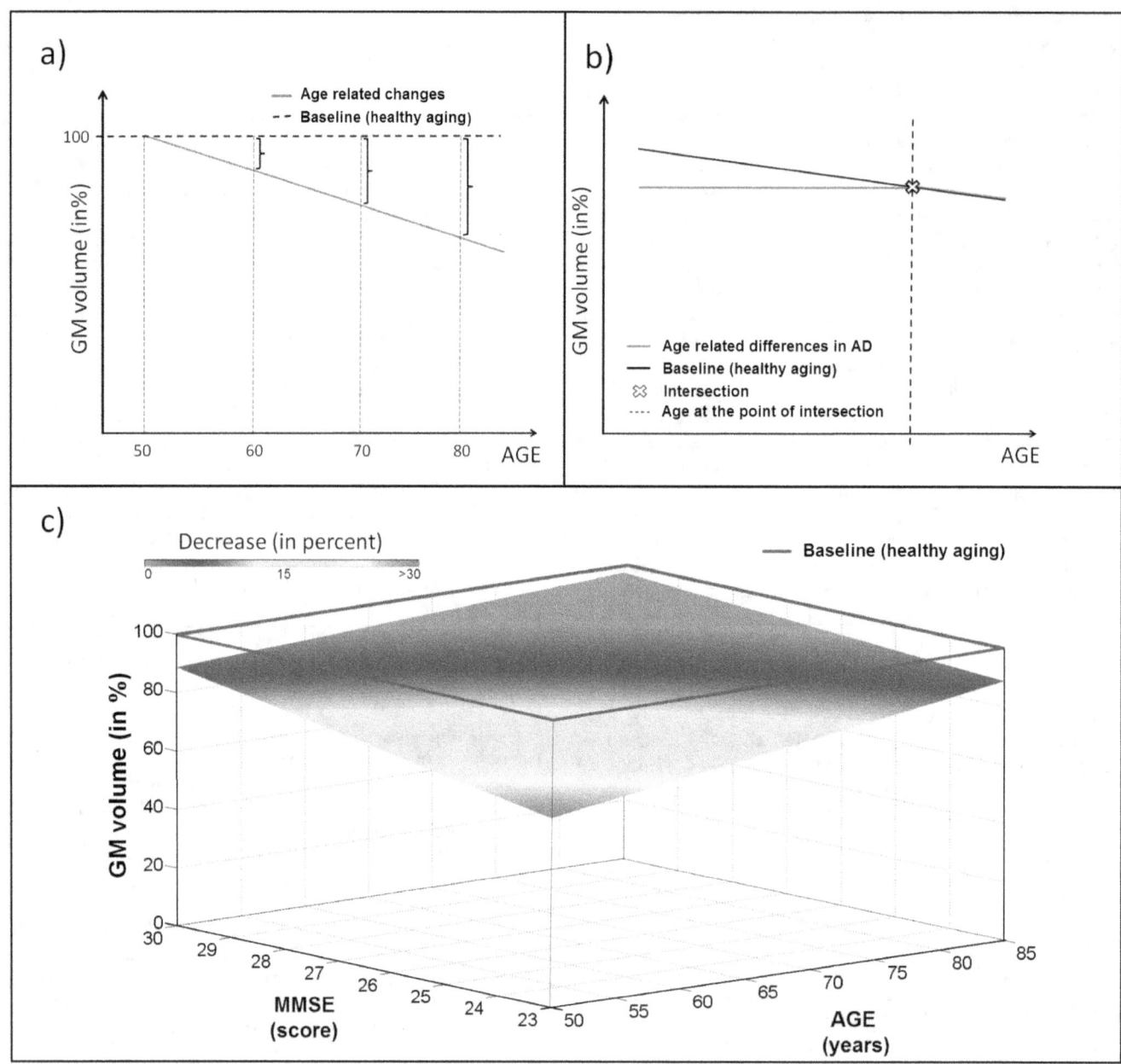

Figure 1. Schematic representation of voxel-wise age- and symptom severity- related models. a) Schematic representation of age-related changes in one voxel (in %) considering GM volume at the age of 50 years as baseline. b) Schematic representation of changes related to healthy aging (black line) and age-related differences in AD (red line) in one voxel. Intersection age (dotted line) represents the age at which healthy aging in this voxel becomes similar to changes observed in AD. The hinge in the red line (aging in AD) at the intersection point indicates that after the intersection age, according to our assumption of the additive impact of AD related processes to healthy aging, the healthy aging model would apply in AD patients as no pathological processes in terms of atrophy or glucose hypometabolism are longer observable after this time point. c) Decrease (in %) in GM volume observed in an exemplary voxel in AD depending on the constellation of age and symptom severity (MMSE) relative to the baseline provided by healthy aging (violet line). AD Alzheimer's disease, GM grey matter, MMSE Mini Mental State Examination.
doi:10.1371/journal.pcbi.1002987.g001

To dissociate healthy aging- and AD-related changes, the variance in glucose utilization and GM atrophy explained by healthy aging was removed by voxel-wise linear regressions from all imaging data used for further models (control subjects and AD patients for both FDG-PET and sMRI; [19]). GLMs with age and symptom severity (as measured by MMSE, [30]) as regressors were built for the AD group separately for both FDG-PET and MRI. To model the interaction of both factors the product of age and symptom severity was also included. The inclusion of the interaction between age and symptom severity accounts for any differential disease progression associated with age in the AD

group. In this model we took the control group mean glucose metabolism and GM volume at each voxel as a baseline. In an effort to define the specific variance attributable to AD explained by aging and symptom severity we removed variance from this baseline that was explained by these factors and their interaction (Figure 1c).

Further, we determined at what age the changes related to normal aging become similar to those found in AD. For this purpose, a third GLM, using age as the only factor, was calculated in the AD cohort for both FDG-PET and sMRI data. The ages at which the separate regressions for normal and AD associated aging intersect (referred to as intersection ages) were calculated on a voxel-wise basis (Figure 1b). To calculate these voxel-wise intersection ages x_{age} the linear regression equations for healthy aging and aging in AD ($y_{Con} = x_{age} \cdot \beta_{Con} + c_{Con}$ and $y_{AD} = x_{age} \cdot \beta_{AD} + c_{AD}$, where y_{Con} and y_{AD} are the predicted voxel-wise grey matter volumes/glucose metabolism, c_{Con} and c_{AD} the corresponding intercepts and β_{Con} and β_{AD} the slopes of regression lines in controls and AD respectively) were set equal and resolved for x_{age}. The intersection age x_{age} is then given by:

$$x_{age} = \frac{c_{Con} - c_{AD}}{\beta_{AD} - \beta_{Con}}.$$

Generally, an early intersection age indicates that a region is relatively spared by AD, if healthy aging affects AD patients similarly to controls. A higher intersection age suggests that the region is predominantly affected by disease-related processes.

All three voxel-based models are based on a previously validated assumption of linearity between healthy aging- and AD symptom severity- related changes with FDG-PET and sMRI data. [16,31]. To exclude a more complex *e.g.*, quadratic relationship between age or symptom severity in the AD cohort we calculated further regression analyses after removing variance explained by healthy aging. These comprised a) including only linear relationships for both age and symptom severity; b) additionally modelling quadratic relationships with age; and c) additionally modelling a quadratic relationship for symptom severity. Gender was included as a covariate for both imaging modalities and total intracranial volume was additionally included as a covariate for the sMRI data. A significance threshold of 0.001 uncorrected at voxel-level and 0.05 family-wise error (FWE)-corrected for non-stationarity of smoothness at cluster level was used for statistical analyses [32].

Statistical analysis of behavioural data

Group comparisons of AD patients and control subjects for age and symptom severity were carried out using T-tests with a significance threshold of p<.05. Group differences regarding gender were evaluated using a chi-square test for independent samples. The statistical analyses were performed with SPSS 17.0 (http://www.spss.com/statistics/). A Pearson's correlation coefficient was calculated (p<.05) in the AD group to investigate the relationship between age and symptom severity.

Results

Subject demographic characteristics

AD patients and control subjects did not differ in age [t(157) = 0.1;p = .887]. As expected MMSE differed significantly between the groups [t(157) = 16.6;p<.001]. The comparison of AD patients and control subjects in relation to sex showed no statistical differences [$\chi^2(1) = 0.06$;p = .811].

Differential pattern of changes related to healthy aging in FDG-PET and sMRI

The generative model for healthy aging based on sMRI reveals a widespread pattern of grey matter volume reductions sparing only bilateral dorsal primary sensorimotor regions, brainstem, lateral thalamus and the dorsal part of caudate nucleus (Figure 2a). We observe the greatest reductions in GM volume, of more than 10% per decade, in right superior parietal lobule, superior and inferior frontal gyrus, inferior frontal sulcus, primary auditory cortex, pars triangularis, and anterior hippocampus. Left-hemispheric reductions are observed in the premotor cortex, and in superior and middle frontal gyri. Bilateral GM volume reductions

are restricted to calcarine gyri, insulae, anterior cingulate cortex, superior temporal sulcus and posterior hippocampus.

The equivalent FDG-PET based model demonstrates a specific pattern of age-related metabolic changes with an age related decrease in glucose utilization of more than 10% per decade in bilateral parietal, occipital, sensorimotor, premotor, dorsolateral prefrontal and anterior insular cortices. Additionally, we see a major reduction in glucose metabolism in bilateral posterior putamina and in the left dorsal caudate nucleus (Figure 1b).

Age- and symptom severity- related changes

We report a negative relationship between symptom severity and both metabolism and GM volume (Figure 3) and (Figure 4). Lesser reductions in glucose utilization and GM volume are associated with greater age in AD patients.

Symptom severity related GM volume changes at age 60 years were detected throughout the brain with greatest degrees of atrophy seen in bilateral parietal, temporal, occipital, dorsolateral prefrontal, posterior cingulate and premotor cortices, the precuneus, dorsal caudate nucleus, amygdala and hippocampus. At 80 years of age, the greatest, bilateral, symptom severity related atrophy was found in parietal, temporal, occipital, primary sensorimotor and dorsolateral prefrontal cortices, the hippocampus and thalamus.

We show symptom severity- related glucose metabolism reductions bilaterally in posterior temporal, parietal, lateral occipital, dorsolateral prefrontal and premotor cortices and in the precuneus. Symptom severity related hypometabolism is less extensive at higher than lower ages.

In general, regional decreases in metabolism and grey matter volumes relative to healthy aging are significantly more pronounced in the lower compared to higher age range in AD. In the model, we observe substantial age-dependant differences in terms of hypometabolism and atrophy in AD patients compared to a healthy aging baseline even at an MMSE score of 30. At the age of 60 years these differences are bilaterally restricted to inferior frontal gyrus, premotor regions, inferior and medial temporal gyrus, cerebellum, rectal gyrus and to left parietal regions. Regions showing an initial difference in this age range do not correspond well to the anatomical pattern observed in later symptom severity stages and remain rather less affected compared to other regions. Initial differences observed at the age of 80 years are located in bilateral parietal, bilateral hippocampal and left sensorimotor regions and in both caudate nuclei.

We observe a more consistent anatomical pattern of initial differences in hypometabolism at a MMSE score of 30. For the whole age range of 60–80 years, initial glucose hypometabolism is observed in bilateral parietal, inferior temporal and posterior cingulate cortices, posterior thalamus and the precuneus. Additionally, at 80 years of age we demonstrate significant differences in bilateral primary sensorimotor and premotor regions and in the anterior temporal lobes. All regions showing initial glucose hypometabolism, except for the posterior thalamus, also show the steepest symptom severity-related metabolic decline. Regions hypometabolic only at age 80 show no specific symptom severity-related decline.

Dissociating healthy aging from Alzheimer's disease

To dissociate brain changes related to healthy aging from AD pathology at specific ages we computed the intersection age of models for healthy aging and aging in AD at the voxel level (Figure 5). With sMRI, we see the highest intersection ages bilaterally in hippocampus, anterior and posterior thalamus, posterior and midcingulate, parietal, temporal, cerebellar, pre-

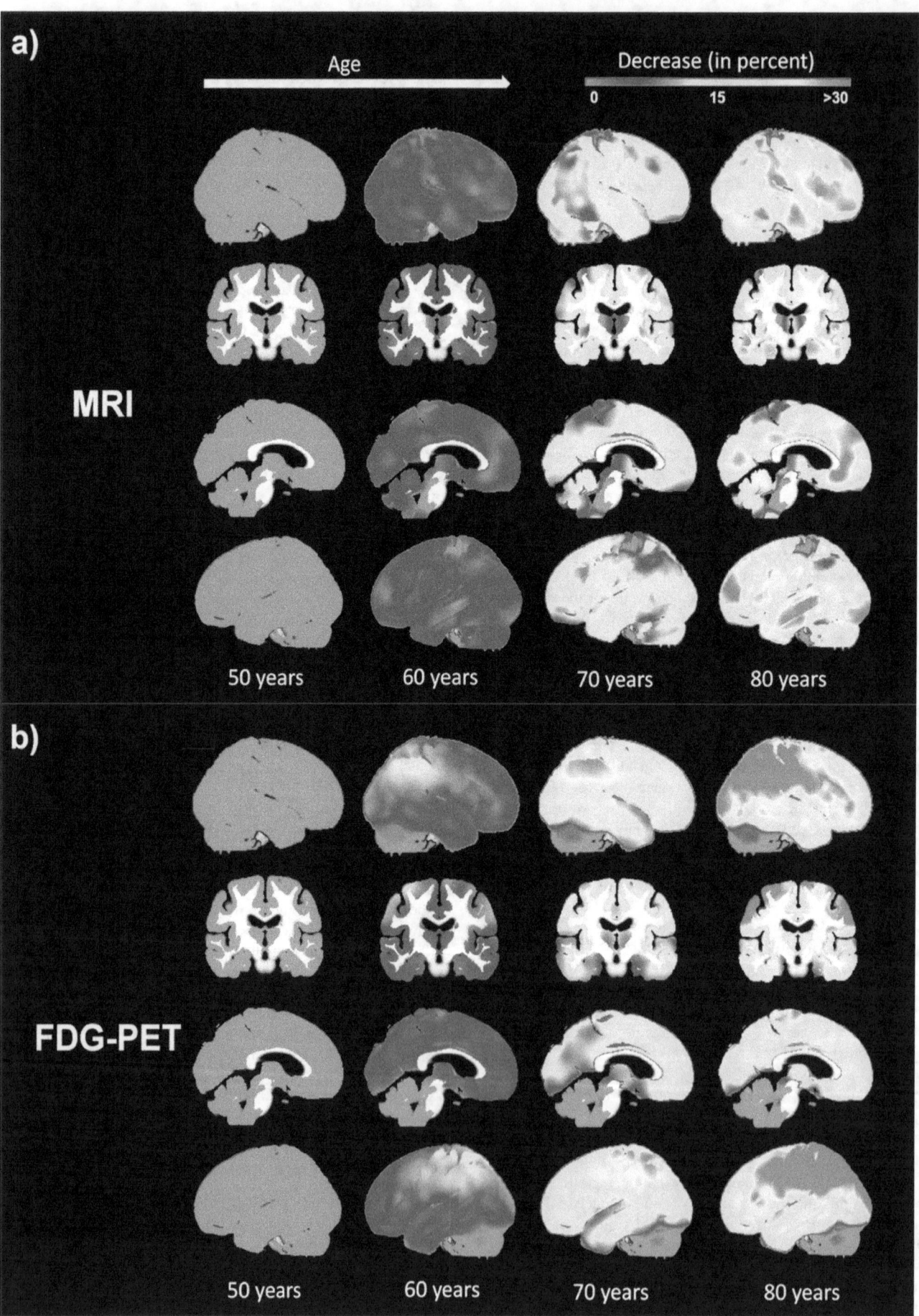

Figure 2. Healthy aging related changes observed in MRI (a) and FDG-PET (b) considering the expression of GM volume and glucose metabolism at the age of 50 years as baseline. FDG-PET [18F]fluorodeoxyglucose positron emission tomography, GM grey matter, MRI structural magnetic resonance imaging.
doi:10.1371/journal.pcbi.1002987.g002

frontal and premotor regions. With FDG-PET, regions with the highest intersection ages are bilaterally restricted to precuneus, cerebellum, anterior and posterior cingulate, posterior parietal, temporal, lateral occipital, primary motor, premotor and prefrontal cortices and the left dorsal caudate nucleus.

Linear relationship between age, symptom severity and imaging results

With sMRI, the linear regression model describing the relationship between age, symptom severity and structural changes in AD showed a significant correlation for each factor with atrophy (Figure 6a). After removing the variance attributable to healthy aging, age correlates positively with GM volume in AD in right premotor and bilaterally in parietal, temporal, occipital and medial and lateral prefrontal regions. Additional significant bilateral positive correlations were observed in anterior cingulate cortex and in the cerebellum. These counter-intuitive positive correlations can be interpreted as reflecting the additional age-specific atrophy needed to produce a similar degree of symptom severity in younger compared to older AD patients. There were no significant negative correlations. Further, we found significant bilateral positive correlations with symptom severity in temporal, lateral and medial prefrontal, inferior parietal, occipital regions and in thalamus as well as the left premotor cortex. Again no negative correlations were observed.

With FDG-PET we found a significant positive correlation between age and glucose metabolism in bilateral temporal and parietal regions. There were no other significant correlations with age or symptom severity.

Inclusion of a quadratic relationship with age or MMSE into the models revealed significant positive correlations of glucose metabolism with a quadratic age coefficient only in left dorsal parietal cortex (Figure 5b). No other significant correlations were observed.

Discussion

In this study we demonstrate that a generative model captures the anatomical and metabolic features associated with AD and

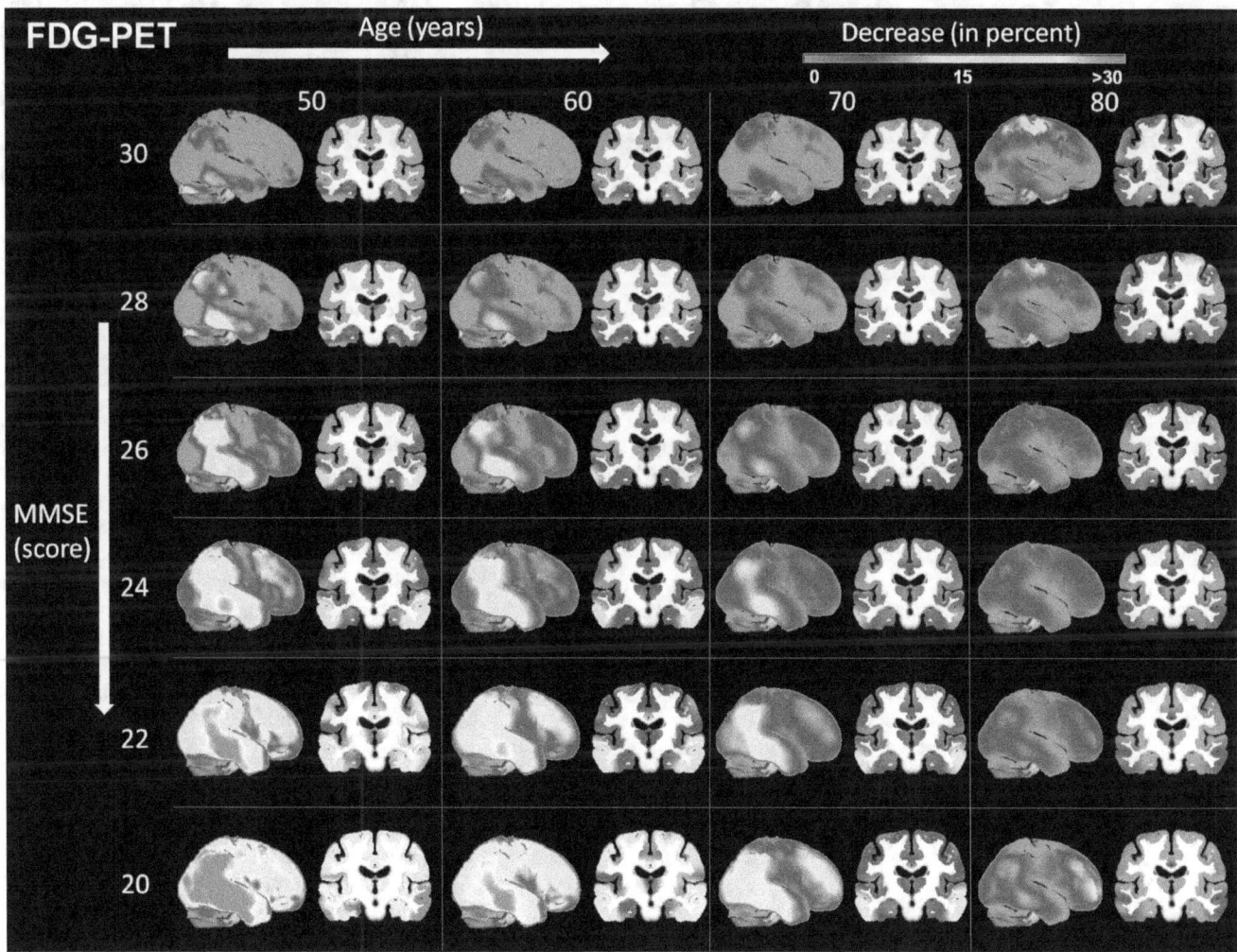

Figure 3. A linear model of age and MMSE related changes observed in AD in FDG-PET considering the healthy control group as baseline. AD Alzheimer's disease, FDG-PET [18F]fluorodeoxyglucose positron emission tomography, MMSE Mini Mental State Examination.
doi:10.1371/journal.pcbi.1002987.g003

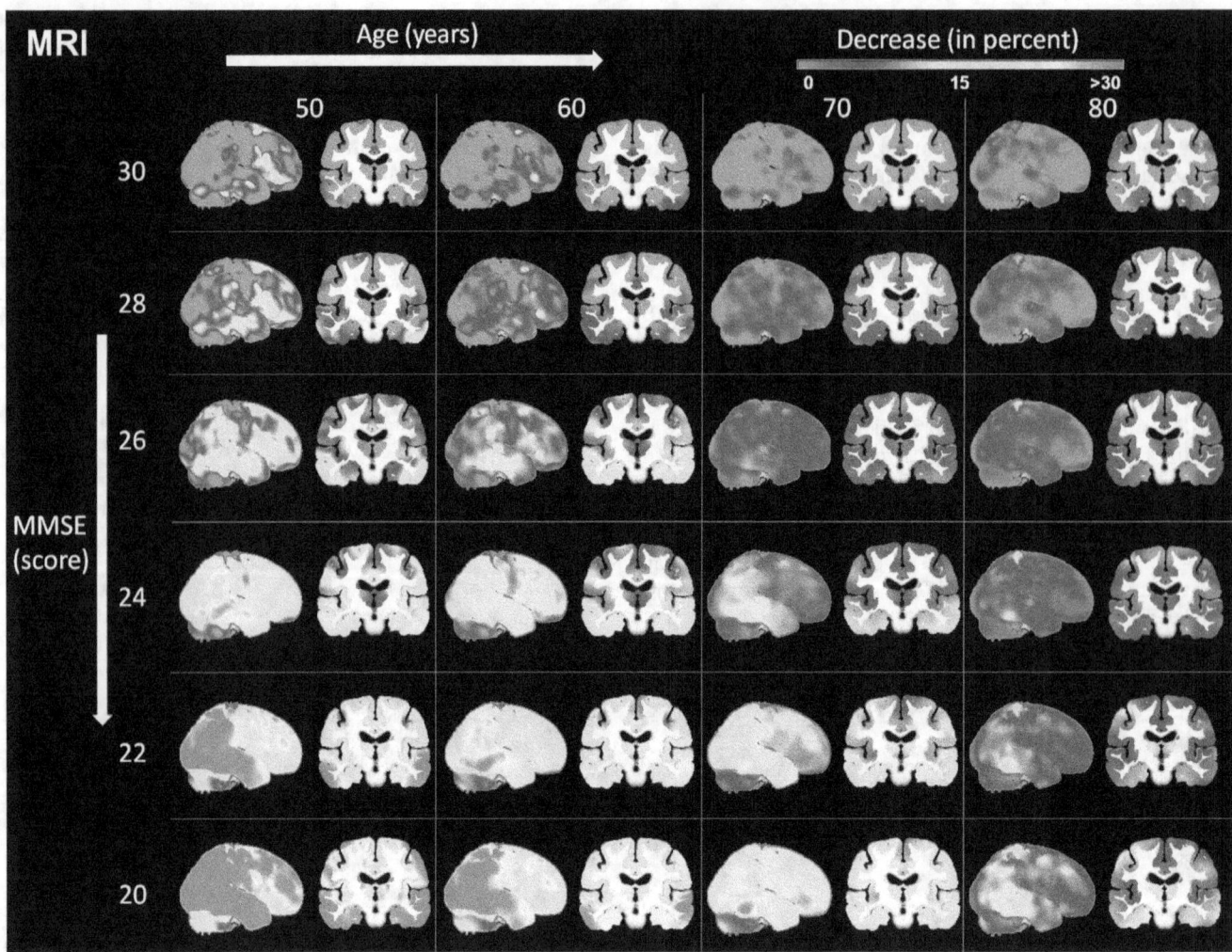

Figure 4. A linear model of age and MMSE related changes observed in AD in MRI considering the healthy control group as baseline. AD Alzheimer's disease, MMSE Mini Mental State Examination, MRI structural magnetic resonance imaging.
doi:10.1371/journal.pcbi.1002987.g004

healthy aging in the age range 60 to 80 years accurately and robustly. The model differentiates between the effects of aging and symptom severity in AD patients. It also provides a means to test for interactions between them, as exemplified here with disease progression and patient age. The age-dependant differential sensitivity of structural and metabolic scanning for the detection of AD pathology we demonstrate emphasises the ability of our generative model to infer expected age- and symptom severity-specific changes recorded with both imaging modalities.

Our study's three main findings support and extend observations made previously. Firstly, the spatial location of changes related to different ages and symptom severities in AD was mostly consistent with regions reported in the literature [33–35]. However we also identified a more widespread network of regions showing age related metabolic decreases and atrophy whilst controlling for potential PVE related changes in FDG-PET. The AD model at lower ages was substantially more extensive in terms of decreases in glucose metabolism and GM volume than at greater ages. This finding is in accordance with previous research [12–14].

Our second result is that in general, the magnitude of healthy aging related imaging changes between 50 and 80 years is comparable to that of changes associated with an increase in AD symptom severity at any age. Substantial regional overlap in both

hypometabolism and atrophy was observed between a network of areas affected by healthy aging and that identified in AD. To interpret this overlap it is important to note that all changes related to age and symptom severity in AD we report here were calculated after removing the variance explained by healthy aging. That means that all age-related differences can be interpreted as an add-on required to normal age-related changes to induce a predefined symptom severity at the corresponding age. In previous research comparing differently aged AD groups with age-matched healthy control subjects a split of AD into different subgroups *e.g.*, early- and late-onset AD, was suggested [12]. In contrast, the results of our study indicate that the anatomically different qualitative and quantitative patterns observed in AD at different ages may be explicable by regionally inhomogeneous, age-related, baseline changes in healthy controls. This notion is supported by the observation of a similar anatomical pattern of structural and metabolic changes across the studied age range in AD patients. Overall, our results suggest a more integrative view of AD indicating that previously reported differences between early- and late-onset AD patients can be explained as an interaction of AD pathology with changes due to healthy aging. More simple, assuming that AD affects parietal and temporal regions, a strong healthy aging related decrease in glucose metabolism e.g. in the parietal cortex with at the same time relatively preserved

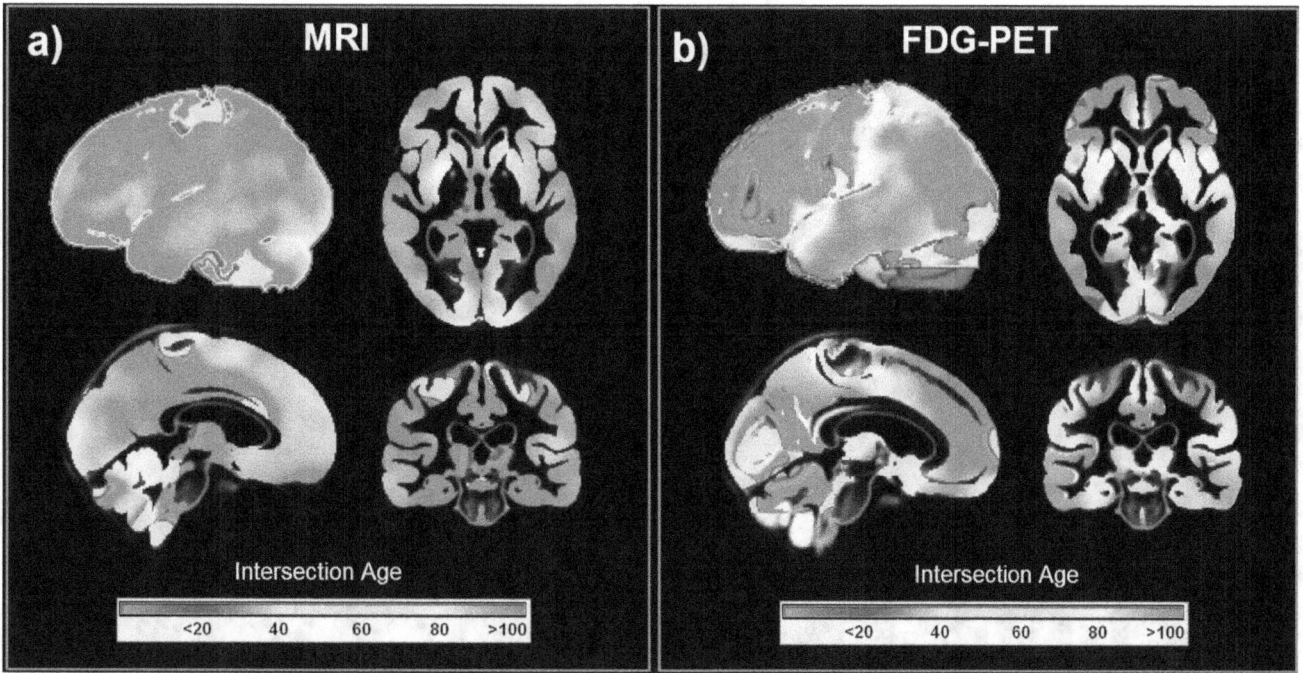

Figure 5. Voxel-wise intersections of healthy aging and changes observed in AD in MRI (a) and FDG-PET (b). Colour bars represent the intersection age. AD Alzheimer's disease, FDG-PET [18F]fluorodeoxyglucose positron emission tomography, MRI structural magnetic resonance imaging.
doi:10.1371/journal.pcbi.1002987.g005

metabolism in the temporal region would lead to an observation of both regions when comparing younger patients to younger controls. Yet, only the temporal region would be detected when comparing older patients to older controls.

A third result is in the dissociation of age- and disease- related processes inferred from the intersection ages of healthy aging and AD models. While in previous research some studies successfully applied whole-brain approaches to discriminate dementia patients from control subjects [6,11,36], sparse solutions based on highly discriminative features have been used in most [4,37–40]. However, there is a problem with feature selection that has been neglected till now. This is the assumption of feature reliability, independent of the expression of possible confounding variables. We decided to investigate this assumption by testing whether a correlation of AD symptom severity with imaging data was also affected by the processes of normal aging as defined in a healthy population. We did this with our described method of model intersections. Our results suggest that features like local atrophy or glucose hypometabolism that discriminate between AD patients and control subjects at the age of 60 are not necessarily observed at age 80. This non-stationarity of features is mainly explained by atrophy and hypometabolism related to healthy aging, which affect some regions similarly to AD. We previously demonstrated that accounting for changes related to healthy aging improves AD detection with support vector machine classification [19]. This study extends that approach and suggests that diagnostic classifier algorithms, like machine learning techniques, when applied to the general population, need to take potential interactions of imaging features with demographic and clinical factors into account. Related to this, our intersection model also provides evidence that the pathological pattern observed in AD in some regions is clearly distinguishable from healthy aging even at very advanced age.

The obtained models could be used to improve early AD detection e.g. by training automated classifiers on age- and

symptom severity- specific pathological AD patterns (features) extracted by thresholding the obtained AD model. They could also be applied directly in clinical assessment by evaluating the similarity of observed pathology in any individual to age- and symptom severity- specific patterns generated using the AD model. Thereby, to enable individual assessment, percent signal difference maps could be calculated between each subject's imaging data and imaging data generated using the healthy aging model. However, both of these approaches require careful evaluation in future studies prior to clinical application.

Nonetheless, a valid interpretation of our results needs to consider the effects of several other assumptions and limitations. First, the sensitivity of the generative model for detecting and predicting AD pathology depends on the accuracy of the model of healthy aging. The age- related, widespread patterns of brain atrophy and hypometabolism we find are consistent with previous findings [16,31,41–43]. The most prominent changes of glucose hypometabolism we observed include large parts of an occipital-parietal-frontal network. The only non-linear (quadratic) relationship between age and metabolic changes we found in an anatomically highly restricted area in the left dorsal parietal cortex. The absence of more complex relationships between these parameters indicates that linear models are very probably a sufficient approximation of the underlying structural and metabolic processes.

A major advantage of our approach is the generalizability of our model to any constellation of age and symptom severity. A further difference to conventional approaches is that the method we propose relies on a voxel-wise group mean, ignoring the variance and so allowing detection of quite minor group differences. This type of analysis, though more flexible than conventional statistics, nevertheless requires caution in the interpretation of results. Minor differences between groups of healthy subjects and AD patients could still be due to random effects unrelated to AD. However, as

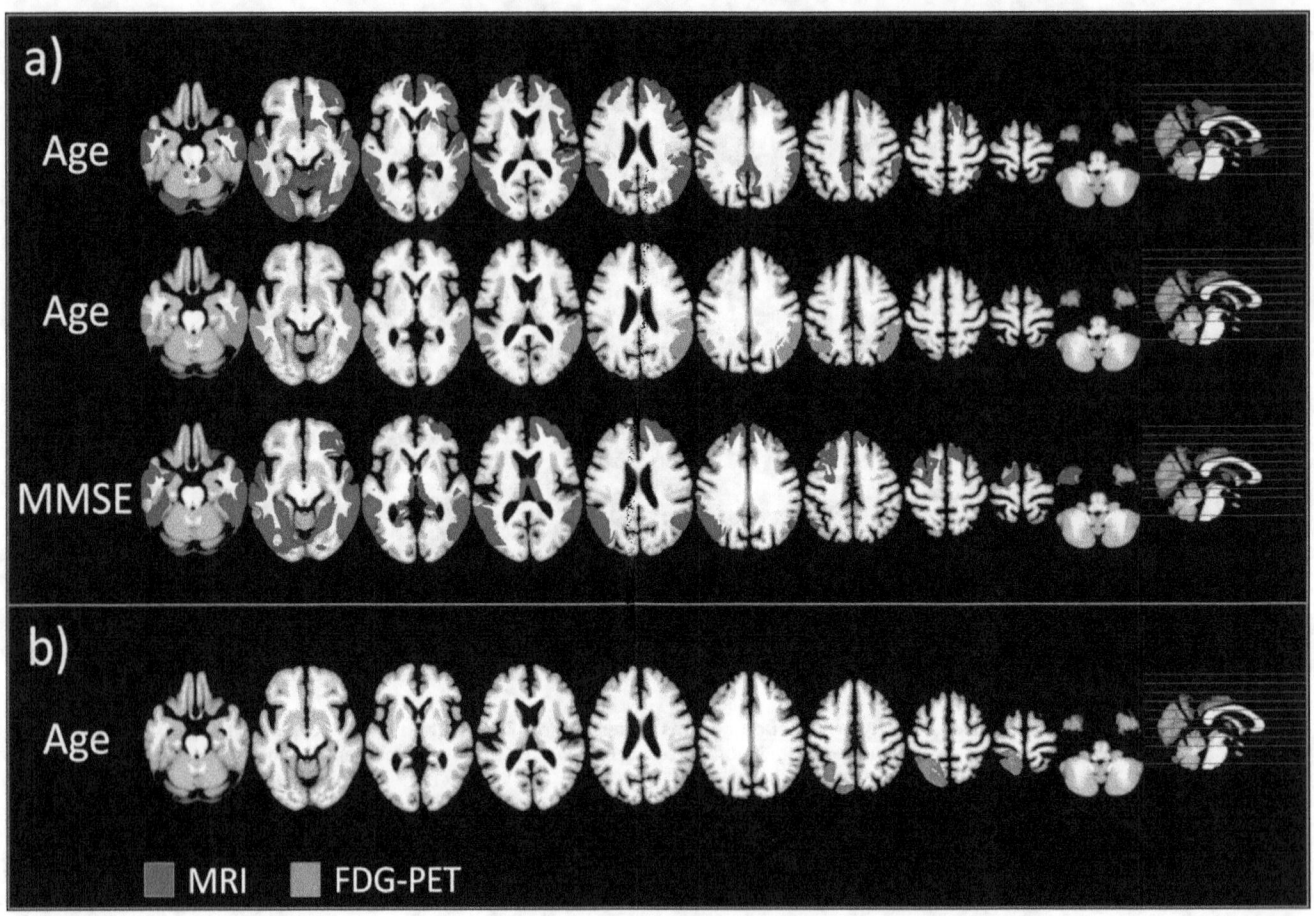

Figure 6. Positive linear (a) or quadratic (b) relationship observed between age and MMSE in MRI (blue) and FDG-PET (red) in AD patients after removing the variance explained by heathy aging. Only clusters are shown exceeding a significance threshold of p = 0.001 uncorrected on voxel level and p = 0.05 FWE-corrected on cluster level. AD Alzheimer's disease, FDG-PET [18F]fluorodeoxyglucose positron emission tomography, MRI structural magnetic resonance imaging.
doi:10.1371/journal.pcbi.1002987.g006

we model disease progression (albeit based on cross-sectional data) we would expect the magnitude of differences to increase with higher symptom severity. This assumption suggests that local differences between AD patients and control subjects that are not so correlated with it are more likely to be due to random artefacts than disease related pathology.

For all three models used in our study, we made the assumption that healthy aging affects AD patients in the same way as healthy subjects in terms of hypometabolic and atrophic changes, with AD pathology additive to changes associated with healthy aging. This assumption is in line with current views that AD as a pathological process is unrelated to healthy aging.

A further issue of interpretation of interactions is the recognised inaccuracy of clinical diagnosis of AD, which may differ in younger vs. older or in mildly vs. severely impaired patients. Any bias towards an alternative diagnosis or co-diagnosis with another dementing condition could lead to a different anatomical or hypometabolic pattern. Such a differential pattern of glucose hypometabolism was seen, for example, in sensorimotor regions only in old AD patients with low symptom severity.

Most of these problems are also common to standard statistical methods of evaluation of group differences. In group statistics one often uses a high significance threshold to avoid false positive results thus minimising their effect on between group differenti-

ations. By contrast, our approach also provides an opportunity to evaluate the impact of possible confounding effects, such as age in this case, on the discrimination between AD patients and control subjects.

Supporting Information

Text S1 Acknowledgment list for ADNI publications. (PDF)

Acknowledgments

We thank Jessica Peters for preparing parts of the data used in this project.

Data used in preparation of this article were obtained from the Alzheimer's Disease Neuroimaging Initiative (ADNI) database (adni.loni.ucla.edu). As such, the investigators within the ADNI contributed to the design and implementation of ADNI and/or provided data but did not participate in analysis or writing of this report. A complete listing of ADNI investigators can be found in Text S1.

Author Contributions

Conceived and designed the experiments: JD MLS RSJF BD. Performed the experiments: JD. Analyzed the data: JD. Contributed reagents/materials/analysis tools: JD FK KM SA. Wrote the paper: JD FK KM SA MLS RSJF BD.

References

1. Mielke R, Pietrzyk U, Jacobs A, Fink GR, Ichimiya A, et al. (1994) HMPAO SPET and FDG PET in Alzheimer's disease and vascular dementia: comparison of perfusion and metabolic pattern. Eur J Nucl Med 21: 1052–1060.

2. Laakso MP, Soininen H, Partanen K, Helkala EL, Hartikainen P, et al. (1995) Volumes of hippocampus, amygdala and frontal lobes in the MRI-based diagnosis of early Alzheimer's disease: correlation with memory functions. J Neural Transm Park Dis Dement Sect 9: 73–86.

3. Silverman DH, Gambhir SS, Huang HW, Schwimmer J, Kim S, et al. (2002) Evaluating early dementia with and without assessment of regional cerebral metabolism by PET: a comparison of predicted costs and benefits. J Nucl Med 43: 253–266.

4. Davatzikos C, Resnick SM, Wu X, Parmpi P, Clark CM (2008) Individual patient diagnosis of AD and FTD via high-dimensional pattern classification of MRI. Neuroimage 41: 1220–1227.

5. Habeck C, Foster NL, Perneczky R, Kurz A, Alexopoulos P, et al. (2008) Multivariate and univariate neuroimaging biomarkers of Alzheimer's disease. Neuroimage 40: 1503–1515.

6. Kloppel S, Stonnington CM, Chu C, Draganski B, Scahill RI, et al. (2008) Automatic classification of MR scans in Alzheimer's disease. Brain 131: 681–689.

7. Sadeghi N, Foster NL, Wang AY, Minoshima S, Lieberman AP, et al. (2008) Automatic classification of Alzheimer's disease vs. Frontotemporal dementia: A spatial decision tree approach with FDG-PET. In: 5th IEEE International Symposium on Biomedical Imaging: From Nano to Macro; 14–17 May 2008; Paris, France. Vols 1–4: 408–411.

8. Haense C, Herholz K, Jagust WJ, Heiss WD (2009) Performance of FDG PET for detection of Alzheimer's disease in two independent multicentre samples (NEST-DD and ADNI). Dement Geriatr Cogn Disord 28: 259–266.

9. Schroeter ML, Stein T, Maslowski N, Neumann J (2009) Neural correlates of Alzheimer's disease and mild cognitive impairment: a systematic and quantitative meta-analysis involving 1351 patients. Neuroimage 47: 1196–1206.

10. Morinaga A, Ono K, Ikeda T, Ikeda Y, Shima K, et al. (2010) A comparison of the diagnostic sensitivity of MRI, CBF-SPECT, FDG-PET and cerebrospinal fluid biomarkers for detecting Alzheimer's disease in a memory clinic. Dement Geriatr Cogn Disord 30: 285–292.

11. Dukart J, Mueller K, Horstmann A, Barthel H, Möller HE, et al. (2011) Combined Evaluation of FDG-PET and MRI Improves Detection and Differentiation of Dementia. PLoS One 6: e18111.

12. Sakamoto S, Ishii K, Sasaki M, Hosaka K, Mori T, et al. (2002) Differences in cerebral metabolic impairment between early and late onset types of Alzheimer's disease. J Neurol Sci 200: 27–32.

13. Ishii K, Kawachi T, Sasaki H, Kono AK, Fukuda T, et al. (2005) Voxel-based morphometric comparison between early- and late-onset mild Alzheimer's disease and assessment of diagnostic performance of z score images. AJNR Am J Neuroradiol 26: 333–340.

14. Frisoni GB, Pievani M, Testa C, Sabattoli F, Bresciani L, et al. (2007) The topography of grey matter involvement in early and late onset Alzheimer's disease. Brain 130: 720–730.

15. Franke K, Ziegler G, Kloppel S, Gaser C (2010) Estimating the age of healthy subjects from T1-weighted MRI scans using kernel methods: exploring the influence of various parameters. Neuroimage 50: 883–892.

16. Good CD, Johnsrude IS, Ashburner J, Henson RN, Friston KJ, et al. (2001) A voxel-based morphometric study of ageing in 465 normal adult human brains. Neuroimage 14: 21–36.

17. Baron JC, Chételat G, Desgranges B, Perchey G, Landeau B, et al. (2001) In vivo mapping of gray matter loss with voxel-based morphometry in mild Alzheimer's disease. Neuroimage 14: 298–309.

18. Teipel SJ, Wegrzyn M, Meindl T, Frisoni G, Bokde AL, et al. (2012) Anatomical MRI and DTI in the Diagnosis of Alzheimer's Disease: A European Multicenter Study. J Alzheimers Dis 31: S33–47.

19. Dukart J, Schroeter ML, Mueller K, Initiative TAsDN (2011) Age Correction in Dementia - Matching to a Healthy Brain. PLoS One 6: e22193.

20. Karow DS, McEvoy LK, Fennema-Notestine C, Hagler DJ, Jennings RG, et al. (2010) Relative capability of MR imaging and FDG PET to depict changes associated with prodromal and early Alzheimer disease. Radiology 256: 932–942.

21. Muller-Gartner HW, Links JM, Prince JL, Bryan RN, McVeigh E, et al. (1992) Measurement of radiotracer concentration in brain gray matter using positron emission tomography: MRI-based correction for partial volume effects. J Cereb Blood Flow Metab 12: 571–583.

22. Jack CR, Knopman DS, Jagust WJ, Shaw LM, Aisen PS, et al. (2010) Hypothetical model of dynamic biomarkers of the Alzheimer's pathological cascade. Lancet Neurol 9: 119–128.

23. McKhann G, Drachman D, Folstein M, Katzman R, Price D, et al. (1984) Clinical diagnosis of Alzheimer's disease: report of the NINCDS-ADRDA Work Group under the auspices of Department of Health and Human Services Task Force on Alzheimer's Disease. Neurology 34: 939–944.

24. Rousset OG, Ma Y, Evans AC (1998) Correction for partial volume effects in PET: principle and validation. J Nucl Med 39: 904–911.

25. Quarantelli M, Berkouk K, Prinster A, Landeau B, Svarer C, et al. (2004) Integrated software for the analysis of brain PET/SPECT studies with partial-volume-effect correction. J Nucl Med 45: 192–201.

26. Ashburner J (2007) A fast diffeomorphic image registration algorithm. Neuroimage 38: 95–113.

27. Dukart J, Mueller K, Horstmann A, Vogt B, Frisch S, et al. (2010) Differential effects of global and cerebellar normalization on detection and differentiation of dementia in FDG-PET studies. Neuroimage 49: 1490–1495.

28. Yanase D, Matsunari I, Yajima K, Chen W, Fujikawa A, et al. (2005) Brain FDG PET study of normal aging in Japanese: effect of atrophy correction. Eur J Nucl Med Mol Imaging 32: 794–805.

29. Salmon E, Collette F, Degueldre C, Lemaire C, Franck G (2000) Voxel-based analysis of confounding effects of age and dementia severity on cerebral metabolism in Alzheimer's disease. Hum Brain Mapp 10: 39–48.

30. Folstein MF, Folstein SE, McHugh PR (1975) "Mini-mental state". A practical method for grading the cognitive state of patients for the clinician. J Psychiatr Res 12: 189–198.

31. Loessner A, Alavi A, Lewandrowski KU, Mozley D, Souder E, et al. (1995) Regional cerebral function determined by FDG-PET in healthy volunteers: normal patterns and changes with age. J Nucl Med 36: 1141–1149.

32. Hayasaka S, Phan KL, Liberzon I, Worsley KJ, Nichols TE (2004) Nonstationary cluster-size inference with random field and permutation methods. Neuroimage 22: 676–687.

33. Willis MW, Ketter TA, Kimbrell TA, George MS, Herscovitch P, et al. (2002) Age, sex and laterality effects on cerebral glucose metabolism in healthy adults. Psychiatry Res 114: 23–37.

34. Zuendorf G, Kerrouche N, Herholz K, Baron JC (2003) Efficient principal component analysis for multivariate 3D voxel-based mapping of brain functional imaging data sets as applied to FDG-PET and normal aging. Hum Brain Mapp 18: 13–21.

35. Kalpouzos G, Chételat G, Baron JC, Landeau B, Mevel K, et al. (2009) Voxel-based mapping of brain gray matter volume and glucose metabolism profiles in normal aging. Neurobiol Aging 30: 112–124.

36. Kloppel S, Stonnington CM, Barnes J, Chen F, Chu C, et al. (2008) Accuracy of dementia diagnosis: a direct comparison between radiologists and a computerized method. Brain 131: 2969–2974.

37. Davatzikos C, Fan Y, Wu X, Shen D, Resnick SM (2008) Detection of prodromal Alzheimer's disease via pattern classification of magnetic resonance imaging. Neurobiol Aging 29: 514–523.

38. Fan Y, Resnick SM, Wu X, Davatzikos C (2008) Structural and functional biomarkers of prodromal Alzheimer's disease: a high-dimensional pattern classification study. Neuroimage 41: 277–285.

39. Mosconi L, Tsui WH, Herholz K, Pupi A, Drzezga A, et al. (2008) Multicenter standardized 18F-FDG PET diagnosis of mild cognitive impairment, Alzheimer's disease, and other dementias. J Nucl Med 49: 390–398.

40. Chaves R, Ramirez J, Gorriz JM, Lopez M, Salas-Gonzalez D, et al. (2009) SVM-based computer-aided diagnosis of the Alzheimer's disease using t-test NMSE feature selection with feature correlation weighting. Neurosci Lett 461: 293–297.

41. Sowell ER, Thompson PM, Toga AW (2004) Mapping changes in the human cortex throughout the span of life. Neuroscientist 10: 372–392.

42. Smith CD, Chebrolu H, Wekstein DR, Schmitt FA, Markesbery WR (2007) Age and gender effects on human brain anatomy: a voxel-based morphometric study in healthy elderly. Neurobiol Aging 28: 1075–1087.

43. Giorgio A, Santelli L, Tomassini V, Bosnell R, Smith S, et al. (2010) Age-related changes in grey and white matter structure throughout adulthood. Neuroimage 51: 943–951.

Evaluating Alzheimer's Disease Progression Using Rate of Regional Hippocampal Atrophy

Edit Frankó[1,2,3]*, Olivier Joly[4,5], for the Alzheimer's Disease Neuroimaging Initiative

1 INSERM U1075, Université de Caen Basse-Normandie, Caen, France, 2 Department of Neurodegenerative Disease, Institute of Neurology, University College London, London, United Kingdom, 3 National Prion Clinic, Institute of Neurology, University College London, London, United Kingdom, 4 NeuroSpin, Gif-sur-Yvette, France, 5 Institute of Neuroscience, Newcastle University, Newcastle upon Tyne, United Kingdom

Abstract

Alzheimer's disease (AD) is characterized by neurofibrillary tangle and neuropil thread deposition, which ultimately results in neuronal loss. A large number of magnetic resonance imaging studies have reported a smaller hippocampus in AD patients as compared to healthy elderlies. Even though this difference is often interpreted as atrophy, it is only an indirect measurement. A more direct way of measuring the atrophy is to use repeated MRIs within the same individual. Even though several groups have used this appropriate approach, the pattern of hippocampal atrophy still remains unclear and difficult to relate to underlying pathophysiology. Here, in this longitudinal study, we aimed to map hippocampal atrophy rates in patients with AD, mild cognitive impairment (MCI) and elderly controls. Data consisted of two MRI scans for each subject. The symmetric deformation field between the first and the second MRI was computed and mapped onto the three-dimensional hippocampal surface. The pattern of atrophy rate was similar in all three groups, but the rate was significantly higher in patients with AD than in control subjects. We also found higher atrophy rates in progressive MCI patients as compared to stable MCI, particularly in the antero-lateral portion of the right hippocampus. Importantly, the regions showing the highest atrophy rate correspond to those that were described to have the highest burden of tau deposition. Our results show that local hippocampal atrophy rate is a reliable biomarker of disease stage and progression and could also be considered as a method to objectively evaluate treatment effects.

Citation: Frankó E, Joly O, for the Alzheimer's Disease Neuroimaging Initiative (2013) Evaluating Alzheimer's Disease Progression Using Rate of Regional Hippocampal Atrophy. PLoS ONE 8(8): e71354. doi:10.1371/journal.pone.0071354

Editor: Karl Herholz, University of Manchester, United Kingdom

Received March 13, 2013; **Accepted** June 28, 2013; **Published** August 12, 2013

Funding: The authors of this study have only been funded by the University of Caen and INSERM. Data collection and sharing for this project was funded by the Alzheimer's Disease Neuroimaging Initiative (ADNI) (National Institutes of Health Grant U01 AG024904). ADNI was funded by the National Institute on Aging, the National Institute of Biomedical Imaging and Bioengineering, and through generous contributions from the following: Abbott, AstraZeneca AB, Bayer Schering Pharma AG, Bristol-Myers Squibb, Eisai Global Clinical Development, Elan Corporation, Genentech, GE Healthcare, GlaxoSmithKilne, Innogenetics, Johnson and Johnson, Eli Lilly and Co., Medpace, Inc., Merck and Co., Inc., Novartis AD, Pfizer Inc, F. Hoffman-La Roche, Schering-Plough, Synarc, Inc., as well as non-profit partners the Alzheimer's Association and Alzheimer's Drug Discovery Foundation, with participation from the U.S. Food and Drug Administration. Private sector contributions to ADNI are facilitated by the Foundation for the National Institutes of Health (www.fnih.org). The grantee organization is the Northern California Institute for Research and Education, and the study is coordinated by the Alzheimer's Disease Cooperative Study at the University of California, San Diego. ADNI data are disseminated by the Laboratory for Neuro Imaging at the University of California, Los Angeles. This research was also supported by NIH grants P30 AG010129, K01 AG030514, and the Dana Foundation. The funders had no role in study design, data collection and analysis, decision to publish, or preparation of the manuscript.

Competing Interests: The authors have declared that no competing interests exist.

* E-mail: e.franko@ucl.ac.uk

Introduction

Alzheimer's disease (AD) is the most common form of dementia in the elderly population [1]. In 2010, the estimated number of patients with AD worldwide was 35.6 million, and this number is predicted to triple by 2050 (World Alzheimer Report, 2010). These numbers highlight a pressing need to develop disease-modifying treatments. Existing treatments are only effective in the early phase of the disease, and even then, their effect is highly variable among patients [2].

At present, the clinical diagnosis of AD requires that the patient has dementia [3], which is already associated with the widespread deposition of amyloid plaques and neurofibrillary tangles in the brain [4]. Indeed, amyloid and tau deposition in the entorhinal cortex has been detected in clinically silent cases [5]. Even in mild AD, these neuropathological changes cause neuronal loss in the entorhinal cortex and hippocampus [6], and these changes result in decreased volume [7]. Many magnetic resonance imaging

(MRI) studies have indeed reported smaller volumes in AD patients than in controls [8–10], which indirectly reflects faster atrophy in AD. However, a more direct way of measuring the atrophy is the use of repeated MRI scans within the same individual. This can then be used to monitor the disease progression in patients. More and more volumetric studies used longitudinal dataset and reported a higher rate of hippocampal volume loss in patients with AD than in elderly controls [11–17] However, global hippocampal volumetry is not always sensitive enough to follow changes within a single population [18], which may reflect conversion from healthy state or disease progression. Therefore, recent studies focus on changes in hippocampal shape. Examining the shape of the hippocampus gives not only more sensitivity to follow the progression of the atrophy, but also allows the evaluation of atrophy in the different parts of the hippocampus. Thompson et al. [19] and Morra et al. [20,21] reported that atrophy indeed varies by hippocampal sub-region. Based on differences in atrophy, they could distinguish healthy subjects from patients with AD and demonstrated correlation between atrophy and cognitive decline. However, their atrophy maps differed notably; Thompson et al. [19] described higher atrophy in the supero-lateral side of the hippocampus in AD compared to controls, whereas Morra et al. [20] found the main difference between groups in the inferior hippocampal surface. Surprisingly, the regions showing significant difference between groups did not correspond to the regions with significant atrophy in AD. These contradictory results ask for further research to find more precise methods to measure the hippocampal deformation during the progression of the disease.

In the present longitudinal study, we examined the hippocampal atrophy rate and compared its topography among healthy people and patients with MCI and AD to identify areas that can distinguish between groups. We found similar patterns of atrophy among the groups. Regional higher atrophy rate was found in AD as compared to controls. These regions also distinguish patients with stable MCI from those who eventually progressed to AD. Finally, the atrophy pattern is in agreement with the known regional anatomic specificity of tau deposition.

Methods

Subjects

Data used in the preparation of this article were obtained from the Alzheimer's Disease Neuroimaging Initiative (ADNI) database (adni.loni.ucla.edu), for up-to-date information, see www.adni-info.org. The data were analysed anonymously, using publicly available secondary data from the ADNI study, therefore no ethics statement is required for this work.

From the ADNI database, a preliminary dataset containing AD and normal subjects were downloaded first while developing the method [22]. From this first dataset, we selected the subjects who had at least 2 scans with at least 200 days apart. This resulted in 90 AD patients and 54 control subjects. Later we expanded the dataset to have similar number of controls as patients and added the MCI group. From the downloaded subjects, we included the first about 90 subjects who fulfilled the inclusion criteria, namely having at least two MRIs with at least 200 days apart. Few control subjects, who turned to MCI or AD during the follow-up period, were then removed from the statistical tests. The final number of subjects included in this study were 85 healthy controls, 102 patients diagnosed with MCI and 90 patients with AD. An overview of the subject groups is provided in Table 1, including the total number of subjects, their age, sex, mini-mental state examination (MMSE) and clinical dementia rating (CDR) scores. The interscan intervals are also shown for each group. We further divided the MCI group into progressive MCI (pMCI, n = 39), containing subjects who converted to AD between the baseline and the last scan (CDR>0.5), and stable MCI (sMCI, n = 44), containing subjects with CDR scores of 0.5 at the time of the last scan. The subjects, whose CDR score was not available at the time of the last scan, were not included into this analysis. Almost all patients with AD (88 out of 90) received medication (cholinesterase inhibitors and NMDA-receptor antagonists), as did 78% of the patients with MCI (80 out of 102) whereas none of the controls.

MRI Acquisitions

Structural brain MRIs were acquired at multiple ADNI sites using 1.5 Tesla MRI scanners manufactured by General Electric Healthcare, Siemens Medical Solutions, and Philips Medical Systems. Sagittal 3D MP-RAGE sequences were acquired using standard ADNI protocols (adni.loni.ucla.edu). MRI acquisition parameters were as follows: repetition time 8–9 ms, echo time 3.9 ms, flip angle 8, and slice thickness 1.2 mm. In-plane resolution differed slightly among subjects: 0.94×0.94 mm, 1.25×1.25 mm, or 1.3×1.3 mm.In this study, we used two scans from each subject. MRI_acq1 was the baseline scan (first scan of the subject), and MRI_acq2 was the last available scan (through December 2011). All subjects included in the analyses had a duration of at least 200 days between the first and last scans.

Hippocampal Segmentation

A template hippocampus (right hemisphere) was manually segmented from the single-subject MNI-T1 template available in SPM (www.fil.ion.ucl.ac.uk/spm). The segmentation followed the description of Franko et al. [23] and Insausti and Amaral [24] and contains the hippocampus proper (cornu ammonis (CA) 1–3 fields), the dentate gyrus and the subiculum. For guided extraction of the subject's hippocampus in MRI_acq1, two sets of seven points were defined in the template and in the MRI_acq1, respectively. The locations of the points are similar to those used by Pluta et al. [25]; three points were placed on coronal slices and four points on sagittal slices. The first point on the coronal view marks the appearance of the hippocampus inferior to the amygdala, the second marks the most medial point of the hippocampus at the level of the hippocampal-amygdaloid transitional area, and the third point indicates the most posterior part of the hippocampus [23]. On the sagittal view, we placed the first point on the most lateral slice of the hippocampus, the second and the third were placed 2–3 mm more medial on the anterior and posterior borders of hippocampus, respectively, and the last point was placed at the end of the intralimbic gyrus lateral to the hippocampal fissure. Finally, to extract the 3D hippocampus from MRI_acq1, the Iterative Closest Point (ICP) algorithm (www.vtk.org) was used to compute the affine transformation between the template and the subject's hippocampus (Fig. 1A).

Measurements of Atrophy

Following the recommendation of Yushkevich et al. [26], we performed an unbiased symmetric deformation field estimation to measure the hippocampal atrophy rate. ANTS software (www.picsl.upenn.edu/ANTS) was used to compute the symmetric deformation field (SyN method) between MRI_acq1 and MRI_acq2 using a normalised cross-correlation metric. The displacement of each voxel in MRI_acq1 was written in the WarpX, WarpY, and WarpZ images of the deformation fields. The parameters of our deformation-based morphometry included isotropic 2 mm (FWHM Gaussian kernel) image smoothing. Finally, for each vertex of the hippocampal surface (MRI_acq1), the dot product between the normal and the deformation field defined the signed displacement of the vertex (in mm) (Fig. 1B). The resulting values (divided by the duration between acquisition MRI_acq1 and MRI_acq2) represent the atrophy rate in mm/year. The texture was displayed on the 3D hippocampus in the radiological convention with visualisation software (anatomist, brainvisa.info/). The 3D mesh together with statistical maps is also available: brainsenses.x10host.com/hc.htm. The hippocampal volume was computed from the volumetric meshes. The technique described here was partly published in abstract form with preliminary results [22].

Statistical Analyses

Statistical analyses were performed using the R software (www.cran.r-project.org). The permutation test was used to assess the significant atrophy rate within each group. Statistical maps are displayed on the 3D hippocampi as -log10(p-value) for above threshold. Group differences were assessed using the Wilcoxon

Table 1. Characteristics of subjects in each group.

Group	Age in years	MMSE	CDR	Interscan time in days
Control (n = 85) F:37 M:48	76 (5)	29.2 (1)	0 (0)	1217 (303)
MCI (n = 102) F:34 M:68	75 (7)	26.8 (1.8)	0.5 (0)	1030 (393)
AD (n = 90) F:42 M:48	75 (7)	23.3 (2.2)	0.83 (0.35)	652 (188)

Mean values are followed by standard deviations (SD). MMSE: mini-mental state examination; CDR: clinical dementia rating; F: female; M:male.
doi:10.1371/journal.pone.0071354.t001

signed-rank test, which does not require the normality of the data. For both type of tests, significance level (p<0.05) was corrected for multiple comparison (number of vertices) using Bonferroni correction.

Hippocampal Subfields

Even though the hippocampal subfields are determined by histology and their boundaries are not visible on MRI, the subfields are often indicated on in vivo MRIs based solely on visual cues derived from histological images. However, a more reliable and unbiased subfield delineation can be achieved by using an independent MRI atlas. Hence, to help localise significant atrophy rates on the hippocampus, we projected the hippocampal subfields as defined from the high-resolution atlas of the human hippocampus [27] computed from post-mortem MRI at 9.4 Tesla (www.nitrc.org/projects/pennhippoatlas) onto our template using ICP algorithm. The borders of the subfields including CA1, CA2–3, the dentate gyrus, and the subiculum are illustrated as outlines on the 3D surface of the right hippocampus in Fig. 2A.

Region of Interest Analysis

To further test for differences between pMCI and sMCI, we performed a Region of Interest (ROI) analysis of the atrophy rate. The ROIs were used to increase the sensitivity to distinguish patients with stable MCI from progressive ones. We defined the ROIs as clusters of vertices with significantly higher atrophy rates in AD than in control subjects; which make them independently defined from the MCI dataset. A total of four ROIs were defined both in the right (R1R-R4R) and left (R1L-R4L) hippocampi. R1 is the cluster of vertices in the medial side of the hippocampal head, R2 corresponds to the cluster in the medial side of the body, R3 represents the cluster in the lateral side of head, whereas R4 contains the clusters along the lateral side of the hippocampal body and tail. The ROIs therefore do not correspond to a specific hippocampal subfield derived from the high-resolution atlas (see section Hippocampal subfields).

Within each region, we computed the average atrophy rate for each MCI patient. The stable and progressive MCI groups were compared statistically using Wilcoxon test (significance level was adjusted for the number of ROIs with Bonferroni correction). Receiver Operating Characteristic (ROC) analysis was then performed using the R package pROC version 1.4.4 [28].

Results

Hippocampal Volume Change

We first examined the difference in hippocampal volume between MRI_acq1 and MRI_acq2. Estimations of hippocampal volumes (in mm3) for MRI_acq1 and the volume change between MRI_acq1 and MRI_acq2 (in mm3/year) are listed in Table 2. We found significant hippocampal volume loss rates in each group (Table 2). However, the loss was greater in patients with AD than

in controls in both hippocampi (right: W = 5390, p-value = 1.501e-06; left: W = 4690, p-value = 0.004927). The volume loss was significantly higher in patients with MCI than in controls in the right hemisphere but not the left (right: W = 5273, p-value = 0.005484; left: W = 4719, p-value = 0.149 n.s.). Similarly, the AD group showed significantly greater volume loss than the MCI group in the right but not in the left hippocampus (right: W = 5507, p-value = 0.008535; left: W = 5190, p-value = 0.05936 n.s.). No significant difference in volume change was found between progressive and stable MCI (right: W = 1025, p-value = 0.06436 n.s.; left: W = 996, p-value = 0.1048 n.s.). Collectively, the volumetric measurements revealed significant loss in all groups and a larger loss in the AD and the MCI groups than in controls, but they failed to show significant difference between pMCI and sMCI.

Mapping the Rate of Atrophy

We computed averaged maps of hippocampal atrophy rates (mm/year) for patients with AD (Fig. 2A), MCI (Fig. 2B), and for controls (Fig. 2C). This mapping revealed a similar pattern of atrophy rates in all groups. Nonetheless, the rate of atrophy was the highest in the AD group (demonstrated by darker blue in Fig. 2), particularly in CA1 and subiculum. To assess atrophy rate significance, statistical maps were derived from a permutation test within each of the three populations (Fig. 3 A–C). Again, a similar pattern was found in the three groups. Significant atrophy occurred in the medial head and body and along the lateral side of the hippocampi. The highest significance was found in the medial head of the right hippocampus in the AD group (Fig. 3A and online 3D mesh, see Methods). Figures 2 and 3 suggest a similar pattern of atrophy rate among the three groups with different magnitudes that were further examined.

Group Differences

The significantly higher rate of atrophy in patients with AD than in controls (Fig. 4A and online 3D mesh, see Methods) was found mainly in the medial part of the head and body and along the lateral side of the hippocampi (Wilcoxon test, p < 0.05 corr.). A higher atrophy rate in the MCI group as compared to controls (Fig. 4B) was found in much smaller regions, mainly on the lateral side of the hippocampal head. Finally, significant differences between the AD and MCI groups (Fig. 4C) were found in a few vertices along the lateral side.

Stable versus Progressive Mild Cognitive Impairment

The difference in atrophy rate between the pMCI and sMCI groups (Fig. 5) was only assessed within the regions showing significantly higher atrophy rate in AD compared with control in order to increase the sensitivity. These comparisons revealed significantly higher rates in pMCI in all but one ROI (Wilcoxon test, R1R: W = 518, p-value = 0.001951; R1L: W = 497, p-value = 0.001004; R2R: W = 563, p-value = 0.007208; R2L:

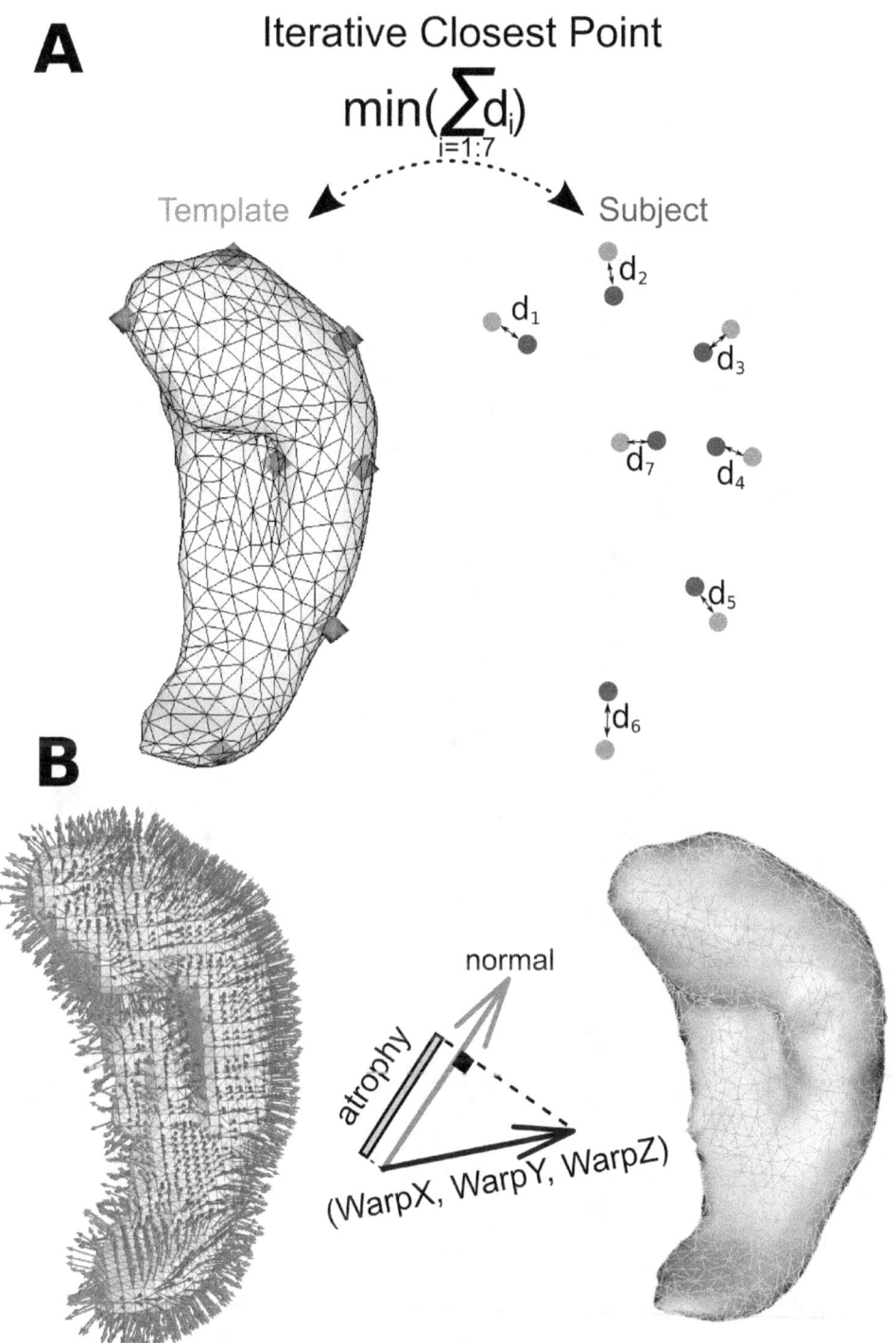

Figure 1. Illustration of the methods. (A) On the left side of this panel, we illustrate the triangulated surface of the template hippocampus and the manually defined seven points (in red). On the right side, the seven points drawn on the subject's hippocampus are shown in blue, and the ICP algorithm is illustrated which minimises the sum of distances (di) between the red and blue points. **(B)** Illustration of the deformation field mapping onto the triangulated hippocampal surface resulting in different colours for inward (blue) and outward (orange) deformation.
doi:10.1371/journal.pone.0071354.g001

W = 570, p-value = 0.00871; R3R: W = 453, p-value = 0.0002236; R3L: W = 519, p-value = 0.002011; R4R: W = 737, n.s; R4L: W = 543, p-value = 0.004110). The largest difference was found in the R3R ROI, which represents the antero-lateral part of the right hippocampus. Within this ROI, we performed an ROC analysis to determine how well the atrophy rate of this region is able to distinguish between pMCI and sMCI. The ROC analysis revealed

72.4% accuracy in discriminating the two groups, with 70.5% specificity and 74.4% sensitivity (area under the curve: 78.1%).

Discussion

In the present study, we used two MRI scans to map the rate of hippocampal atrophy in patients with AD and MCI and in healthy elderly controls. We also measured the total hippocampal volume

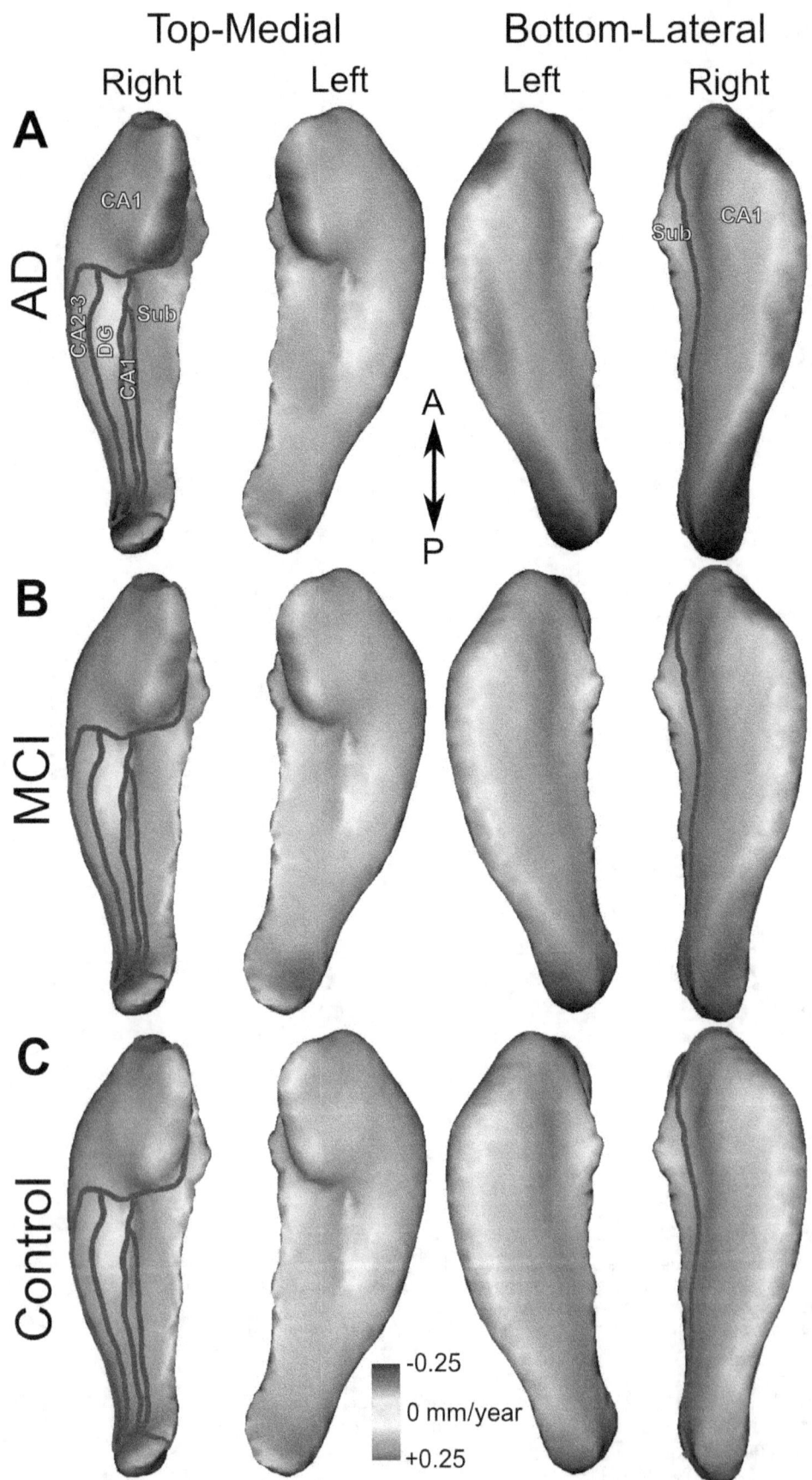

Figure 2. Mean atrophy rate. Mean atrophy rate in mm/year for the left and right hippocampi in patients with AD (**A**), MCI (**B**) and controls (**C**). On the right hippocampus, projected borders of subfields CA1, CA2–3, dentate gyrus (DG) and subiculum (Sub) are indicated with grey outlines.
doi:10.1371/journal.pone.0071354.g002

Table 2. Summary of hippocampal volumetry.

Group	Volume MRI_acq1 (R/L)	Volume change per year (R/L)	Statistics and p-value (R/L)
2*Control (n = 85)	2402 (476)/	−9 (30)/	V = 774, p-value = 1.975e-06/
	2059 (404)	−6 (22)	V = 992, p-value = 0.0001267
2*MCI (n = 102)	2181 (468)/	−20 (31)/	V = 815, p-value = 2.079e-09/
	1946 (431)	−10 (30)	V = 1360, p-value = 3.115e-05
2*AD (n = 90)	2129 (446)/	−28 (41)/	V = 479, p-value = 1.403e-10/
	1805 (397)	−14 (34)	V = 978, p-value = 8.489e-06

Average hippocampal volume in mm3 (SD) at the first scan, average volume loss in mm3/year between the two scans for right and left (R/L) hippocampi (SD), and the statistical tests on volume loss (Wilcoxon test) in each group.
doi:10.1371/journal.pone.0071354.t002

and compared its decrease among the three groups. We found the lowest baseline volume in the AD group, and the greatest in the group of healthy elderlies. The average hippocampal volume of patients with MCI was in between the other two groups. Looking at the volume loss over time, we found the fastest loss in the AD group. This was significantly higher than the loss in the normal group both in the left and the right hippocampi. The difference in volume loss between the AD and MCI groups was significant only in the right side. Similarly, only the right hippocampus showed greater volume loss in the MCI group than in controls. Comparison of the atrophy rates among the three subject groups revealed similar patterns. The regions with the highest rate of atrophy were located on the medial side of the hippocampal head and body and along the lateral side. These regions also showed significantly higher atrophy rates in patients with AD compared with controls. The difference in hippocampal atrophy rate between MCI and controls was located at the lateral side of the right hippocampal head, whereas the higher atrophy rate in AD compared to MCI was mainly found on the lateral side of the right hippocampal body and tail. To relate these regions to the histological subparts of the hippocampus, we used the atlas of the human hippocampus segmented from high-resolution MRIs [27]. Based on this atlas, the fastest atrophy occurred in the CA1 zone. Similarly, the strongest differences between the groups were localised in the CA1 zone and in the subiculum.

Our volumetric measurements are in accordance with previous studies measuring the hippocampal volume in different populations, namely sequential decrease in volume among healthy elderlies, MCI and AD patients [29]. We also found smaller volume in the left side compared to the right, as did many groups previously [30–32]. Our results are also in line with studies examining the volume loss over time [11,31,33–37]. They reported the greatest annual percent change in the hippocampal volume in patients with AD. This was significantly higher than that in patients with MCI and in normal subjects. Leung et al. [37] showed that the volume loss was even accelerating in the MCI group over time.

Although the difference in hippocampal volume had the same trend in many studies previously, the volume itself differed substantially. Groups, using the ADNI database of patients with AD and MCI and healthy elderly controls, reported hippocampal volumes in AD varying between 1600 [35] and 3000 mm3 [20]. In the present study, the hippocampal volume of AD patients was about 2000 mm3. The remarkable difference among studies might derive from the segmentation of the template hippocampus used to extract the structure in each individual. There are different recommendations for hippocampal segmentation which include different amount of the subiculum and the tail of the hippocampus

[38]. It can also differ how far anterior the hippocampus is segmented inferior to the amygdala. Here we followed the recommendations of Franko et al. [23] and Insausti and Amaral [24]. These studies described landmarks visible on MRI which are based on the histological examination and post-mortem MRI of the same brains.

Recently, several studies have focused on 3D shape analyses and detailed hippocampal atrophy mapping, and compared these maps among healthy controls and patients with MCI and AD [20,21,32,39–43]. Most of them used a single MRI scan and looked for differences in the hippocampal shape between healthy elderly and patients [20,39,40,44–47], referring to this shape difference as atrophy. However, this requires the assumption that the patient group had the same hippocampal shape as the control group prior to the disease process, which might not be the case if the number of subjects is not sufficiently high. Importantly, more and more studies measure the atrophy using a longitudinal MRI dataset, allowing the visualisation of the hippocampal atrophy within each single subject over time [15,19,21,32,42]. This method does not require a template hippocampus computed by averaging of healthy subjects' brains, therefore it is more robust for individual variability in the hippocampal shape. However, the methods could be biased by asymmetric deformation mapping [26,48], which could explain the contradicting findings in the previous studies. We therefore examined the hippocampal atrophy performing an unbiased symmetric deformation field estimation.

One of the first studies comparing the hippocampal atrophy rate in patients with AD to that in healthy subjects was performed by Thompson et al. [19]. They reported similar atrophy rate patterns between the two groups but found significantly higher atrophy rates on the lateral side of the left hippocampal head in AD patients. We also found similar atrophy rate patterns among the groups; however, we found significantly higher rates in AD patients compared to controls not only on the lateral side of the head but also on the medial part of the head and body and the lateral side of the hippocampal body and tail. The hippocampal atrophy rate maps reported by other groups [21,32,42] differ more from our results. Morra et al. [21] mainly found atrophy on the superior and inferior parts of the body and on the tail of the hippocampus of AD patients, whereas in our study, the atrophy rate was higher on the lateral and medial sides relatively sparing the superior and inferior surfaces. However, when comparing the patients to healthy controls, the significantly different atrophy was located mainly on the inferior part of the head and on the lateral and medial sides of the hippocampus, which is closer to our findings. However, another study from the same group [20] reported significant difference between AD patients and controls on almost the entire surface of the hippocampus sparing only a line

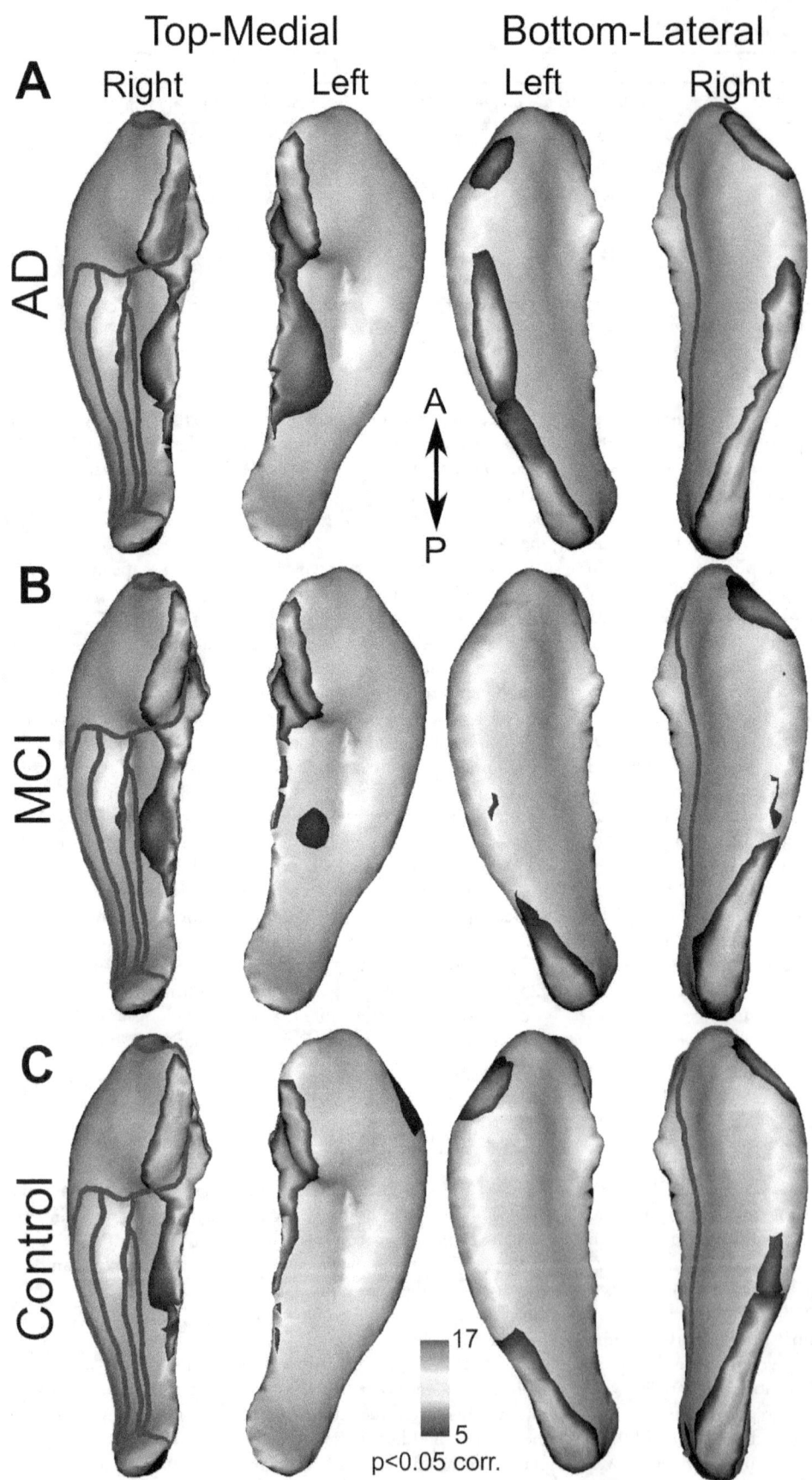

Figure 3. Significant atrophy rates. Statistical maps showing the -log(p-values) for significant (p < 0.05 corr.) atrophy rates for the left and right hippocampi in patients with AD (**A**), MCI (**B**) and controls (**C**). Significance level (p < 0.05 corr.) is indicated in the colour bar.
doi:10.1371/journal.pone.0071354.g003

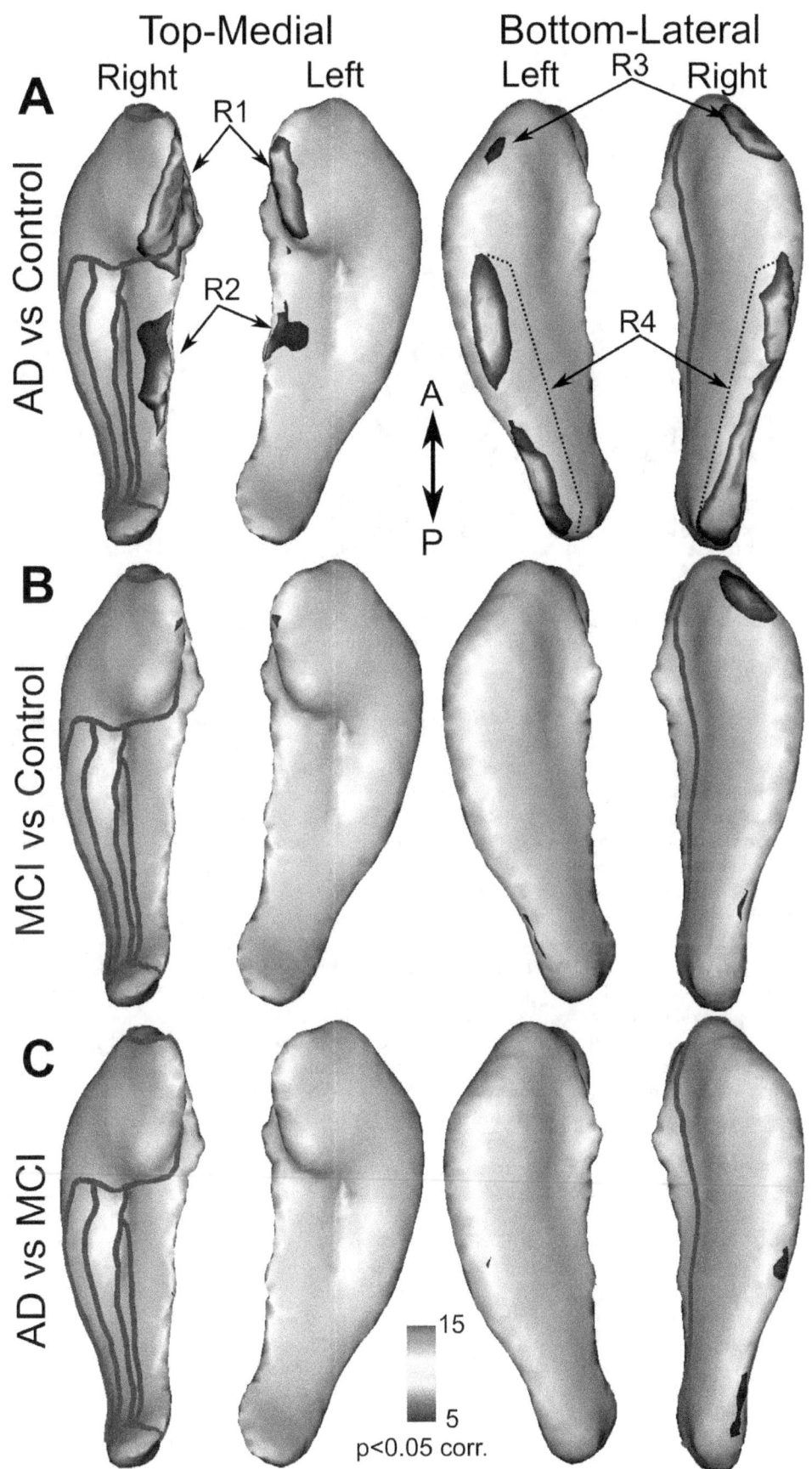

Figure 4. Statistical maps of atrophy rate differences among groups. Statistical maps showing significantly higher atrophy rate in AD versus control (**A**), MCI versus control (**B**), and AD versus MCI (**C**). Significance level (p < 0.05 corr.) is indicated in the colour bar.
doi:10.1371/journal.pone.0071354.g004

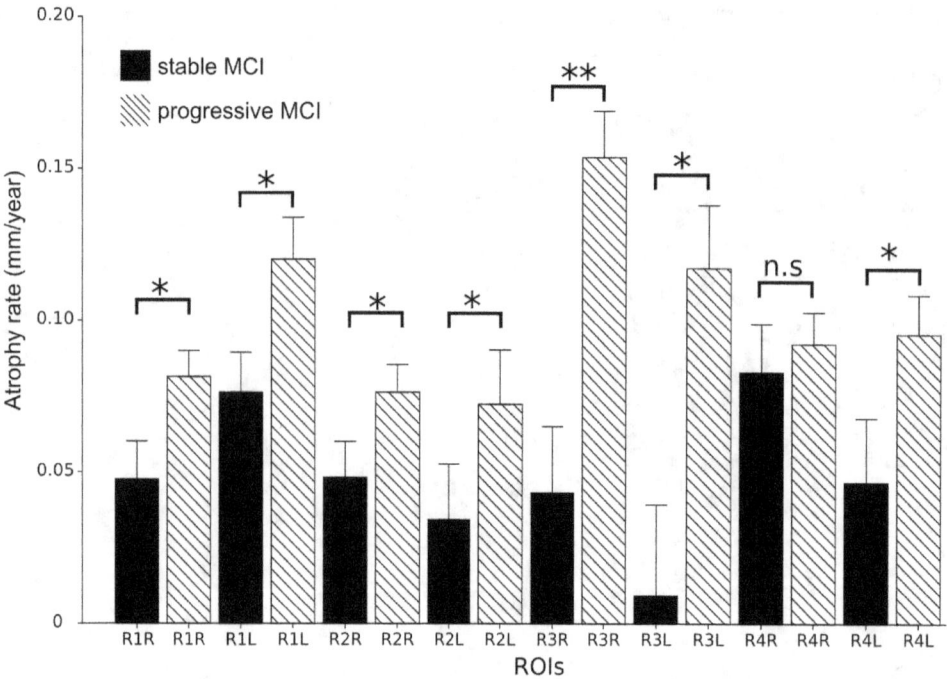

Figure 5. ROI analysis of atrophy rates in progressive and stable MCI. Bar plots of atrophy rates in the left and right hippocampal ROIs (shown in Figure 4) for pMCI (n = 39) and sMCI (n = 44). *: p < 0.05, **: p < 0.001 Bonferroni adjusted p-values.
doi:10.1371/journal.pone.0071354.g005

along the middle of the superior and inferior surfaces. Wang et al. [32,39] compared patients with MCI (CDR = 0.5) to healthy controls. They found more inward deformation in patients on the superior side of the head and the inferior and lateral parts of the hippocampal body and tail. They also reported the inward deformation of these regions to predict conversion from healthy state to MCI [49]. Apostolova et al. [42] compared subjects who remained cognitively normal with those who converted to MCI or AD and showed significant differences in hippocampal atrophy rate in all parts of the hippocampus without subfield specificity (CA1–3 subfields and subiculum).

Although Gerardin et al. [40] used a single scan to examine the hippocampal shape, the topography of atrophy found in the present study is the most like their results. They found morphological differences between the hippocampi of patients with AD and those of controls, predominantly on the medial part of the head and the lateral part of the body and tail. However, the use of a single scan prevented the investigation of atrophy evolution. Our data suggest that the morphological differences among groups in their study may be the consequence of different atrophy rates. Costafreda et al. [43] also used a single scan to predict conversion from MCI to AD using a baseline atrophic phenotype. Similarly to our findings, the atrophy of the anterior part of the CA1 field best predicted the conversion, with 80% accuracy. We also found the lateral side of the hippocampal head (corresponding to CA1) to be the best predictor of the progression to AD from MCI based on the atrophy rate. Although the accuracy is slightly lower, our method can be used to identify patients at high risk of progression. This can help identify patients most likely to be helped by treatments that are mainly effective in the early phase of AD.

We found similar patterns of atrophy rate among the three subject groups which might suggest that certain hippocampal subregions are more prone to atrophy caused by normal or pathological ageing. However, the current method cannot

distinguish between different sources of atrophy (underlying mechanisms of cell death). Therefore, we cannot speculate whether the similarity in atrophy pattern in AD compared to the controls would indicate that the disease simply accelerates the normal ageing. Braak and Braak [5] found that tau (neurofibrillary tangle and neuropil thread) deposition in the hippocampus first occurs on the medial and lateral side of the CA1 field in the early phase of AD (stage II, their Fig. 4); these regions are also more affected in the later phases than the middle portion of the CA (superior portion of the 3D hippocampus, see Methods) or the subiculum (infero-medial portion of the 3D hippocampus). Importantly, these regions that have the highest burden of neurofibrillary tangle and neuropil thread deposition correspond to those showing the highest atrophy rate in our study. This good correspondance between our results and the well-established neuropathology in AD supports a biological interpretation of the current mapping of atrophy rate.

Longitudinal studies are also necessary to evaluate atrophy progression at the individual level, which is the best way to objectively measure treatment effects. Jack and colleagues previously demonstrated that higher annual hippocampal volume loss correlated with worsening of the clinical status [11]. However, when comparing treated and untreated AD patients, Fox et al. [34] reported non-significant hippocampal volume change. Similarly, Wang et al. [41] did not find significant differences in hippocampal volume or surface deformation between treated and untreated MCI patients. Their method of averaging the deformation within each subfield assumes homogeneous atrophy. This might decreases the sensitivity to mild treatment effects. The present method is more sensitive to local deformation, which makes it more appropriate for use in clinical trials.

Beside its high sensitivity to local deformation, our method is also free of biases arising from asymmetric global normalization [26]. In a very recent study, Lorenzi and colleagues [48] developed another local symmetric registration algorithm robust to intensity bias. Their method will be useful for future longitudinal studies. Even though we used a semi-automated segmentation of the hippocampus at baseline, this step could be replaced with a fully-automated method. Several groups have developed fully-automated hippocampal segmentation tools [50–52] and some are recently available using FIRST/FSL and FreeSurfer softwares. Although our method is more time-consuming for large cohorts of patients and requires anatomical knowledge, it enabled us to use hippocampal boundaries as described by Insausti and Amaral [24].

In conclusion, our MRI-based regional hippocampal atrophy maps are in high agreement with the known AD histopathology. This shows that longitudinal MRI and particularly the measurement of local hippocampal atrophy rate are reliable methods to investigate AD. Additionally, we describe an unbiased method to objectively evaluate AD progression that can be used in clinical trials to test novel disease-modifying drugs and measure their efficacy.

Acknowledgments

The authors are indebted to T.E Cope for comments on earlier versions of the manuscript.

Data used in preparation of this article were obtained from the Alzheimers Disease Neuroimaging Initiative (ADNI) database (adni.loni.u-cla.edu). As such, the investigators within the ADNI contributed to the design and implementation of ADNI and/or provided data but did not participate in analysis or writing of this report. A complete listing of ADNI investigators can be found at: http://adni.loni.ucla.edu/wp-content/uploads/how_to_ apply/ADNI_Acknowledgement_List.pdf.

Author Contributions

Conceived and designed the experiments: EF OJ. Performed the experiments: EF OJ. Analyzed the data: EF OJ. Contributed reagents/materials/analysis tools: EF OJ. Wrote the paper: EF OJ.

References

1. Ferri CP, Prince M, Brayne C, Brodaty H, Fratiglioni L, et al. (2005) Global prevalence of dementia: a delphi consensus study. Lancet 366: 2112–7.
2. Cummings JL (2004) Treatment of alzheimer's disease: current and future therapeutic approaches. Rev Neurol Dis 1: 60–9.
3. McKhann G, Drachman D, Folstein M, Katzman R, Price D, et al. (1984) Clinical diagnosis of alzheimer's disease: report of the nincds-adrda work group under the auspices of department of health and human services task force on alzheimer's disease. Neurology 34: 939–44.
4. Braak H, Braak E, Bohl J (1993) Staging of alzheimer-related cortical destruction. Eur Neurol 33: 403–8.
5. Braak H, Braak E (1995) Staging of alzheimer's disease-related neurofibrillary changes. Neurobiol Aging 16: 271–8; discussion 278–84.
6. Price JL, Ko AI, Wade MJ, Tsou SK, McKeel DW, et al. (2001) Neuron number in the entorhinal cortex and ca1 in preclinical alzheimer disease. Arch Neurol 58: 1395–402.
7. Bobinski M, Wegiel J, Wisniewski HM, Tarnawski M, Bobinski M, et al. (1996) Neurofibrillary pathology–correlation with hippocampal formation atrophy in alzheimer disease. Neurobiol Aging 17: 909–19.
8. Juottonen K, Laakso MP, Insausti R, Lehtovirta M, Pitkänen A, et al. (1998) Volumes of the entorhinal and perirhinal cortices in alzheimer's disease. Neurobiol Aging 19: 15–22.
9. Convit A, de Asis J, de Leon MJ, Tarshish CY, De Santi S, et al. (2000) Atrophy of the medial occipitotemporal, inferior, and middle temporal gyri in non-demented elderly predict decline to alzheimer's disease. Neurobiol Aging 21: 19–26.
10. Chetelat G, Baron JC (2003) Early diagnosis of alzheimer's disease: contribution of structural neuroimaging. Neuroimage 18: 525–41.
11. Jack CR, Petersen RC, Xu Y, O'Brien PC, Smith GE, et al. (2000) Rates of hippocampal atrophy correlate with change in clinical status in aging and ad. Neurology 55: 484–489.
12. Fox NC, Cousens S, Scahill R, Harvey RJ, Rossor MN (2000) Using serial registered brain magnetic resonance imaging to measure disease progression in alzheimer disease: power calculations and estimates of sample size to detect treatment effects. Arch Neurol 57: 339–44.
13. van de Pol LA, Barnes J, Scahill RI, Frost C, Lewis EB, et al. (2007) Improved reliability of hippocampal atrophy rate measurement in mild cognitive impairment using uid registration. Neuroimage 34: 1036–1041.
14. Misra C, Fan Y, Davatzikos C (2009) Baseline and longitudinal patterns of brain atrophy in mci patients, and their use in prediction of short-term conversion to ad: results from adni. Neuroimage 44: 1415–1422.
15. Risacher SL, Shen L, West JD, Kim S, McDonald BC, et al. (2010) Longitudinal mri atrophy biomarkers: relationship to conversion in the adni cohort. Neurobiol Aging 31: 1401–1418.
16. Wolz R, Heckemann RA, Aljabar P, Hajnal JV, Hammers A, et al. (2010) Measurement of hippocampal atrophy using 4d graph-cut segmentation: application to adni. Neuroimage 52: 109–118.
17. Leung KK, Barnes J, Ridgway GR, Bartlett JW, Clarkson MJ, et al. (2010) Automated crosssectional and longitudinal hippocampal volume measurement in mild cognitive impairment and alzheimer's disease. Neuroimage 51: 1345–1359.
18. Henneman WJP, Sluimer JD, Barnes J, van der Flier WM, Sluimer IC, et al. (2009) Hippocampal atrophy rates in alzheimer disease: added value over whole brain volume measures. Neurology 72: 999–1007.
19. Thompson PM, Hayashi KM, De Zubicaray GI, Janke AL, Rose SE, et al. (2004) Mapping hippocampal and ventricular change in alzheimer disease. Neuroimage 22: 1754–66.
20. Morra JH, Tu Z, Apostolova LG, Green AE, Avedissian C, et al. (2009) Automated 3d mapping of hippocampal atrophy and its clinical correlates in 400 subjects with alzheimer's disease, mild cognitive impairment, and elderly controls. Hum Brain Mapp 30: 2766–88.
21. Morra JH, Tu Z, Apostolova LG, Green AE, Avedissian C, et al. (2009) Automated mapping of hippocampal atrophy in 1-year repeat mri data from 490 subjects with alzheimer's disease, mild cognitive impairment, and elderly controls. Neuroimage 45: S3–15.
22. Frankó E, Joly O (2010) Mapping changes in the hippocampal shape over time in alzheimer's disease. Program No 75620 2010 Neuroscience Meeting Planner San Diego, CA: Society for Neuroscience, 2010 Online.
23. Frankó E, Insausti AM, Artacho-Pérula E, Insausti R, Chavoix C (2012) Identification of the human medial temporal lobe regions on magnetic resonance images. Hum Brain Mapp : In Press, DOI: 10.1002/hbm.22170.
24. Insausti R, Amaral D (2004) Hippocampal formation. The human nervous system: 871–914.
25. Pluta J, Avants BB, Glynn S, Awate S, Gee JC, et al. (2009) Appearance and incomplete label matching for diffeomorphic template based hippocampus segmentation. Hippocampus 19: 565–71.
26. Yushkevich PA, Avants BB, Das SR, Pluta J, Altinay M, et al. (2010) Bias in estimation of hippocampal atrophy using deformation-based morphometry arises from asymmetric global normalization: an illustration in adni 3 t mri data. Neuroimage 50: 434–45.
27. Yushkevich PA, Avants BB, Pluta J, Das S, Minkoff D, et al. (2009) A high-resolution computational atlas of the human hippocampus from postmortem magnetic resonance imaging at 9.4 t. Neuroimage 44: 385–98.
28. Robin X, Turck N, Hainard A, Tiberti N, Lisacek F, et al. (2011) proc: an open-source package for r and s+ to analyze and compare roc curves. BMC Bioinformatics 12: 77.
29. Convit A, Leon MJD, Tarshish C, Santi SD, Tsui W, et al. (1997) Specific hippocampal volume reductions in individuals at risk for alzheimer's disease. Neurobiol Aging 18: 131–138.
30. Jack CR, Twomey CK, Zinsmeister AR, Sharbrough FW, Petersen RC, et al. (1989) Anterior temporal lobes and hippocampal formations: normative volumetric measurements from mr images in young adults. Radiology 172: 549–554.
31. Laakso MP, Lehtovirta M, Partanen K, Riekkinen PJ, Soininen H (2000) Hippocampus in alzheimer's disease: a 3-year follow-up mri study. Biol Psychiatry 47: 557–561.
32. Wang L, Swank JS, Glick IE, Gado MH, Miller MI, et al. (2003) Changes in hippocampal volume and shape across time distinguish dementia of the alzheimer type from healthy aging. Neuroimage 20: 667–82.
33. Jack CR, Shiung MM, Gunter JL, O'Brien PC, Weigand SD, et al. (2004) Comparison of different mri brain atrophy rate measures with clinical disease progression in ad. Neurology 62: 591–600.
34. Fox NC, Black RS, Gilman S, Rossor MN, Griffith SG, et al. (2005) Effects of abeta immunization (an1792) on mri measures of cerebral volume in alzheimer disease. Neurology 64: 1563–1572.
35. Schuff N, Woerner N, Boreta L, Kornfield T, Shaw LM, et al. (2009) Mri of hippocampal volume loss in early alzheimer's disease in relation to apoe genotype and biomarkers. Brain 132: 1067–1077.
36. Macdonald KE, Bartlett JW, Leung KK, Ourselin S, Barnes J, et al. (2012) The value of hippocampal and temporal horn volumes and rates of change in predicting future conversion to ad. Alzheimer Dis Assoc Disord.
37. Leung KK, Bartlett JW, Barnes J, Manning EN, Ourselin S, et al. (2013) Cerebral atrophy in mild cognitive impairment and alzheimer disease: Rates and acceleration. Neurology 80: 648–654.

38. Konrad C, Ukas T, Nebel C, Arolt V, Toga AW, et al. (2009) Defining the human hippocampus in cerebral magnetic resonance images–an overview of current segmentation protocols. Neuroimage 47: 1185–95.

39. Wang L, Miller JP, Gado MH, McKeel DW, Rothermich M, et al. (2006) Abnormalities of hippocampal surface structure in very mild dementia of the alzheimer type. Neuroimage 30: 52–60.

40. Gerardin E, Chételat G, Chupin M, Cuingnet R, Desgranges B, et al. (2009) Multidimensional classification of hippocampal shape features discriminates alzheimer's disease and mild cognitive impairment from normal aging. Neuroimage 47: 1476–86.

41. Wang L, Harms MP, Staggs JM, Xiong C, Morris JC, et al. (2010) Donepezil treatment and changes in hippocampal structure in very mild alzheimer disease. Arch Neurol 67: 99–106.

42. Apostolova LG, Mosconi L, Thompson PM, Green AE, Hwang KS, et al. (2010) Subregional hippocampal atrophy predicts alzheimer's dementia in the cognitively normal. Neurobiol Aging 31: 1077–88.

43. Costafreda SG, Dinov ID, Tu Z, Shi Y, Liu CY, et al. (2011) Automated hippocampal shape analysis predicts the onset of dementia in mild cognitive impairment. Neuroimage 56: 212–9.

44. Gutman B, Wang Y, Morra J, Toga AW, Thompson PM (2009) Disease classification with hippocampal shape invariants. Hippocampus 19: 572–578.

45. Frisoni GB, Sabattoli F, Lee AD, Dutton RA, Toga AW, et al. (2006) In vivo neuropathology of the hippocampal formation in ad: a radial mapping mr-based study. Neuroimage 32: 104–110.

46. Frisoni GB, Ganzola R, Canu E, Rb U, Pizzini FB, et al. (2008) Mapping local hippocampal changes in alzheimer's disease and normal ageing with mri at 3 tesla. Brain 131: 3266–3276.

47. Pluta J, Yushkevich P, Das S, Wolk D (2012) In vivo analysis of hippocampal subfield atrophy in mild cognitive impairment via semi-automatic segmentation of t2-weighted mri. J Alzheimers Dis 31: 85–99.

48. Lorenzi M, Ayache N, Frisoni GB, Pennec X, for the Alzheimer's Disease Neuroimaging Initiative (ADNI) (2013) Lcc-demons: A robust and accurate diffeomorphic registration algorithm. Neuroimage.

49. Csernansky JG, Wang L, Swank J, Miller JP, Gado M, et al. (2005) Preclinical detection of alzheimer's disease: hippocampal shape and volume predict dementia onset in the elderly. Neuroimage 25: 783–792.

50. Leemput KV, Bakkour A, Benner T, Wiggins G, Wald LL, et al. (2009) Automated segmentation of hippocampal subfields from ultra-high resolution in vivo mri. Hippocampus 19: 549–557.

51. Chupin M, Mukuna-Bantumbakulu AR, Hasboun D, Bardinet E, Baillet S, et al. (2007) Anatomically constrained region deformation for the automated segmentation of the hippocampus and the amygdala: Method and validation on controls and patients with alzheimer's disease. Neuroimage 34: 996–1019.

52. Chupin M, Grardin E, Cuingnet R, Boutet C, Lemieux L, et al. (2009) Fully automatic hippocampus segmentation and classification in alzheimer's disease and mild cognitive impairment applied on data from adni. Hippocampus 19: 579–587.

Other titles by iMedPub:

- *Social Medicine in the 21st Century* by Samuel Barrack.
- *World Health Report 2012: No Health Without Research* by Samuel Barrack.
- *Quality design in Anatomical Pathology* by Anil Malleshi Betigeri.
- *Escherichia coli infections* by Viroj Wiwanitkit.
- *Atlas of Biomarkers for Alzheimer's disease* by Manuel Menendez.